Diabetes

The book explains the underlying pathophysiology of the disease and covers in detail all its main forms and complications. Separate chapters consider the range of treatment options, together with summaries of key clinical trials. Coverage also includes epidemiology and classification, as well as diagnosis, screening, limiting risk, and other aspects of disease management and patient care. The book is illustrated throughout by explanatory diagrams, graphs, tables, and photos.

Key Features:

- Builds on its strength of having excellent content on long-term management of hyperglycemia by including pancreas and islet transplantation.
- Contains invaluable information on glucose monitoring for healthcare professionals interested in diabetes.

Clinician's Desk Reference Series

Parkinson's Disease: Clinician's Desk Reference
By Donald Grosset, Hubert Fernandez, Katherine Grosset, Michael Okun

Asthma: Clinician's Desk Reference
By J Graham Douglas, Kurtis S Elward

Diabetes: Clinician's Desk Reference, Second Edition
By M Cecilia Lansang, Richard David Leslie, Tahseen A Chowdhury, Keren Zhou

For more information about this series, please visit: https://www.routledge.com/Clinicians-Desk-Reference-Series/book-series/CRCCLIDESREF

CLINICIAN'S DESK REFERENCE

Diabetes

Second Edition

M. Cecilia Lansang
MD, MPH

Professor of Medicine
Cleveland Clinic Lerner College of Medicine of the
Case Western Reserve University
Director of Endocrinology
Cleveland Clinic Main Campus
Cleveland, OH, USA

Richard David Leslie
MD, FRCP, FAoP

Professor of Diabetes and Autoimmunity
Honorary Consultant Physician
Blizard Institute, Barts and the Royal London
Medical School
University of London
London, UK

Tahseen A. Chowdhury
MD, FRCP

Honorary Professor of Diabetes
Barts and the London School of Medicine and
Dentistry
Consultant in Diabetes
Department of Diabetes and Metabolism
The Royal London Hospital
London, UK

Keren Zhou
MD

Clinical Assistant Professor
Cleveland Clinic Lerner College of Medicine of the
Case Western Reserve University
Director of Research
Cleveland Clinic
Cleveland, OH, USA

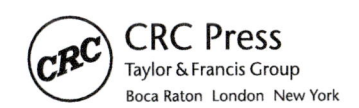

CRC Press
Taylor & Francis Group
Boca Raton London New York

CRC Press is an imprint of the
Taylor & Francis Group, an **informa** business

Second edition published 2023
by CRC Press
6000 Broken Sound Parkway NW, Suite 300, Boca Raton, FL 33487-2742

and by CRC Press
4 Park Square, Milton Park, Abingdon, Oxon, OX14 4RN

CRC Press is an imprint of Taylor & Francis Group, LLC

© 2023 Taylor & Francis Group, LLC

This book contains information obtained from authentic and highly regarded sources. While all reasonable efforts have been made to publish reliable data and information, neither the author[s] nor the publisher can accept any legal responsibility or liability for any errors or omissions that may be made. The publishers wish to make clear that any views or opinions expressed in this book by individual editors, authors or contributors are personal to them and do not necessarily reflect the views/opinions of the publishers. The information or guidance contained in this book is intended for use by medical, scientific or health-care professionals and is provided strictly as a supplement to the medical or other professional's own judgement, their knowledge of the patient's medical history, relevant manufacturer's instructions and the appropriate best practice guidelines. Because of the rapid advances in medical science, any information or advice on dosages, procedures or diagnoses should be independently verified. The reader is strongly urged to consult the relevant national drug formulary and the drug companies' and device or material manufacturers' printed instructions, and their websites, before administering or utilizing any of the drugs, devices or materials mentioned in this book. This book does not indicate whether a particular treatment is appropriate or suitable for a particular individual. Ultimately it is the sole responsibility of the medical professional to make his or her own professional judgements, so as to advise and treat patients appropriately. The authors and publishers have also attempted to trace the copyright holders of all material reproduced in this publication and apologize to copyright holders if permission to publish in this form has not been obtained. If any copyright material has not been acknowledged please write and let us know so we may rectify in any future reprint.

Except as permitted under U.S. Copyright Law, no part of this book may be reprinted, reproduced, transmitted, or utilized in any form by any electronic, mechanical, or other means, now known or hereafter invented, including photocopying, microfilming, and recording, or in any information storage or retrieval system, without written permission from the publishers.

For permission to photocopy or use material electronically from this work, access www.copyright.com or contact the Copyright Clearance Center, Inc. (CCC), 222 Rosewood Drive, Danvers, MA 01923, 978-750-8400. For works that are not available on CCC please contact mpkbookspermissions@tandf.co.uk

Trademark notice: Product or corporate names may be trademarks or registered trademarks and are used only for identification and explanation without intent to infringe.

ISBN: 978-1-032-14647-8 (hbk)
ISBN: 978-1-032-14645-4 (pbk)
ISBN: 978-1-003-24034-1 (ebk)

DOI: 10.1201/9781003240341

Typeset in Garamond
by SPi Technologies India Pvt Ltd (Straive)

To Hubert and Annella, thank you for filling my life with love and laughter. To mom and dad, my gratitude for introducing me to the world of endocrinology and diabetes.
M. Cecilia Lansang

To my family and my two boys, Nico and Alexander.
Richard David Leslie

Dedicated to my wife, Shawarna, children Aisha (and husband Sybghat), Nasser and Amber, mother Najma and father, Ismail (deceased), all of who have supported me throughout my career. Thank you for all your love and support.
Tahseen A. Chowdhury

To my parents, Aiqing and Hua, and my husband, Cory, for their love and support.
Keren Zhou

Contents

Preface ix

Acknowledgements ix

Author biographies x

Abbreviations xi

CHAPTER 1
The nature of diabetes 1

What is diabetes? 1
Forms of diabetes 7
Clinical presentations of diabetes 9
Complications of diabetes 9
The cost of diabetes 10

CHAPTER 2
Glucose, insulin, and diabetes 12

The role and regulation of glucose 12
The role and regulation of insulin 18

CHAPTER 3
Type 1 diabetes 25

Epidemiology 25
Causes of type 1 diabetes 26
Development of type 1 diabetes 31
Mortality 31
Screening for potential type 1 diabetes 32

CHAPTER 4
Type 2 diabetes 34

Epidemiology 34
Causes of type 2 diabetes 35
Associated conditions 37
Metabolic syndrome and obesity 40
Development of type 2 diabetes 42
Incretin hormones 44
The role of amylin 44
Glucotoxicity and lipotoxicity 45
Screening and prevention 46

CHAPTER 5
Diabetes screening and patient care 49

Management overview 49
Risk factors 49
Annual examination 50
Screening for complications 50
Treating children 52
The elderly person with diabetes 56
Ethnic minorities 58
Patient education and community care 59
Living with diabetes 60

CHAPTER 6
Diabetes and vascular disease 64

Macrovascular disease 64
Pathogenesis of macrovascular complications 65
Treatment and management principles for macrovascular disease 66
Glucose-lowering drugs and cardiovascular disease 67
Microvascular disease 73
Pathogenesis of microvascular complications 73
Treatment and management principles for microvascular disease 77
Reducing the risk of vascular disease 78

CHAPTER 7
Diabetic neuropathy 85

Prevalence and classification 85
Diagnosis 86
Chronic sensory polyneuropathy 87
Acute sensory neuropathy 89
Acute motor neuropathy 90
Autonomic neuropathy 90
Treatment and management 92

CHAPTER 8
Diabetic eye disease 95

Overview 95

Natural history 95
Nonproliferative diabetic retinopathy 96
Proliferative diabetic retinopathy 98
Diabetic maculopathy 99
Cataracts 99
Glaucoma 100
Ocular nerve palsies 100
Treatment and management 100

CHAPTER 9
Diabetic kidney disease 103

Overview 103
Natural history 103
Diagnosis of nephropathy 106
Urinary tract infections 106
Treatment and management 107
Newer glucose-lowering drugs in diabetic kidney disease 108
Renal replacement therapy 115
Pancreas transplant or islet cell implantation 117

CHAPTER 10
Skin and musculoskeletal complications of diabetes 118

Skin manifestations of diabetes 118
Musculoskeletal conditions associated with diabetes 124
Diabetic foot 128
Charcot's arthropathy 134

CHAPTER 11
Infections and diabetes 136

Overview 136
Pathophysiology 136
Infections 137
COVID-19 and diabetes 144
Glycemic control and infection outcomes 145

CHAPTER 12
Severe diabetic metabolic disturbances 146

Diabetic ketoacidosis 146
Acute management 150
Hyperosmolar hyperglycemic state or hyperosmolar nonketotic state 153

Brittle diabetes mellitus 155
Recurrent ketoacidosis 156
Lactic acidosis 156

CHAPTER 13
Long-term management of hyperglycemia 157

Overview 157
Targets of treatment 158
Dietary management 159
Calorie intake 160
Carbohydrates 161
Fats 161
Protein 161
Prescribing a diet 162
Exercise 162
Remission of type 2 diabetes 164

CHAPTER 14
Noninsulin therapies 166

Overview 166
Oral agents 167
Non-insulin injections 178

CHAPTER 15
Insulin treatment and pancreatic/islet cell transplantation 181

Overview 181
Indications for insulin treatment 181
Classes of insulin 182
Insulin delivery systems 184
Insulin regimen: type 1 diabetes 186
Continuous glucose monitors (CGMs) 190
Insulin regimen: type 2 diabetes 191
Metabolic instability on insulin 195
Complications: hypoglycemia 196
Treating hypoglycemia 199
Other complications or adverse effects from insulin treatment 200
Pancreas transplantation 201
Islet cell transplant 202

CHAPTER 16
Special management considerations 205

Inpatient diabetes considerations 205
Diabetes and surgery 206

Conception, contraception, and pregnancy 208
Neonatal problems 217

References 220

Resources: Research and support organizations 228
Glossary 230
Index 238

Preface

The aim of this book is to provide clinicians and other health professionals with an easily readable and clinically applicable text on diabetes. The joint European and American authorship indicates the widespread international agreement on the best way to manage diabetes, both in terms of limiting the disease risk and of treating complications once they develop. The book integrates the physiology and anatomy of the disease with clinical and laboratory analysis. Summaries of key clinical trials emphasize the knowledge base underlying the practical recommendations. A range of treatment options is provided, reflecting the need for customized treatment strategies. The authors have sought to provide a clear and concise guide to the optimal treatment approach. The text is intended for clinicians with an interest in diabetes at all levels, including primary-care physicians, medical students, nurse specialists, physician assistants, diabetes educators and those in postgraduate training.

Acknowledgements

The authors would like to thank Dr. Aaron Hoschar and Dr. Keith Lai for the slide used for the front cover, and the contributors of photos acknowledged in the specific chapters. They would also like to recognize the authors of the first edition – Drs. Richard David Leslie, M. Cecilia Lansang, Simon Coppack and Laurence Kennedy – for the backbone provided by their previous work

Author biographies

M. Cecilia Lansang is Professor of Medicine at the Cleveland Clinic Lerner College of Medicine of the Case Western Reserve University, and Director of Endocrinology at the Cleveland Clinic Main Campus, Ohio, USA. She had her endocrine clinical and research fellowship training at the Brigham and Women's Hospital, where she stayed on as staff before moving to the University of Florida, and then to the Cleveland Clinic. She obtained her Master of Public Health degree at the Harvard School of Public Health. She is active in research and medical education, serves on journal editorial boards and focuses clinical work on kidney transplant, inpatient diabetes and technology.

Richard David Leslie is Professor of Diabetes and Autoimmunity at the Blizard Institute, University of London, and Honorary Consultant Physician at St Bartholomews and the Royal London Hospitals, London, UK, as well as Lead Professor on the International Medical Faculty, Campus Biomedico, University of Rome, Italy. He has published 12 books and more than 250 peer-reviewed papers, He was Principle Investigator of three major EU programmes, Wellcome Trust Senior Fellow in Clinical Science and formerly President of the Association of Physicians of Great Britain and Ireland. He has held Visiting Chairs in USA (Chicago and Kansas) and is Emeritus Professor in China (Central South University).

Tahseen Chowdhury is a clinician in the Department of Diabetes and Metabolism at the Royal London Hospital, in the East End of London. He runs a large specialist diabetes and metabolism unit, dealing with diabetes particularly amongst the Bangladeshi community of Tower Hamlets. He has a research / clinical interest in diabetes in South Asians and diabetic kidney disease, and has authored many publications, including books entitled *Diabetes in South Asian people: Explained*, *Fatty Liver* and *Diabetes Management in Clinical Practice*. He is Honorary Professor at Barts and the London School of Medicine and Dentistry in London, where he runs the metabolism programme for medical students. He qualified from the University of Birmingham and trained in Birmingham and Manchester before becoming a consultant physician in 2000.

Keren Zhou completed her medical degree at Case Western Reserve University. She subsequently trained in internal medicine and endocrinology at the Cleveland Clinic in Ohio, USA, where she is currently staff in the Endocrinology and Metabolism Institute and a clinical assistant professor at the Cleveland Clinic Lerner College of Medicine of the Case Western Reserve University. She serves as Research Director for the Institute and a principal investigator on a number of studies related to diabetes and diabetes technology.

Abbreviations

AACE	American Association of Clinical Endocrinologists	CSII	continuous subcutaneous insulin infusion
ABX	Abciximab	CT	computed tomography
ACEI	angiotensin-converting enzyme inhibitor	CVD	cardiovascular disease
acyl-CoA	acyl-coenzyme-A	DAN	diabetic autonomic neuropathy
ADA	American Diabetes Association	DNA	deoxyribonucleic acid
ADP	adenosine diphosphate	DCCT	Diabetes Control and Complications Trial
AGE	advanced glycation endproducts	DIGAMI	Diabetes Mellitus Insulin Glucose Infusion in Acute Myocardial Infarction (study)
AGI	a-glucosidase inhibitor		
ALLHAT	Anti-Hypertensive and Lipid-Lowering Treatment to Prevent Heart Attacks Trials	DKA	diabetic ketoacidosis
		DPP	Diabetes Prevention Program
AMPK	AMP-activated protein kinase	DPP	dipeptidyl peptidase
ARB	angiotensin-receptor blocker	DREAM	Diabetes REduction Assessment with ramipril and rosiglitazone Medication (trial)
ATP	adenosine triphosphate		
AUC	area under the curve	DSME	diabetes self-management education
BARI	Bypass Angioplasty Revascularization Investigation (trial)	DVLA	Driver and Vehicle Licensing Agency
BENEDICT	Bergamo Nephrologic Diabetes Complications Trial	EASD	European Association for the Study of Diabetes
BMI	body mass index	ECD	expanded criteria donor
BP	blood pressure	ECG	Electrocardiogram
BUN	blood urea nitrogen	ED50	effective dose of insulin that produces 50% of maximal effect
C4	complement 4		
CABG	coronary artery bypass grafting	eGFR	estimated glomerular filtration rate
CAD	coronary artery disease		
cAMP	cyclic adenosine monophosphate	EGIR	European Group for the Study of Insulin Resistance
CAPD	continuous ambulatory peritoneal dialysis	eNOS	endothelial nitric oxide synthase
CARDS	Collaborative Atorvastatin Diabetes Study	EPIC	Evaluation of Platelet IIb/IIIa Inhibition for Prevention of Ischemic Complications (trial)
CARE	Cholesterol and Recurrent Events (trial)	EPILOG	Evaluation of PTCA to Improve Long-term Outcome by c7E3 GP IIb/IIIa Receptor Blockade (trial)
CHF	congestive heart failure		
CK-MB	creatine kinase, muscle-brain type		
CNS	central nervous system	EPISTENT	Evaluation of Platelet IIb/IIIa Inhibitor for Stenting (trial)
CRP	C-reactive protein	ESR	erythrocyte sedimentation rate
CSF	cerebrospinal fluid	ESRD	end-stage renal disease

ETDRS	Early Treatment Diabetic Retinopathy Study	IDF	International Diabetes Federation
FDA	Food and Drug Administration	IDNT	Irbesartan Type 2 Diabetic Nephropathy Trial
FEV1	forced expiratory volume in 1 second	IEC	International Expert Committee
FFA	free fatty acids	IFCC	International Federation of Clinical Chemistry
FIELD	Fenofibrate Intervention and Event Lowering in Diabetes (study)	IFG	impaired fasting glycemia
		IGF	insulin-like growth factor
FPG	fasting plasma glucose	IgG	immunoglobulin G
FSH	follicle-stimulating hormone	IGT	impaired glucose tolerance
FTO	fused-toe gene	IPF-1	insulin promoter factor-1
		IR	immunoreactive (insulin)
GAD	glutamic acid decarboxylase	IRMA	intraretinal microvascular abnormalities
GADA	glutamic acid decarboxylase antibody	IRMA-2	Irbesartan in Patients with Type 2 Diabetes and Microalbuminuria (study)
GBM	glomerular basement membrane		
GDM	gestational diabetes mellitus	KATP	ATP-sensitive potassium (channel)
GFAT	glutamine:fructose-6 phosphate amidotransferase	K_m	Michaelis constant
GFR	glomerular filtration rate	KPD	ketosis-prone diabetes
GIP	glucose-dependent insulinotrophic peptide	LADA	latent autoimmune diabetes of adults
GIR	glucose infusion rate	LDL	low-density lipoprotein
GLP	glucagon-like peptide	LDL-C	low-density lipoprotein cholesterol
GLUT	glucose transporter protein		
HAPO	Hyperglycemia and Adverse Pregnancy Outcome (study)	LH	luteinizing hormone
		LIFE	Losartan Intervention for Endpoint Reduction (study)
HbA1c	glycated hemoglobin	LIPID	Long-Term Intervention with Pravastatin in Ischemic Disease (trial)
HDL	high-density lipoprotein		
HGO	hepatic glucose output		
HLA	histocompatibility leukocyte antigen	MDI	multiple daily insulin injections
H/Ma	hemorrhages or microaneurysms	MDRD	Modification of Diet in Renal Disease (formula)
HNF	hepatic nuclear factor	MHC	major histocompatibility complex
HONK	hyperosmolar nonketotic hyperglycemia	Micro-HOPE	Micro-Heart Outcomes Prevention Evaluation (study)
HOT	Hypertension Optimal Treatment (trial)	MODY	maturity onset diabetes of the young
HHS	hyperosmolar hyperglycemic state	MNT	medical nutrition therapy
		MRFIT	Multiple Risk Factor Intervention Trial
IAA	insulin autoantibody	MRI	magnetic resonance imaging
IA-2	insulinoma-associated antigen-2		
IADPSG	International Association of the Diabetes and Pregnancy Study Groups	NAD	nicotinamide adenine dinucleotide
IAPP	islet amyloid polypeptide	NADPH	nicotinamide adenine dinucleotide phosphate

NAVIGATOR	Nateglinide and Valsartan in Impaired Glucose Tolerance Outcomes Research (trial)	TRIPOD	Troglitazone in the Prevention of Diabetes (study)
NCEP	National Cholesterol Education Program	TZD	Thiazolidinedione
NDDG	National Diabetes Data Group	UDP	uridine diphosphate
NEFA	nonesterified fatty acids	UGDP	University Group Diabetes Program
NFKB	nuclear factor-kappa B	UKPDS	UK Prospective Diabetes Study
NICE	National Institute for Health and Clinical Excellence	VA-HIT	Veterans Affairs HDL Intervention Trial
NICE-SUGAR	Normoglycaemia in Intensive Care Evaluation and Survival Using Glucose Algorithm Regulation (study)	VB	venous beading
		VCAM	vascular cell adhesion molecule
NIDDM	noninsulin-dependent diabetes mellitus	VEGF	vascular endothelial growth factor
NIMGU	noninsulin-mediated glucose uptake	VIP	vasoactive intestinal peptide
NPDR	nonproliferative diabetic retinopathy	VISEP	Efficacy of Volume Substitution and Insulin Therapy in Severe Sepsis (study)
NPH	neutral protamine Hagedorn	VLDL	very low-density lipoprotein
NVD	neovascularization near the optic disk	VLDLR	very low density lipoprotein receptor
NVE	neovascularization elsewhere	VSMC	vascular smooth muscle cell
OGTT	oral glucose tolerance test	WESDR	Wisconsin Epidemiologic Study of Diabetic Retinopathy
OECD	Organisation for Economic Co-operation and Development	WHO	World Health Organization
OHA	oral hypoglycemic agents	XENDOS	XENical in the Prevention of Diabetes in Obese Subjects (study)
PARP	poly(ADP-ribose) polymerase		
PDE5	phosphodiesterase type-5	ZnT8	zinc transporter 8
PDR	proliferative diabetic retinopathy		
PKC	protein kinase C		
PKC-b	protein kinase C-beta		
PPAR	peroxisome proliferator-activated receptor		
PTCA	percutaneous transluminal coronary angioplasty		
RAGE	advanced glycation endproduct receptor		
RENAAL	Reduction of Endpoints in NIDDM with the Angiotensin II Antagonist Losartan (trial)		
RIA	radio-immunoassay		
ROS	reactive oxygen species		
RNA	ribonucleic acid		
SGLT	sodium–glucose co-transporter		
SMBG	self-monitored blood glucose		
STOP-NIDDM	Study to Prevent NIDDM (trial)		
SU	Sulfonylurea		

CHAPTER 1

The nature of diabetes

What is diabetes?

Overview

- Diabetes mellitus is a serious chronic hormonal condition in which the body is unable to properly use the energy from food.
- The name 'diabetes mellitus' differentiates the condition from the more uncommon diabetes insipidus. Both of these conditions cause an increase in urine production. The word mellitus has its derivation from "honey", referring to sweetness in the urine (whereas the urine in diabetes insipidus is insipid). Diabetes mellitus will be referred to simply as diabetes in this book.
- The two major pathologies leading to diabetes are insulin deficiency and insulin resistance, where insulin is ineffective in enabling glucose to enter the body's cells for use as energy. When glucose cannot enter the cells, its levels in the blood increase, resulting in hyperglycemia.
- Genetic and environmental factors both appear to be involved in the development of diabetes.
- There are two main types of diabetes:
  - *Type 1* (insulin-dependent) diabetes, where the beta (β)-cells of the pancreas (Figure 1.1) suffer autoimmune destruction so that little or no insulin is produced. This type is most often diagnosed in children or young adults. Patients with type 1 diabetes have to use insulin to control blood glucose levels; however, some adults have a more insidious onset called latent autoimmune diabetes in adults (LADA), where need for insulin is much later on. In a small proportion of patients with type 1 diabetes, there is no autoimmune process found.

Diabetes occurs as a result of insulin deficiency and/or insulin resistance.

  - *Type 2* (noninsulin-dependent) diabetes, where some insulin is produced but is not fully taken up by the tissues. Type 2 diabetes is associated

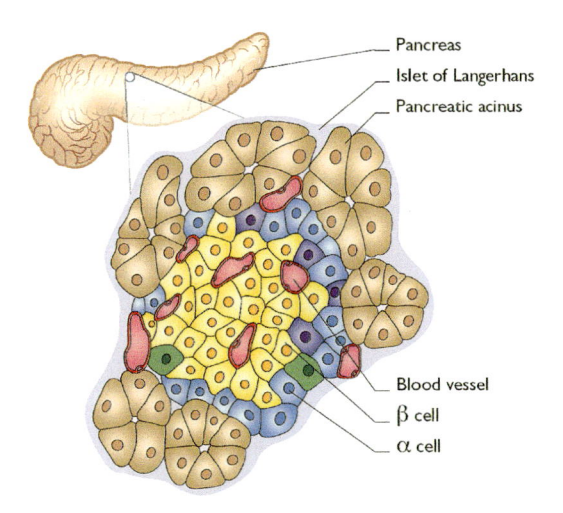

Figure 1.1 Beta cells. Beta cells contained within the islets of Langerhans produce the hormone insulin, which controls glucose levels in the blood. Type 1 diabetes is caused in the majority of cases by autoimmune destruction of these cells, whereas in type 2 diabetes their function deteriorates over time. Alpha cells produce glucagon – a counter-regulatory hormone.

DOI: 10.1201/9781003240341-1

with obesity and is most commonly diagnosed in adults. This type of diabetes could possibly be controlled with lifestyle changes (healthier meals and exercise) but often needs medication, insulin or noninsulin.
  ◇ These two types of diabetes differ in their pathogenesis and metabolic features.
◆ Long-term complications in blood vessels, kidneys, eyes, and nerves occur in both types of diabetes and are the major causes of morbidity and death.

Epidemiology
◆ Diabetes is the most common metabolic disorder, with 5–10% of adult populations living affluent, westernized lifestyles developing the condition at some time in their lives.
◆ According to the International Diabetes Federation (IDF) there were approximately 537 million adults with diabetes in 2021, with this number projected to rise to 643 million by 2030 and 783 million by 2045. In comparison, data from the IDF in 2011 showed a figure of 366 million predicted to rise to 552 million by 2030, so the numbers continue to escalate beyond previous projections.
◆ The rates of both type 1 and type 2 diabetes are increasing:
  ◇ With the epidemic of obesity, the burden of type 2 diabetes at all ages is increasing exponentially.
  ◇ The incidence of type 1 diabetes has also been increasing for many years for reasons that are much less apparent.
◆ There is a wide variation in the prevalence of diabetes worldwide, with the greatest expected increase in Africa, and in the Middle East/North Africa (see map, Figure 1.2).
◆ The predicted increase in incidence is, to a large extent, related to the increasing numbers of people living to more than 65 years of age. Diabetes is more prevalent in men, but there are more women than men with diabetes, as more women than men survive to old age in most societies.
◆ Population screening programs typically reveal that up to half of the subjects found to have type 2 diabetes had previously been undiagnosed.
◆ As of 2017, it was estimated that 9 million people in the world had type 1 diabetes.
◆ The incidence of type 2 diabetes in children and adolescents is also rising, with obesity being a major contributor, as well as the hormonal changes and insulin resistance seen around puberty.
◆ It is difficult to obtain accurate figures for deaths related to diabetes, because people with diabetes most often die from cardiovascular and renal disease, and it is these that are recorded on death certificates. The IDF estimates diabetes and its complications to comprise 12.2% of global (all cause) mortality in 2021.

Definitions and classification
◆ Diabetes mellitus is characterized by increased blood glucose concentrations.
  ◇ Such glucose concentrations vary as a continuum in different people and so the definition of diabetes is somewhat arbitrary, but the cutoff points were chosen in relation to levels of glycemia associated with specific diabetic complications such as retinopathy.
◆ Historically we define diabetes by either a raised fasting glucose or a raised glucose following oral glucose challenge. Random glucose levels can also be used if the patient has symptoms typical of hyperglycemia, such as thirst and polyuria.
◆ The WHO had been revising the diagnostic criteria to define diabetes, with the update in 1999 reflecting a better understanding of 'milder' glucose intolerance and its impact on vascular disease.
◆ The WHO criteria for diagnosis are shown in Tables 1.1 and 1.2.
  ◇ WHO criteria only consider fasting and 120-minutes values in the oral glucose tolerance test (OGTT).

The nature of diabetes

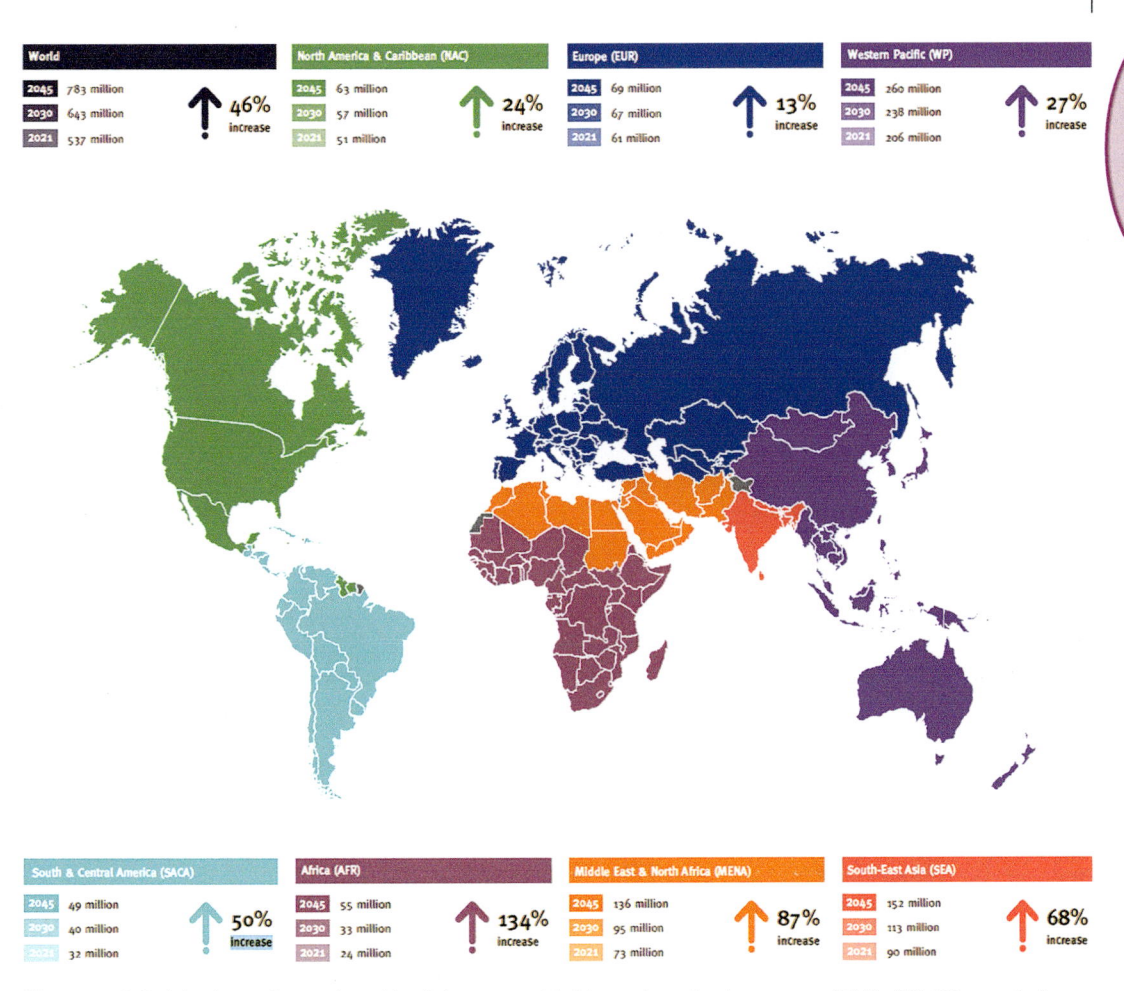

World
2045 783 million
2030 643 million
2021 537 million
↑ 46% increase

North America & Caribbean (NAC)
2045 63 million
2030 57 million
2021 51 million
↑ 24% increase

Europe (EUR)
2045 69 million
2030 67 million
2021 61 million
↑ 13% increase

Western Pacific (WP)
2045 260 million
2030 238 million
2021 206 million
↑ 27% increase

South & Central America (SACA)
2045 49 million
2030 40 million
2021 32 million
↑ 50% increase

Africa (AFR)
2045 55 million
2030 33 million
2021 24 million
↑ 134% increase

Middle East & North Africa (MENA)
2045 136 million
2030 95 million
2021 73 million
↑ 87% increase

South-East Asia (SEA)
2045 152 million
2030 113 million
2021 90 million
↑ 68% increase

Figure 1.2 Number of people with diabetes worldwide and projection up to 2045 (20–79 years) *Source: International Diabetes Federation. IDF Diabetes Atlas, 10th edn. Brussels, Belgium: International Diabetes Federation, 2021. http://www.diabetesatlas.org.*

Table 1.1 Diagnostic criteria for diabetes. In the absence of unequivocal hyperglycemia, these criteria should be confirmed by repeat testing on a different day. In 2011 the WHO accepted the use of the HbA1c test in diagnosing diabetes, with 48 mmol/mol (6.5%) recommended as the cutoff point.

WHO diagnostic criteria	
1	Symptoms of diabetes plus casual plasma glucose concentration of 11.1 mmol/L (200 mg/dL) *(Casual is defined as any time of day without regard to time since last meal. Symptoms of diabetes include polyuria, polydipsia, and unexplained weight loss)*
OR 2	Fasting plasma glucose 7.0 mmol/L (126 mg/dL) *(Fasting is defined as no caloric intake for at least 8 h)*
OR 3	2 h post-load glucose 11.1 mmol/L (200 mg/dL) during an OGTT*

Note: (The test should be performed as described by WHO, using a glucose load containing the equivalent of 75 g anhydrous glucose dissolved in water. Not recommended for routine clinical use.)

Table 1.2 Diagnostic glucose values. For epidemiological or population screening purposes, the fasting or 2 h value after 75 g oral glucose may be used alone. For clinical purposes, the diagnosis of diabetes should always be confirmed by repeating the test on another day, unless there is unequivocal hyperglycemia with acute metabolic decompensation or obvious symptoms. Glucose concentrations should not be determined on serum unless red cells are immediately removed, otherwise glycolysis will result in an unpredictable underestimation of the true concentrations. Note that glucose preservatives do not totally prevent glycolysis. If whole blood is used, the sample should be kept at 0–4°C or centrifuged/assayed immediately.

	Fasting plasma glucose	Two-hour glucose post 75 g oral glucose tolerance test	Glycated hemoglobin
Normal (ADA)	<100 mg/dL (5.6 mmol/L)	<140 mg/dL (7.8 mmol/L)	<5.7% (39 mmol/mol)
Normal (IEC)	<110 mg/dL (6.0 mmol/L)	<140 mg/dL (7.8 mmol/L)	<6.0% (42 mmol/mol)
Impaired Fasting Glucose (IFG) (ADA)	100–125 mg/dL (5.6–6.9 mmol/L)	<140 mg/dL (7.8 mmol/L)	-
Impaired Fasting Glucose (IFG) (WHO)	110–125 mg/dL (6.1–6.9 mmol/L)	<140 mg/dL (7.8 mmol/L)	-
Impaired Glucose Tolerance (IGT)	<126 mg/dL (7.0 mmol/L)	140–199 mg/dL (7.8–11.0 mmol/L)	-
Prediabetes (ADA)	-	-	5.7–6.4% (39–47 mmol/mol)
Prediabetes (IEC)	-	-	6.0–6.4% (42–47 mmol/mol)
Diabetes	≥126 mg/dL (7.0 mmol/L)	≥200 mg/dL (11.1 mmol/L)	≥6.5% (48 mmol/mol)

- Intermediate time points are used in the National Diabetes Data Group (NDDG) criteria.
  ◇ The reproducibility of the OGTT leaves much to be desired (the coefficient of variation of 120-minutes plasma glucose concentrations is reported to be up to 50%).
- Even if a subject fulfils the WHO criteria for diabetes, subsequent improvement in glucose tolerance can possibly occur (for example, as a result of weight loss or spontaneously), but such individuals are considered to have a lifelong tendency to diabetes.
- Impaired glucose tolerance (IGT) and impaired fasting glycemia (IFG) are metabolic states intermediate between normal glucose tolerance and diabetes mellitus (Table 1.2). People with IFG or IGT are at high risk of progression to diabetes and/or cardiovascular disease.
- Diagnostic criteria based on glycated hemoglobin or hemoglobin A1c (HbA1c) also show gradations of hyperglycemia. Reflecting average glycemia over 2–3 months, this gives equal or almost equal sensitivity and specificity to glucose measurement.
  ◇ HbA1c can be expressed as a percentage, as in the DCCT (Diabetes Control and Complications Trial). Alternatively it can be expressed as mmol/mol, which is recommended by the International Federation of Clinical Chemistry (IFCC) and is now the standard in the UK. A level of HbA1c of 5.7–6.4% (39–47 mmol/mol) is considered as prediabetes, and 6.5% (48 mmol/mol) or higher broadly equates with the diagnosis of diabetes.
- Some changes in diagnostic criteria were made in recognition of the increased cardiovascular risk evident at even

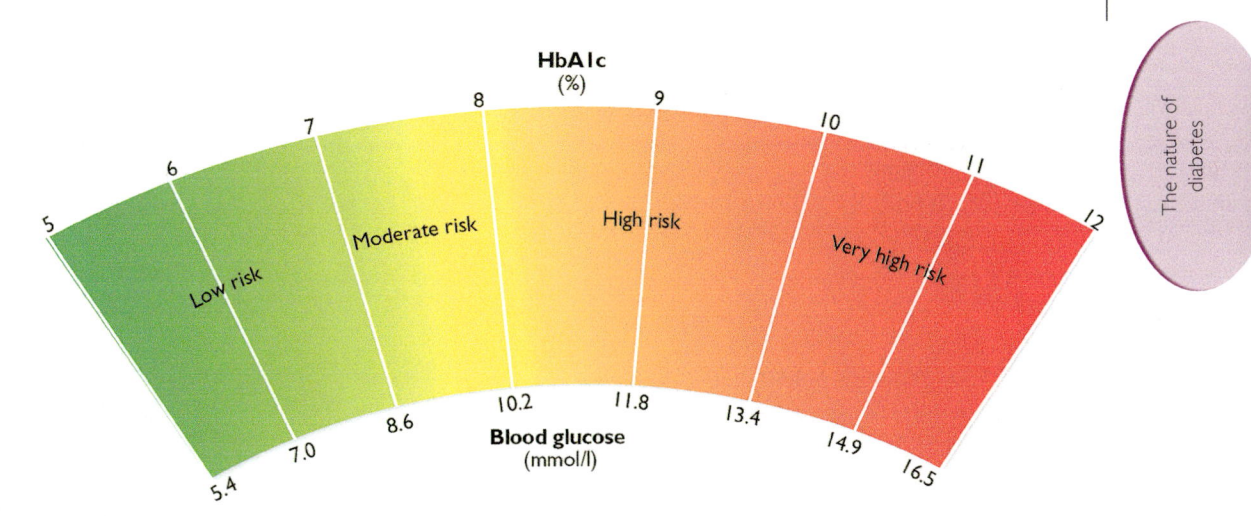

Figure 1.3 HbA1c and diabetes risk. The higher the HbA1c the higher the risk of diabetic complications.

modest levels of fasting hyperglycemia (~6.0 mmol/L or 100–110 mg/dL in some studies) (Figure 1.3).
- ◇ However, the blood glucose threshold for cardiovascular effects is almost certainly lower than the threshold for the microvascular complications (nephropathy, retinopathy, neuropathy) unique to diabetes mellitus. Some people diagnosed as having diabetes therefore may not suffer these microvascular complications, which have traditionally characterized the disease and determined its management.

◆ Diabetes represents a group of metabolic disorders, all of which are characterized by hyperglycemia. Type 1 diabetes is the most florid; type 2 diabetes is the most common.
- ◇ The other forms, although less common, are important because they may need distinct therapy.
- ◇ Some forms of diabetes are 'secondary' to another disease. Secondary diabetes accounts for 1–2% of all new cases.

◆ Type 1 diabetes (insulin-dependent diabetes mellitus) and type 2 diabetes (noninsulin-dependent diabetes mellitus) represent two distinct disease processes, but clinically this distinction can be unclear.
- ◇ In normal physiology, increased insulin secretion usually compensates for reductions in insulin sensitivity. Decreased insulin sensitivity is a feature of both major types of diabetes, but it is more severe in type 2 diabetes.

◆ Several classifications of diabetes have been proposed, such as that of the ADA (Table 1.3). It should be recognized that unanimity in nomenclature has yet to be achieved.

Table 1.3 Classification categories. There are four major categories of diabetes: type 1 diabetes and type 2 diabetes are the most common.

Etiological classification of diabetes
I TYPE 1 DIABETES (β-cell destruction, usually leading to absolute insulin deficiency)
Immune-mediated

(Continued)

Table 1.3 (Continued)

Etiological classification of diabetes			
Idiopathic			
II TYPE 2 DIABETES (may range from predominantly insulin resistance with relative insulin deficiency to a predominantly secretory defect with insulin resistance)			
III OTHER SPECIFIC TYPES			
Genetic defects of β-cell function	Chromosome 12, HNF-1 α (MODY3) Chromosome 7, glucokinase (MODY2) Chromosome 20, HNF-4α (MODY1) Chromosome 13, insulin promoter factor-1 (IPF-1;MODY4) Chromosome 17, HNF-1α (MOOY5) Chromosome 2, NeuroD1 (MODY6) Mitochondrial DNA Others	**Drug- or chemical-induced***	Vacor Pentamidine Nicotinic acid Glucocorticoids Thyroid hormone Diazoxide β-adrenergic agonists Thiazides Dilantin α-interferon Others
Genetic defects in insulin action	Type A insulin resistance Leprechaunism Rabson–Mendenhall syndrome Lipoatrophic diabetes Others	**Infections***	Congenital rubella Cytomegalovirus Others
Diseases of the exocrine pancreas*	Pancreatitis Trauma/pancreatectomy Neoplasia Cystic fibrosis Hemochromatosis Fibrocalculous pancreatopathy Others	**Uncommon forms of immune-mediated diabetes***	'Stiff-man' syndrome Anti-insulin receptor antibodies Others
Endocrinopathies*	Acromegaly Cushing's syndrome Glucagonoma Pheochromocytoma Hyperthyroidism Somatostatinoma Aldosteronoma Others	**Other genetic syndromes sometimes associated with diabetes**	Down's syndrome Klinefelter's syndrome Turner's syndrome Wolfram's syndrome Friedreich's ataxia Huntington's chorea Laurence–Moon–Biedl syndrome Myotonic dystrophy Porphyria Prader–Willi syndrome Others

IV GESTATIONAL DIABETES MELLITUS (GDM)

Statistical risk classes (subject with normal glucose tolerance but substantially increased risk of developing diabete

Previous abnormality of glucose tolerance
Potential abnormality of glucose tolerance

Note: Causes marked with an asterisk are termed 'secondary' diabetes.

Source: American Diabetes Association. Diagnosis and classification of diabetes mellitus. Diabetes Care. 2013 Jan;36 Suppl 1(Suppl 1):S67–74.

Diabetes is characterized by hyperglycemia.

Forms of diabetes

Type 1 diabetes (see also Chapter 3)

- Type 1 diabetes is the result of severe insulin deficiency leading to insulin-dependent diabetes. Though the incidence is highest during childhood or young adulthood, it can also occur at later ages.
  - In developed countries, most patients have the autoimmune-mediated form of the disease, where the body produces antibodies that destroy the insulin-producing cells of the pancreas. It is not clear what triggers this form of type 1 diabetes, but it is believed that both genetic and environmental factors (e.g. viruses) may be involved.
  - Idiopathic diabetes, where no cause can be found, is rare.
- Type 1 diabetes is the second most common chronic disease of childhood after asthma.

Type 2 diabetes (see also Chapter 4)

- Type 2 diabetes occurs as a result of relative insulin deficiency, where the pancreas does not produce enough insulin; and insulin resistance, where the body's cells do not react normally to insulin. Type 2 diabetes is more prevalent than type 1 diabetes.
- The exact causes of type 2 diabetes are not understood, but risk factors include obesity, having a close relative with type 2 diabetes, being of south Asian, African-Caribbean or Middle Eastern descent, and being over 40 years of age. Though more common in adults, type 2 diabetes is increasing in incidence among children.

Maturity onset diabetes of the young (MODY)

- This is a group of monogenic disorders (unlike type 1 and type 2 that are polygenic) that lead to diabetes. Though initially named numerically, they are now often named by the gene affected. Inheritance is mostly autosomal dominant, hence the strong family history. Onset is usually in childhood or adolescent years. In the main, they do not present with ketosis and weight loss as in type 1 and there is no strong linkage with obesity as for type 2. MODY is a group of diabetes conditions distinct from type 1 and type 2 (Table 1.4).
- MODY should be considered in young people presenting with a typical family history (diabetes affecting a parent and 50% expression of the disease in the family).

MODY 3, which results from a defect in hepatocyte nuclear factor 1 alpha (HNF1α) gene, and MODY 2, which results from a defect in the glucokinase (GCK) gene, are the most common.

Mutations in the ABCC8 (MODY 12) and KCNJ1 (MODY 13) genes are also associated with neonatal diabetes (Table 1.5).

Gestational diabetes mellitus (GDM) (see also Chapter 16)

- GDM occurs when abnormal glucose tolerance develops during pregnancy in a woman not known to have diabetes before pregnancy, unless she has had GDM in a previous pregnancy.
- The abnormal glucose tolerance usually resolves after delivery, but women with GDM are quite likely to develop it again in a subsequent pregnancy and are at considerably increased risk of developing type 2 diabetes sometime in the future.
- Risk factors for GDM include obesity, older age, first-degree relatives with

Table 1.4 Differential diagnosis. The distinction between the common types of diabetes and MODY is not always simple.

Differential diagnosis between diabetes types 1 and 2 and MODY

	TYPE 1 DIABETES	TYPE 2 DIABETES	MODY
Pathophysiology	β-cell failure	β-cell dysfunction and insulin resistance	β-cell dysfunction
Age of onset	Peak at 10–14 years old, but increasingly recognized in adults	Predominantly in middle to old age, but increasingly recognized in children	Typically childhood to young adulthood
Inheritance	Polygenic heterogeneous	Polygenic; heterogeneous	Autosomal dominant
Role of environment	Considerable	Considerable	Minimal
Gender ratio	Males and females equally affected	Females affected more than males	Males and females equally affected
Association with obesity	<24% overweight	85% overweight	Uncommonly associated with obesity
Treatment required	Insulin required in >95%	Insulin required in 17–37% of children, but less frequent initially in adults	Insulin may be required but infrequently
Diabetes-specific autoantibodies status	Usually positive	Negative	Negative

Table 1.5 Some forms of MODY.

	MODY 1	MODY 2	MODY 3	MODY 4	MODY 5	MODY 6
Gene defect	HNF4α	glucokinase	HNF1α	PDX1	HNF1β	NEUROD1
Penetrance	High	Moderate	High	High	High	
Complications	Vascular	Uncommon	Vascular	Pancreatic agenesis	Urogenital	Neurologic
Treatment	Sulfonylurea, GLP-1 receptor agonist	Diet and exercise	Sulfonylurea, GLP-1 receptor agonist			Insulin

diabetes, a history of poor pregnancy outcome, a history of large for gestational age babies, and belonging to an ethnic/racial group with a known high prevalence of type 2 diabetes.

Neonatal diabetes

◆ Neonatal diabetes develops in neonates shortly after birth and within the first two years of life. It can be transient or permanent. It is due to a defect in the potassium channel of insulin-secreting cells, as a result of gene mutations that limit potassium channel closure and thus insulin secretion.

◆ The gene mutations can be rectified by sulfonylureas, which enable activation of the potassium channel, so that children treated with insulin can switch to sulfonylurea treatment with an improvement in glucose control.

Secondary diabetes

◆ This book is not intended to be an authoritative account of the diagnosis and management of the multiple conditions that may cause secondary diabetes or glucose intolerance. Such conditions are listed in Table 1.3.

Clinical presentations of diabetes

- Patients with diabetes present either with symptoms due to the high glucose level or with the complications of diabetes (Figure 1.4).
- The classic triad of symptoms directly due to high blood glucose is:
  - Polyuria – due to the osmotic diuresis that results when blood glucose levels exceed the renal threshold.
  - Thirst – due to the resulting loss of fluid and electrolytes.
  - Weight loss – due to fluid depletion and the accelerated breakdown of fat and muscle secondary to insulin deficiency; this is less prevalent in those with type 2 diabetes.
- Florid symptoms are most often seen in children with type 1 diabetes. Ketoacidosis may be a presenting feature.
- Patients with type 1 diabetes often, but not always, present with severe symptoms of hyperglycemia.
  - The severity of the condition may be reflected in raised blood ketone levels and weight loss.
- Other, nonosmotic symptoms are the consequences of high blood glucose:
  - Lack of energy.
  - Visual blurring (due to glucose-induced changes in refraction).
  - Fungal infections causing pruritus vulvae and balanitis.
  - Bacterial infections causing staphylococcal skin infections.
  - Retinopathy.
  - Polyneuropathy causing tingling and numbness in the feet or erectile dysfunction.
- Subjects with IGT are at risk of macrovascular disease and some already have arterial disease on presentation, including myocardial infarction and gangrene.
- A fraction of cases present without symptoms, either on routine blood screening or with glycosuria.
  - Glycosuria is not diagnostic of diabetes but indicates the need for further investigation.
  - About 1% of the population have renal glycosuria, inherited as an autosomal dominant or recessive trait associated with a low renal threshold for glucose.
- As a common disease that can have multiple consequences, diabetes may be discovered 'fortuitously' in patients being investigated for a wide range of symptoms.

The classic symptoms directly due to hyperglycemia are polyuria, thirst, and weight loss.

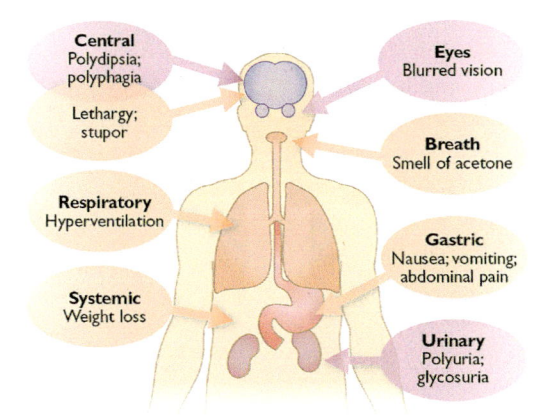

Figure 1.4 Symptoms of diabetes. Those symptoms in orange are typically confined to patients with type 1 diabetes.

- Central: Polydipsia; polyphagia
- Lethargy; stupor
- Respiratory: Hyperventilation
- Systemic: Weight loss
- Eyes: Blurred vision
- Breath: Smell of acetone
- Gastric: Nausea; vomiting; abdominal pain
- Urinary: Polyuria; glycosuria

Complications of diabetes

- If diabetes is not well managed or controlled, the high blood glucose levels can lead to damage to blood vessels, nerves, and organs. Even non-symptomatic, mild hyperglycemia can have damaging effects in the long term. High blood sugar levels can also reduce the efficiency of white blood cells in fighting infections.

Macrovascular complications (see also Chapter 6)

- Macrovascular problems associated with diabetes mellitus include heart disease, stroke, and peripheral vascular disease (which can lead to ulcers, gangrene, and amputation). Prolonged, poorly controlled hyperglycemia increases the likelihood of atherosclerosis. An individual with diabetes is approximately five times more likely to suffer heart disease and stroke than someone without diabetes.

Diabetes dramatically increases an individual's risk of heart disease and stroke.

Microvascular complications

- These include retinopathy, neuropathy, and nephropathy (see also Chapters 6, 7, 8, 9, 10).
- Very small blood vessels can become blocked or leaky as a result of hyperglycemia. The blood vessels most frequently affected are in the eye, the kidney, and nerve sheaths. This microvascular disease is specific to diabetes, and may occur in any type of diabetes.
    - ◇ Damage to the blood vessels of the retina can result in loss of vision.
    - ◇ Damage to blood vessels in the kidneys can result in kidney failure.
    - ◇ Damage to blood vessels in nerve sheaths can result in numbness or tingling. If nerves to the digestive system are affected, the individual may suffer associated symptoms, e.g. nausea or constipation. Loss of sensation in the feet can lead to the development of ulcers.

Acute metabolic complications

- These include hypoglycemia, ketoacidosis, hyperosmolar nonketotic hyperglycemia (see also Chapter 12).
- Hypoglycemia most commonly results from treating diabetes with exogenous insulin or insulin secretagogues.
    - ◇ In a person without diabetes, endogenous production of insulin decreases and counter-regulatory hormones (mostly epinephrine and glucagon) increase in response to hypoglycemia. This fine-tuned system is dysregulated in patients with diabetes, and patients have to resort to intake of carbohydrates to raise the blood glucose back up to normal.
    - ◇ Symptoms range from mild to moderate (palpitations, diaphoresis) to severe (convulsions, coma).
- Diabetic ketoacidosis and hyperosmolar hyperglycemic nonketotic state occur as a result of insulin deficiency during episodes of stress, when counter-regulatory hormones are in excess.
    - ◇ Patients are dehydrated, and frequently present with altered sensorium. Treatment includes hydration to correct the fluid deficit, insulin administration, and correction of the underlying disease.

The cost of diabetes

- The cost of diabetes is substantial and increasing as the cost of therapies rises and the disease frequency increases.
- There is a strong commercial argument, quite apart from a humanitarian one, for primary prevention of diabetes complications.
    - ◇ The cost of effectively treating the complications of diabetes is high, and preventive care in limiting progression to diabetic complications has a definite impact.
- There are striking differences in cost estimates between different countries (Figure 1.5). Many studies have shown that indirect costs (loss of financial output through illness or death, etc.) approximately equal direct costs (treatment, diagnosis, medical care, etc.). In the US, however, direct costs account for about three-quarters of the cost of diabetes, and

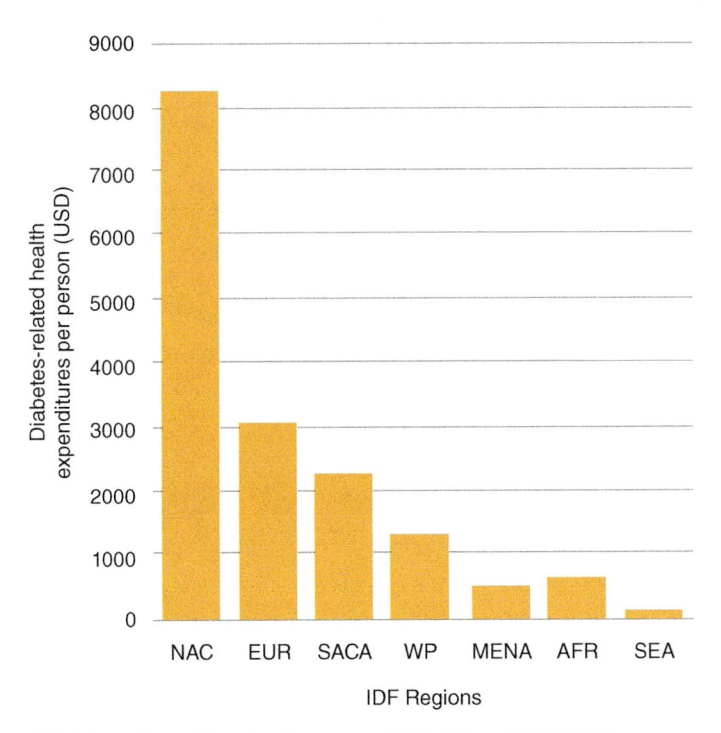

Figure 1.5 Diabetes-related health expenditure (USD) per person with diabetes (20–79 years) in 2021 by IDF Region. *From International Diabetes Federation.* IDF Diabetes Atlas, 10th ed. *Brussels, Belgium: 2021.*

IDF: International Diabetes Federation; AFR: Africa; EUR: Europe; WP: Western Pacific; MENA: Middle East and North Africa; NAC: North America and Caribbean; SACA: South and Central America; SEA: South-East Asia;

about one in four US health care dollars is spent on patients with diabetes.

- The total estimated cost of diabetes in the US in 2007 was $174 billion, with direct medical costs amounting to $116 billion. In 2017, these numbers were $245 billion and $176 billion, respectively. In the UK, the direct cost of diabetes in 2010–2011 was £9.8 billion, and indirect cost was £9 billion.

CHAPTER 2

Glucose, insulin, and diabetes

The role and regulation of glucose

- A vital metabolic fuel glucose is the main source of energy in many tissues. It is metabolized during the process of cellular respiration, which breaks it down to release adenosine triphosphate (ATP).
  - It is a monosaccharide, or simple sugar, with the formula $C_6H_{12}O_6$. Its six carbon atoms can be arranged in open-chain or ring forms.
  - Red blood cells and brain cells use glucose almost exclusively for energy production, whereas other cells in the body can metabolize fats for energy if necessary.
  - Most glucose in the body comes from digested carbohydrates, but it can also be synthesized in the liver.
- The importance of glucose is reflected in the strict control of blood glucose levels (homeostasis [Figure 2.1]). This contrasts with the relative laxity of regulation of other circulating metabolic fuels such as ketone bodies and nonesterified fatty acids (NEFA) (also known as free fatty acids [FFA]) – the form in which stored body fat is transported from adipose tissue to sites of utilization.
- Of all the hormones known to influence blood glucose concentration, insulin is the only one able to lower it. Glucagon, on the other hand, is a hormone that counteracts the effects of glucose. Glucagon stimulates the liver to break down glycogen to release glucose into the blood (glycogenolysis), and also to convert amino acids into glucose (gluconeogenesis).
- Glucose is also important in the formation of glycoproteins, making up the carbohydrate groups on proteins which play key roles in the normal functioning of enzymes and in protein binding.

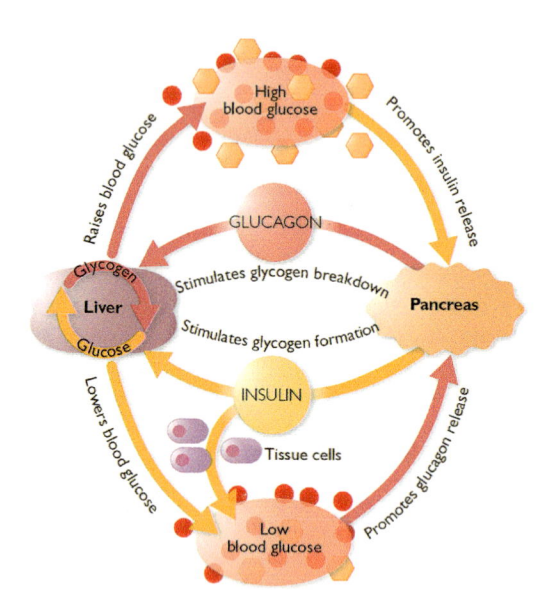

Figure 2.1 Glucose homeostasis. The concentration of glucose in the blood is controlled by the antagonistic actions of two hormones: insulin and glucagon, produced in the β cells and α cells of the pancreatic islets, respectively. High blood glucose causes the pancreas to release more insulin and less glucagon; the excess glucose is converted to glycogen and stored in the liver. If glucose levels are low, then the pancreas releases more glucagon and less insulin, stimulating the breakdown of glycogen back to glucose, which re-enters the bloodstream.

Glucose is the main source of energy for human body cells.
Insulin is the only hormone able to lower blood glucose concentration.

Glucose levels and diabetes

- Diabetes is defined by an increase in blood glucose levels above normal values. To understand how hyperglycemia may occur, we should consider factors that maintain blood glucose within a strict range.
- In healthy people, blood glucose concentrations are maintained within very close limits (Figure 2.2), with a strictly maintained postabsorptive (e.g. fasted overnight) blood glucose concentration of 4.5–5.2 mmol/L (81–94 mg/dL).
  ◇ Inter-individual coefficients of variation (assuming similar times since previous meal, meal composition, levels of activity, etc.) are <5%, so a fasting glucose of 6.0 mmol/L (108 mg/dL) is 4–5 standard deviations above the mean in most healthy populations.
  ◇ Glucose concentrations increase after meals, but typical meals will not raise blood glucose above ~8 mmol/L (144 mg/dL), and normoglycemia is usually restored within 2–4 hours in healthy people.
  ◇ Reductions in glycemia can be produced by severe, sudden, unaccustomed exercise or prolonged fasting (or both), by various pathological conditions (usually hepatic or gastroenterological), and by pharmacological means, but are not commonly encountered in healthy adults in developed countries.
- Strict avoidance of low blood sugars is necessary to avoid the neurological and other consequences of hypoglycemia (see also Chapter 15).
  ◇ Neuroglycopenia (glucose depletion in neural tissue) starts at concentrations around 3.0–3.5 mmol/L (54–63 mg/dL) and counter-regulatory mechanisms are set to respond to maintain glycemia comfortably above this level.
- Prior to reaching neuroglycopenia, insulin secretion decreases at plasma glucose levels of around 4.4–4.7 mmol/L (80–85 m/dL) and glucagon levels increase at

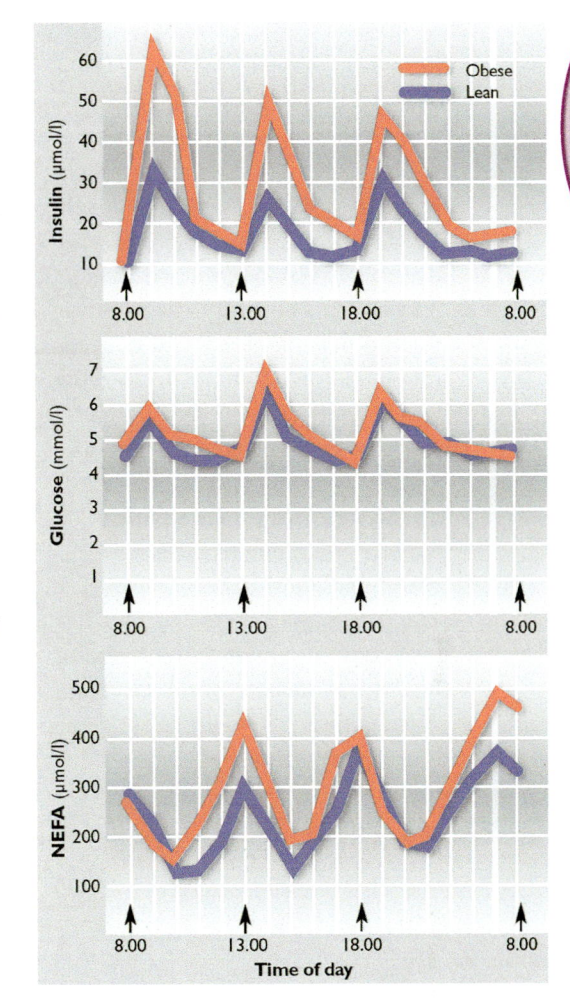

Figure 2.2 Postprandial metabolic responses.
Insulin, glucose, and NEFA concentrations in normal and obese subjects eating three meals a day (arrows). Normal insulin response to meals is rapid and relatively short-lasting. As the insulin concentration rises in response to a meal, NEFA response is suppressed. Insulin resistance in obese individuals means that higher insulin levels are required to maintain normoglycemia.
From Reaven 1985.

plasma glucose levels of 3.6–3.9 mmol/L (65–70 mg/dL).
- ◆ The reason for the strict avoidance of hyperglycemia is less immediately apparent.
  - ◇ Symptoms of hyperglycemia are florid (in subjects used to relative normoglycemia) at blood glucose concentrations of 12–13 mmol/L (216–234 mg/dL) and may commence at concentrations below 10 mmol/L (180 mg/dL). The metabolic consequences of severe hyperglycemia, at levels usually above 20 mmol/L (360 mg/dL), are discussed in the section on diabetic emergencies (Chapter 12).
  - ◇ In contrast, mild hyperglycemia (glucose 6–9 mmol/L [108–162 mg/dL]) is usually asymptomatic. The value of the strict avoidance of mild hyperglycemia is thus not so apparent, except in terms of avoiding the consequences of prolonged hyperglycemia: long-term diabetic complications or tissue damage.
  - ◇ Increased susceptibility to infection may be seen acutely with moderate hyperglycemia.

Normal glucose metabolism

- ◆ Glucose enters the circulation from three main sources:
  - ◇ The gut—as the result of hydrolysis or hepatic conversion of a variety of ingested carbohydrates.
  - ◇ Hepatic and other glycogen stores (glycogenolysis).
  - ◇ New synthesis from precursors (gluconeogenesis) (Figure 2.3).
- ◆ *Gluconeogenesis* takes place in the liver (~75–90%) and kidneys (~10–25%). Glucagon stimulates gluconeogenesis.
  - ◇ The breakdown of fat (from glycerol), muscle glycogen (from lactate), and amino acids (such as alanine) creates two 3-carbon molecules which combine to form the 6-carbon glucose molecule.
  - ◇ In the resting postabsorptive state, hepatic glucose output is ~2.0 mg/kg

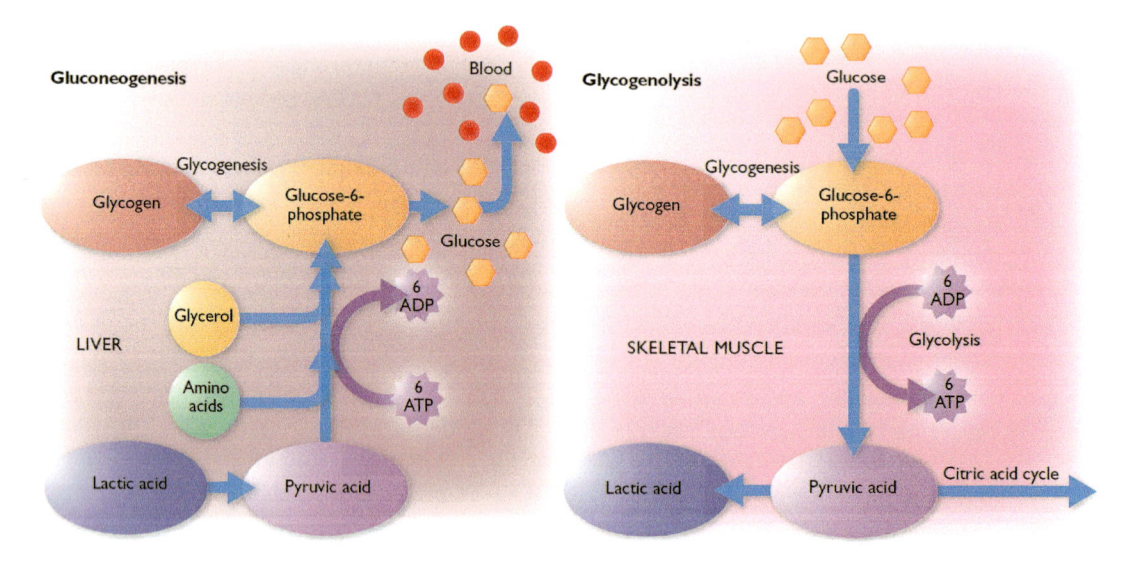

Figure 2.3 Gluconeogenesis and glycogenolysis. Gluconeogenesis is the synthesis of glucose in the liver from noncarbohydrate sources, including lactic acid from the muscles. In glycogenolysis, glycogen reserves in the liver and muscles are converted back into glucose-6-phosphate to begin the glycolytic process, the end results of which are pyruvic acid and, via the citric acid cycle, ATP.

bodyweight/min or 200–300 g during the average day (depending on the availability of glucose from food and the body's requirements).
- ◇ Glycemia is determined by the balance of glucose influx into the circulation (principally from hepatic glucose production) and peripheral clearance.
- ◆ *Glycogenesis* converts excess glucose into glycogen via glucose-6-phosphate, for storage in the liver and muscles. *Glycogenolysis* is the process by which it is converted back again.

  Glucagon inhibits glycogenesis and promotes glycogenolysis.
  - ◇ Glycogen is synthesized from both glucose and the gluconeogenic precursors.
  - ◇ A 70 kg man typically has a total of 700–1000 g of (hydrated) glycogen, mostly stored in the liver (60–125 g) and skeletal muscle (400–600 g).
  - ◇ Glycogen in skeletal muscle can provide local fuel but does not provide a source of glucose for release into the circulation.
- ◆ *Glucose homeostasis* is accomplished predominantly by the liver, which absorbs and stores glucose (as glycogen) in the postabsorptive state and releases it into the circulation between meals.
  - ◇ To maintain homeostasis, the rate of glucose utilization by peripheral tissues must match the rate of glucose production.
  - ◇ The balancing of glucose production and utilization depends partly upon mass action, but also crucially upon endocrine regulation by insulin and its counter-regulatory hormones (see Figure 2.1).
- ◆ Glucose provides approximately 40–60% (on a typical western diet) of the total fuel expenditure of the body during a 24-hour period.
  - ◇ Glucose provides almost all the energy of the central nervous system.
- ◇ During high-intensity exercise and during the 4–6 hours postprandially, glucose is the predominant fuel of the whole body.
- ◇ Glucose is the most efficient fuel for oxidation in terms of the liberation of energy (112.2 kcal or 6 mole ATP per mole of oxygen consumed).
- ◇ Many tissues can use ketone bodies, fatty acids, or glucose for their energy supply, depending upon their relative availability in the circulation.
- ◆ Glucose is fully oxidized to carbon dioxide and water in the brain, liver, skeletal muscle, and some other tissues.
  - ◇ The brain accounts for most of the glucose oxidized in the fasting state (100–125 g/24 hours).
  - ◇ In the fasted state, resting skeletal muscle takes up 10–20% of hepatic glucose output: this is not all oxidized but can be converted to lactate, pyruvate, glycerol, or amino acids, some of which subsequently returns to the liver as gluconeogenic precursors.
  - ◇ Fatty acids (or their partial oxidation products, ketone bodies) are the major fuel of resting muscle, and the heart and liver.
  - ◇ Other tissues such as red blood cells, skin, adipose tissue, and the renal medulla derive most energy from glycolysis to lactate and pyruvate. Glycolysis to lactate is an anaerobic process to which many cells may resort when faced with hypoxia; for example, skeletal muscle during high-intensity exercise.
  - ◇ Glucose taken up by fat tissue is used as a source of energy and to form the glycerol component of triglyceride stores.
- ◆ In resting, postabsorptive subjects, approximately 70% of the body's glucose metabolism occurs independently of the action of insulin. However, these insulin-independent mechanisms cannot maintain normoglycemia for very long.

- Insulin-independent (as well as insulin-dependent) glucose clearance is impaired in subjects with type 2 diabetes and also in normoglycemic subjects with a family history of diabetes. This suggests that abnormalities in insulin-independent glucose disposal manifest at a very early stage of disease evolution.
    - This phenomenon of 'glucose resistance' appears to be quantitatively important: as much as half of an intravenous glucose load is cleared by virtue of the effect of hyperglycemia on insulin-independent glucose disposal in normal subjects.

Glucose transporters

- Glucose is a hydrophilic molecule unable to penetrate the lipid bilayer of cell membranes.
    - Its uptake into cells is achieved by an energy-independent process of facilitated diffusion mediated by a family of glucose transporter proteins (GLUTs).

    In addition, there are also sodium-glucose linked transporters or co-transporters (SGLTs).
    - GLUT transporters allow the uptake of glucose into cells from the interstitial fluid into which glucose diffuses from the bloodstream. Differences in kinetics, tissue and subcellular expression profiles, and substrate specificities enable specific functions such as glucose sensing (GLUT2) and insulin-dependent glucose uptake (GLUT4) (Table 2.1).
- The various sugar transporters recognized to date are classified into those having high glucose affinity (class I, comprising GLUT1–4), high fructose affinity (class II, e.g. GLUT5), and novel transporters whose physiology is not yet fully understood (GLUT6–14) (Table 2.1).
- The different functions of the class I GLUTs are related to their differing K_m values (K_m, the Michaelis constant, is the substrate concentration that produces half the maximum enzyme/transporter activity).
    - GLUT1, GLUT3, and GLUT4 have K_m values of approximately 1–5 mmol/L (36–90 mg/dL) but GLUT2 has a K_m value of approximately 20 mmol/L (450 mg/dL). This variation in K_m permits high rates of glucose entry into essential cells (e.g. the central nervous system) even during relative hypoglycemia via the low-Km GLUT3, but at the same time permits the pancreatic β cells to sense increments in blood glucose over a range well exceeding normality via the high-Km GLUT2.
    - The central nervous system is relatively protected from neuroglycopenia by the low K_m of its GLUT3 transporters.
- GLUT1 and GLUT3 transporters are present in the cell membrane at all times and allow cells to take up glucose independently of insulin action (a process sometimes termed noninsulin-mediated glucose uptake, NIMGU).
- In contrast, GLUT4 transporters are stored in the cell cytoplasm. In the presence of insulin, GLUT4 moves from these storage compartments to the cell membrane, increasing transporter numbers 6–10-fold. When insulin concentrations decline, GLUT4 is removed from the cell membrane by endocytosis and rapidly recycled back into storage (Figure 2.4).
- Dysfunction of the insulin-regulated GLUT4 translocation process appears to play a part in insulin resistance, and mutations of several transporters (e.g. GLUT1, GLUT2) have been associated with inborn errors of carbohydrate metabolism.

The entry of glucose into cells is mediated by a group of transporter proteins known as GLUTs.

Table 2.1 Glucose transporter proteins. GLUT family members are tissue-specific. In addition, their differing kinetic properties allow a range of functions.

Characteristics of the main glucose transporters			
TRANSPORTER	TISSUES	KINETICS	TRANSPORT TYPE
GLUT1	Ubiquitous, erythrocyte, placenta, colon, kidney	Low K_m (~2 mmol/L, 18–36 mg/dL)	Facilitated diffusion
GLUT2	Liver, small intestine, kidney, β cells	High K_m (~20 mmol/L, 450 mg/dL), high V_{max}	Facilitated diffusion, bidirectional
GLUT3	Ubiquitous, brain, placenta, kidney	Low K_m (~1 mmol/L, 18–36 mg/dL), low V_{max} (6–7 mmol/L, 108–126 mg/dL)	Facilitated diffusion
GLUT4	Skeletal muscle, adipocyte, heart	K_m ~5 mmol/L (36–180 mg/dL)	Facilitated diffusion, insulin responsive
GLUT5	Jejunum		Facilitated diffusion of fructose
Na+-glucose co-transporter(s)	Intestine, kidney tubules	Moves glucose against concentration gradient	Active transport, symport using Na+ gradient

Characteristics of the main sodium-glucose linked transporters (SGLTs)		
Transporter	Tissues	Function
SGLT1	Small intestine	Intestinal glucose absorption
	Proximal tubule of kidneys	Reabsorption of 3% of the filtered glucose by the kidney tubules
SGLT2	Proximal convoluted tubule of kidneys	Reabsorption of 90% of the filtered glucose by the kidney tubules
SGLT3	Intestine, testes, uterus, lung, brain, thyroid	Control of glucose levels in intestine and brain
SGLT4	Intestine, kidney, liver, brain, lung, uterus, pancreas	

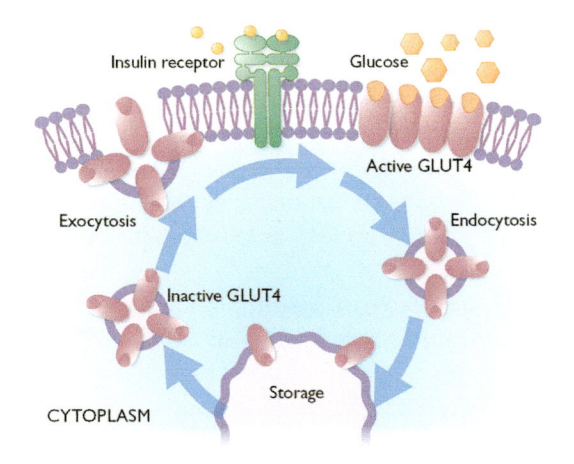

Figure 2.4 Insulin-dependent glucose uptake.
When insulin is present, or there is muscle activity, GLUT4 molecules move from storage within the cell to the plasma membrane, where they contribute to glucose transport.

◇ The insulin-sensitizing agents metformin and the thiazolidinediones appear to increase cell surface expression of GLUT4, as does physical exercise.

◆ Glucose can be moved against a concentration gradient – necessary in the special circumstances of the renal tubule and intestinal epithelium – by using a family of SGLTs.

◇ At least one of these co-transporters (SGLT3) appears to have some glucose concentration–sensing function.

◇ Mutations of SGLT1 are associated with the glucose-galactose malabsorption syndrome, which can cause fatal infantile diarrhea unless these sugars are removed from the diet.

- ◇ A reduced function mutation of SGLT2 has been associated with renal tubular glucose spillage.
- ◆ To trap glucose within the cell (since GLUTs are potentially bidirectional), glucose is phosphorylated on entry by a family of hexokinases.
  - ◇ Hexokinase types I–III are expressed widely and have low K_m.
  - ◇ Hexokinase type IV (also called glucokinase and predominantly expressed in liver and β cells) has a much higher K_m of up to 15 mmol/L (270 mg/dL), permitting it to function as a glucose sensor beyond the physiological range of blood glucose.
  - ◇ Since glucokinase action is also a rate-limiting step in glucose metabolism, it thus becomes a crucial determinant of the rate of insulin secretion from β cells.
- ◆ Loss-of-function mutations of glucokinase are responsible for one form of maturity onset diabetes of the young (MODY 2) (see Chapter 1).
- ◆ Dephosphorylation of glucose (the reverse reaction) is catalyzed by glucose-6-phosphatase. This process is required for the export of glucose (from gluconeogenesis) by hepatic and renal cells in hypoinsulinemic situations.
  - ◇ Overactivity of glucose-6-phosphatase contributes to the increased and relatively insulin-insensitive hepatic glucose production in type 2 diabetes.
  - ◇ Metformin and the thiazolidinediones (see Chapter 14) appear to reduce the activity of this enzyme, although it is not clear whether their effects are direct or mediated through some other upstream action.

The role and regulation of insulin

- ◆ Insulin is the predominant hormone regulating blood glucose concentration. It is the key hormone involved in both the storage and the controlled release of energy.
- ◆ Diabetes occurs as a result of a failure of insulin production and secretion (insulin deficiency) and/or the loss of response to insulin (insulin resistance).
- ◆ Insulin is coded for by genes on chromosome 11 and is synthesized and secreted by the β cells of the islets of Langerhans in the pancreas. Complex cellular events trigger the release of insulin from the secretory granules of these cells.

Hormones called **incretins** are peptides secreted by the gut in response to a meal and stimulate the secretion of insulin. Of these, **glucagon-like peptide**-1 (GLP-1, produced by the lower intestine) and glucose-dependent insulinotropic polypeptide (GIP, produced by the upper intestine) are the better-studied incretins.

- ◆ After secretion, insulin enters the portal circulation, which takes it to the liver, a prime target organ of insulin action.
- ◆ Although insulin is the major regulator of intermediary metabolism, its actions are modified by other hormones, e.g. glucagon, epinephrine (adrenalin), cortisol, and growth hormone. Such counter-regulatory hormones increase glucose production from the liver and, for a given level of insulin, reduce utilization of glucose in adipose tissue and muscle.
- ◆ Insulin concentrations rise after a meal so that postprandial insulin can orchestrate the distribution of energy from food (see Figure 2.2).
  - ◇ During fasting, insulin levels are low, but after eating insulin secretion rapidly increases in healthy subjects.

The structure of insulin
- ◆ Insulin is a peptide hormone, with 51 amino acids arranged in two chains linked by two disulfide bonds.
  - ◇ Some of these amino acids are different in patients with diabetes associated with mutant insulins, others are different in other mammalian species (cattle, pigs), and still others have

- been modified in therapeutic insulin analogs (e.g. Lantus, Humalog).
◆ In the synthesis of insulin translation of mRNA yields preproinsulin, a prohormone containing 110 amino acids, which undergoes post-translational modification prior to the release of the mature insulin molecule.
  ◇ Removal of 24 amino acids from preproinsulin yields proinsulin, with 86 amino acids, which is then stored in secretory granules within the β cell.
  ◇ In healthy subjects, over 90% of proinsulin is converted to mature insulin by the removal of the metabolically inert C-peptide component (Figure 2.5).
◆ C-peptide is only partially extracted by the liver, so levels of this protein can be used as an index of insulin secretion. In healthy subjects only small amounts (<10% of mature insulin output) of proinsulin and partially split proinsulin are released.
  ◇ These ratios are characteristically disturbed in certain pathological states, including autonomous insulin secretion from an insulinoma and in type 2 diabetes, and will be low or undetectable in cases of surreptitious administration of exogenous insulin.
  ◇ Assay of these substances may therefore, in some circumstances, prove helpful in the differential diagnosis of hypoglycemia.
  ◇ Proinsulin may accumulate in renal failure and is elevated in familial hyperproinsulinemia.
◆ Substances stimulating the synthesis and storage of insulin include glucose, mannose, leucine, arginine, hormones such as GLP-1, and a variety of metabolizable sugars or sugar derivatives. Most of these also promote secretion and these factors are collectively termed secretagogues.

Normal insulin secretion and kinetics
◆ The mechanisms regulating insulin release are the focus of much research.
◆ It is known that there is an ATP–dependent, sulfonylurea-sensitive potassium (K^+) channel whose closure is a late

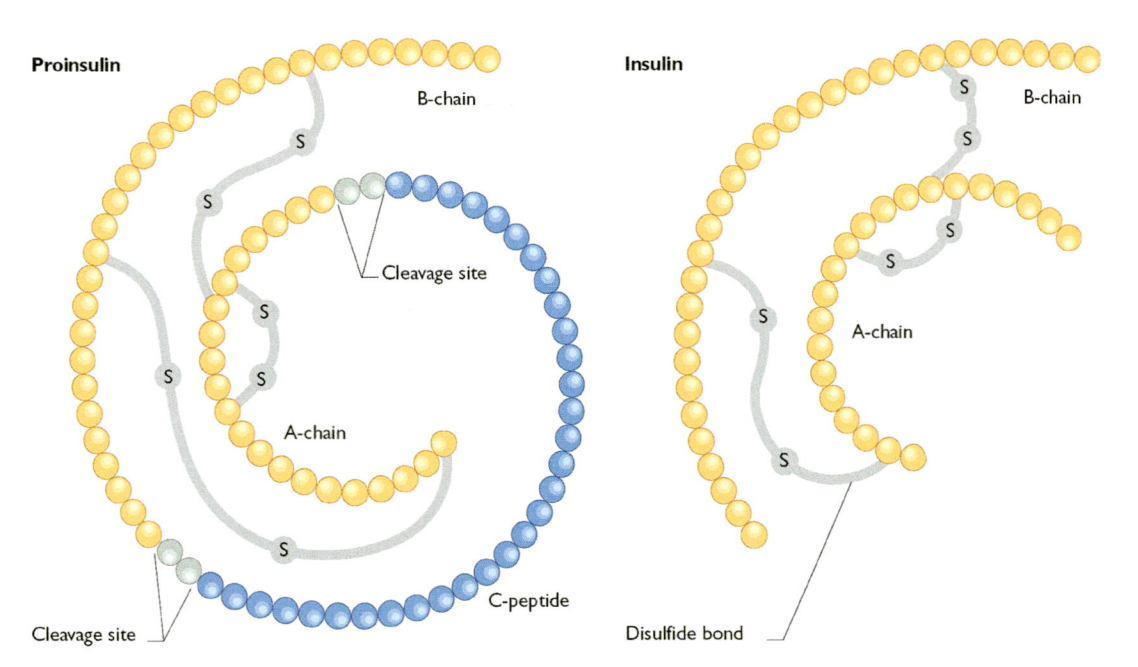

Figure 2.5 Structure of insulin and proinsulin. Proinsulin synthesized in the pancreatic β cells is converted to insulin by the removal of the 31 amino acids that form the C-peptide protein in the center of the sequence; the two other ends (the B chain and A chain) remain connected by disulfide bonds.

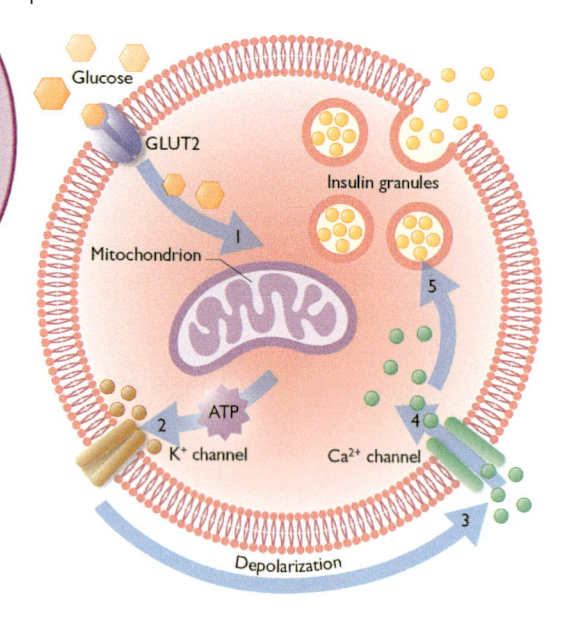

Figure 2.6 Insulin secretion. Extracellular glucose is transported into the β cell via the GLUT2 receptor where it is converted into glucose-6-phosphate by the enzyme glucokinase (1). Glycolysis within the mitochondrion generates ATP, which leads to the closure of ATP–sensitive potassium channels (2) and depolarization of the cell membrane (3). This opens the voltage-dependent calcium channels (4) and allows the influx of calcium and the subsequent release of insulin (5).

event in the intracellular signaling mechanism within the β cell. Potassium channel closure triggers calcium influx and exocytosis (Figure 2.6).

- A wide range of secretagogues will stimulate closure of the K+ channel. The most important of these stimulants is hyperglycemia.
  - ◇ Other secretagogues include mannose, lactate, some amino acids, glucagon, glucose-dependent insulinotropic peptide (GIP), cholecystokinin, vasoactive intestinal peptide (VIP), ghrelin, glucagon-like peptide-1 (GLP-1), sulfonylureas, and parasympathetic cholinergic (muscarinic) nerve activity; many have synergistic effects.
- Conversely, insulin secretion is inhibited by both neural sympathetic tone and circulating catecholamines.

- A combination of cephalic and gastric effects makes oral glucose a more potent stimulus to insulin secretion than an equivalent amount of intravenous glucose. This is known as the 'incretin' effect and is, at least in part, attributable to gut-derived hormones such as GIP and GLP-1.
- In healthy adults, insulin is secreted in pulses with a periodicity of 11–15 minutes.
  - ◇ Stimuli of insulin secretion increase the frequency and amplitude of these pulses.
  - ◇ Approximately 30–40 units (240 pmol) of insulin are secreted every 24 hours in healthy subjects of normal weight.
  - ◇ Insulin secretion is basal (0.25–1.0 U/hours) when glycemia is below a threshold level of about 5 mmol/L (90 mg/dL) and insulin output is maximal at glycemia of 15–20 mmol/L (270–360 mg/dL).
- Insulin is secreted into the portal venous system and must traverse the liver prior to reaching the systemic circulation.
  - ◇ The liver is thus exposed to insulin concentrations approximately three times higher than other tissues when insulin is secreted endogenously.
  - ◇ About 50% of secreted insulin is extracted and degraded in the 'first pass' through the liver; much of the residue is broken down by the kidneys.
- The pulsatile pattern of insulin secretion and clearance is controlled not only by prevailing blood glucose concentration, but also by the secretagogues mentioned earlier.
  - ◇ It is not hard to appreciate the difficulty in replicating the physiological manifestation of insulin with the subcutaneous administration of exogenous insulin.

Hyperglycemia is the most important stimulant for secretion of insulin.

- Autocrine and paracrine regulation of insulin secretion by pancreatic and gut hormones (which may reach very high concentrations within the islet) are incompletely understood. Increased secretion of insulin involves recruitment of more β cells to the secreting mode.
- Fasting peripheral insulin concentrations vary between 3 and 15 mU/L (~20–100 pmol/L), as measured by radio immunoassays in healthy subjects, with the higher values associated with increasing age and obesity.
  ◇ After a typical mixed meal (700–800 kcal), the peak plasma insulin concentration will be 40–80 mU/L (~280–560 pmol/L) in young, lean adults.
- The half-life of insulin injected into a peripheral vein is 2–6 minutes, with the liver clearing most of this insulin. Smaller amounts are cleared in other tissues that have insulin receptors, such as skeletal muscle, although there is also nonreceptor-mediated clearance by a variety of tissue proteases.

The insulin receptor
- Insulin's main glucoregulatory effects are mediated by the insulin receptor – a transmembrane receptor coded by chromosome 19 and found on insulin-sensitive cells. This receptor is a glycoprotein, comprising four peptide subchains – two α and two β subunits – linked by disulfide bridges.
- There are two receptor isoforms, IR-A and IR-D, formed by alternate splicing.
- The DNA sequence and amino acid structure of the insulin receptor show homology with those of the insulin-like growth factor-1 (IGF-1) receptor.
- When insulin binds to the extracellular domain of the α subunit of the insulin receptor, an enzyme (tyrosine kinase) on the intracellular domain of the β subunit is activated; the signal is thus transferred across the membrane. Activation of other intracellular enzymes follows (Figure 2.7).

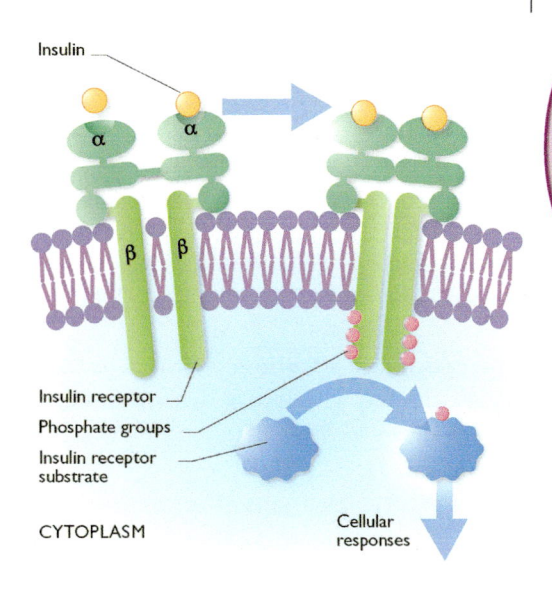

Figure 2.7 Insulin receptor action. When insulin binds to the two extracellular α subunits of the receptor the transmembrane β subunits transmit a signal that activates their protein kinase domain. Phosphorylation of the insulin receptor substrate triggers further reactions, leading to the uptake of glucose.

- After activation, the insulin-receptor complex is internalized by endocytosis. The receptor is later recycled to the cell surface. Internalization of the insulin receptor is important (and possibly essential) for insulin signals to reach the nucleus and influence cell growth and protein synthesis. Internalization is also a route by which insulin is cleared from the circulation and degraded.
- Rare DNA mutations of the insulin receptor have been identified:
  ◇ Leprechaunism and Rabson-Mendenhall syndrome result in severe glucose intolerance with resistance to exogenous insulin and profoundly disordered growth, unlike the 'typical' insulin resistance. These mutations are usually lethal in infancy and adolescence, respectively.
- There are also commoner, 'milder' polymorphisms of the insulin receptor gene, but these appear to explain only a small proportion of the marked variance in

population insulin sensitivity and are considered a rare (<5%) cause of type 2 diabetes.
◇ Most recognized insulin receptor gene mutations are not sufficient alone to cause diabetes, but render it more common in the presence of other risk factors.

The actions of insulin

◆ Insulin has widespread actions, both inhibitory and stimulatory (Figure 2.8, Table 2.2).
  ◇ The mechanisms of the glucoregulatory action of insulin have been the subject of extensive research. These glucoregulatory and antilipolytic effects of insulin are rapid, occurring within a few minutes.
  ◇ Insulin has effects on growth regulation and catabolism (synthesis of new proteins), which occur over hours or days. Much less is known about other possible actions, including effects on blood vessels (vascular smooth muscle proliferation, vasodilatation), the central nervous system (CNS) (appetite, learning, memory), and the immune response (apoptosis and anti-inflammation).
◆ There are individual dose-response curves for the different actions of insulin in different tissues. For example:
  ◇ *Antilipolytic action in adipose tissue:* the ED_{50} (the effective dose or concentration of insulin that produces 50% of the maximal effect) is <20 mU/L (~140 pmol/L) (and for some adipose depots <70 pmol/L).
  ◇ *Inhibition of hepatic glucose output (HGO):* ED_{50} of 30–50 mU/L (~210–350 pmol/L).
  ◇ *Stimulation of glucose uptake into skeletal muscle:* ED_{50} of 50–70 mU/L (~350–490 pmol/L).
  ◇ A doubling of insulin concentration inhibits hepatic glucose output by around 80% and increases peripheral glucose utilization by around 20%.

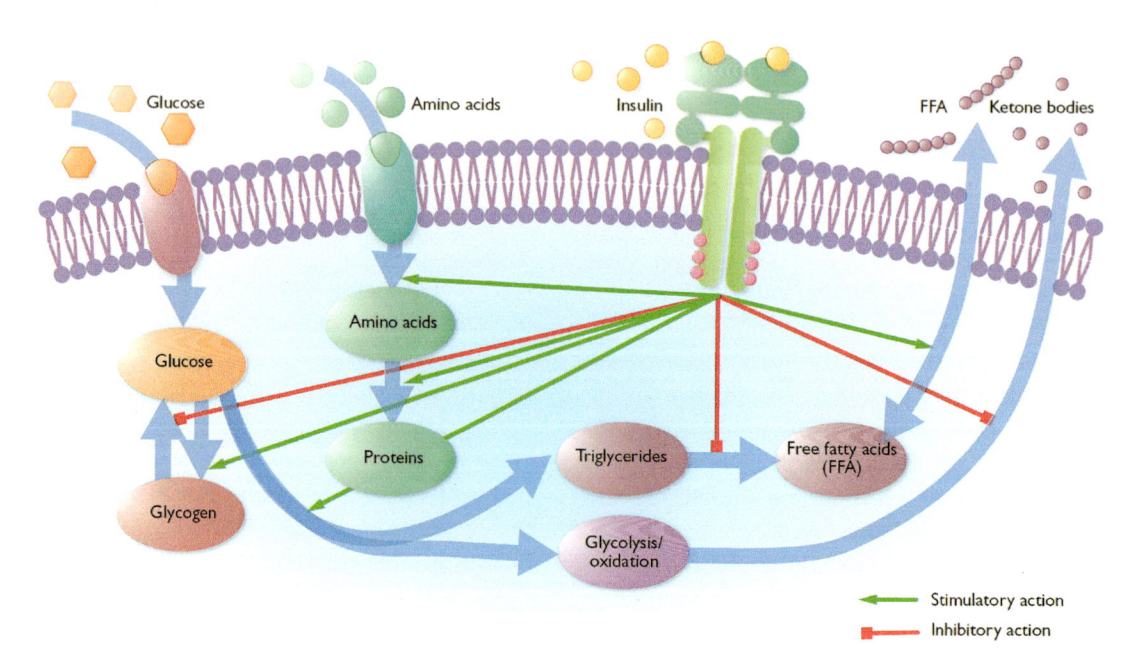

Figure 2.8 Actions of insulin. As well as promoting the uptake of glucose and inhibiting gluconeogenesis, insulin is significant in the metabolism of lipids, promoting synthesis of free fatty acids in the liver and inhibiting the breakdown of fats in adipose tissues. The insulin receptor facilitates uptake of amino acids and glucose across the cell membrane and activates protein, glycogen, and triglyceride synthesis.

Table 2.2 Actions of insulin. Insulin affects virtually every tissue in the body.

Actions of insulin		
TISSUES	**ACTIONS**	**SUGGESTED MECHANISM**
Liver	Inhibition of hepatic glucose output	Limitation of substrate supply
	Stimulation of hepatic glycogen storage	Inhibition of glycogenolysis
	Stimulation of hepatic glycolysis for intermediary metabolism	Inhibition of gluconeogenesis; stimulation of glycogen synthase
	Stimulation of hepatic lipogenesis	Simulation of phosphofructokinase
	Stimulation of hepatic glucose oxidation	Stimulation of pyruvate dehydrogenase
Skeletal muscle	Stimulation of glucose transport	Activation of glucose transporter (GLUT4)
	Stimulation of muscle glycogen synthesis	Simulation of glycogen synthase
	Stimulation of muscle glycolysis	Stimulation of phosphofructokinase
Adipose tissue	Inhibition of lipolysis (stored lipid)	Inhibition of hormone sensitive lipase
	Promotion of re-esterification	Increased supply of glycerol 3-phosphate
	Stimulation of lipolysis (circulating lipid)	Stimulation of lipoprotein lipase
	Increased glucose uptake	Several (probably as for muscle/liver)
Central nervous system	Satiety	Uncertain
	Changes in sympathetic tone	Uncertain
	Postprandial thermogenesis	Uncertain
Other	Promotes DNA synthesis	Uncertain
	Promotes RNA synthesis	Various
	Stimulation of amino acid uptake	Uncertain
	Na^+, K^+-ATPase stimulation	Increase in intracellular energy availability
	Na^+/H^+ antiport activation	Uncertain
	Na^+ retention	Probably several mechanisms

◆ These differential effects on lipolysis, HGO, and glucose uptake are probably responsible for the fact that most individuals with type 2 diabetes retain sufficient insulin action to avoid the development of ketoacidosis for many years, despite the clear defect in glucoregulation.

Insulin is significant in carbohydrate, protein, and lipid metabolism.

◆ The different actions of insulin have different time courses:
  ◇ Glucoregulatory and antilipolytic actions occur within a few minutes, while growth regulation and synthesis of new proteins occur over periods of hours or days.
  ◇ Intravenous injection of insulin typically has little effect on blood glucose for 2–5 minutes; the maximal hypoglycemic action occurs after 5–15 minutes.

- ◇ Insulin stimulation of skeletal muscle glucose uptake declines with a half-life of 10–20 minutes after the insulin stimulus is removed.
- ◆ Proinsulin and partially split proinsulin have metabolic activity generally similar to that of insulin, although plasma half-life is three to five times longer and biological potency is only 8–15% that of insulin. Proinsulin may be relatively more potent in terms of hepatic activity and less potent in terms of peripheral glucose uptake.
  - ◇ In sum, proinsulin has a limited role in general peripheral glucose metabolism but may have a relatively more important role in hepatic metabolism.

Second messenger systems

- ◆ Insulin can have multiple actions even on a single responsive cell and hence there are several different intracellular pathways mediating these actions (see Figure 2.8).
  - ◇ Glucoregulatory and antilipolytic responses are rapid and probably mediated via serine and threonine kinases and cyclic adenosine monophosphate (cAMP).
  - ◇ Stimulation of lipid and protein synthesis, inhibition of proteolysis, the nuclear transcription of RNA, and the replication of DNA are slower and act via different second messenger systems.
  - ◇ As a result of these second messenger cascades, GLUT proteins are translocated to the surface membrane of the cell, where they increase glucose flux into the cytoplasm.
- ◆ The actions of insulin in stimulating DNA transcription and mRNA translation do not depend upon the insulin receptor kinase activity and second messenger systems discussed previously, nor on the IGF receptors described next, but involve direct effects within the nucleus and ribosome.

Insulin-like growth factors (IGFs)

- ◆ In addition to its acute effects on glucose uptake and release and on lipid metabolism, insulin has growth-promoting activity in a variety of tissue-culture models.
  - ◇ Two protein hormones, IGF-1 and IGF-2, have actions that partially resemble these actions of insulin. The amino acid sequences of these proteins and the base sequences of their coding DNA are known and show homology with those of insulin.
- ◆ IGFs are weak agonists for the insulin receptor and have weak glucoregulatory and antilipolytic effects. In addition, they have growth-promoting effects mediated by two IGF receptors.
- ◆ Insulin is a weak agonist of IGF receptors.

Abnormalities of insulin synthesis and secretion

- ◆ The most common abnormality is the progressive loss of normal pulsatility, delayed insulin response to hyperglycemia, and gradual loss of insulin secretory capacity seen as obese individuals move toward type 2 diabetes. The progressive loss of insulin secretion in type 1 diabetes has a different natural history.
- ◆ However, there are also some rarer, genetic abnormalities of insulin structure involving mutations of the DNA code for insulin and hence altered amino acid sequences. Consequences include the inability to cleave insulin from proinsulin, and impaired receptor binding.
  - ◇ For these variants, there is reduced biological activity of the secretory product. This gives a propensity to diabetes, although individuals who can sustain a compensatory hypersecretion may avoid it.
- ◆ There are also recognized polymorphisms that affect the insulin secretory mechanism (e.g. calpain 10, a molecule that promotes the fusion of the secretory granule with the cell membrane) and are associated with diabetes.

CHAPTER 3

Type 1 diabetes

Epidemiology

- Type 1 diabetes is associated with insulin deficiency usually leading to insulin-dependent diabetes. It is one of the most common chronic diseases of childhood but is most commonly adult onset. There is immunogenetic and clinical heterogeneity within type 1A diabetes.
- Highest incidence rates of type 1A (autoimmune) diabetes are in Finland and the island of Sardinia. The frequency of type 1A diabetes in Europe is comparatively high compared with the rest of the world, higher in temperate zones and developed countries, correlating with gross national product as an index of wealth.
- Type 1B (idiopathic) diabetes has been noted in Japanese patients, who progress rapidly to insulin dependence in adult life without diabetes-associated antibodies but with increased serum amylase consistent with a subacute pancreatitis. Other causes include pancreatic disease and genetic disorders, which can each lead to insulin-dependent diabetes.
- The incidence of type 1 diabetes is increasing (Figure 3.1), particularly in children under 5 years of age. The peak incidence is reached around the time of puberty, but it can present at any age.

Type 1 diabetes can present at any age.

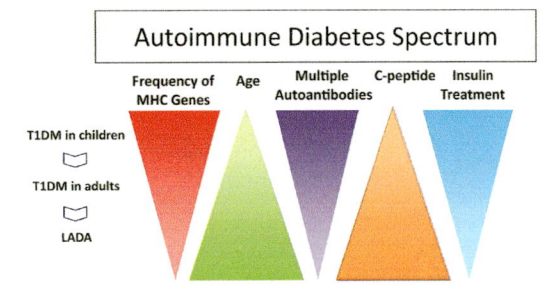

Figure 3.1 Type 1 diabetes subtypes seen in adulthood. The differential characteristics of these forms of type 1 diabetes overlap in part, reflecting their complex and diverse pathogenesis. With increasing age, individuals tend to have less genetic risk, fewer autoantibodies, more C-peptide (a proxy for insulin secretion) and less need for early insulin treatment. *From Leslie, RD (2010).*

Incidence of childhood type 1 diabetes. There is enormous variation in the incidence of type 1 diabetes, from 0.1/100,000 per year in China and Venezuela to 36.8/100,000 per year in Sardinia and 36.5/100,000 per year in Finland. Results from 37 studies in 27 countries during 1960 to 1996 showed that the overall annual increase in incidence was around 3.0%. Some 70,000 children worldwide are expected to develop type 1 diabetes each year. Nevertheless, the disease is most prevalent in adults. In China, despite low childhood incidence, the frequency of autoimmune diabetes is similar to that in Europe. The average rate of new cases of diabetes among under-20s compared with 20—64 years of age in the USA was 34.3 and 18.6 per 100,000 respectively each year for type 1 diabetes but only 5.3 per 100,000 for type 2 diabetes.

- Slow progression to insulin deficiency occurs in about 5–10% of adult patients who present initially with noninsulin-dependent diabetes. This is often called latent autoimmune diabetes of adults (LADA) or in Japan, slowly progressive insulin dependent diabetes (SPIDDM), though it appears to be a slowly progressive form of type 1 diabetes.
  - ◇ LADA, that is, adult-onset autoimmune diabetes, is characterized by the presence of diabetes-associated antibodies, including glutamic acid decarboxylase antibody (GADA). However, some patients appear to have features of both type 1 and type 2 diabetes (called double-diabetes) and some ethnic groups, including those of Hispanic or African origin, may present with ketoacidosis which later passes through a period of not requiring insulin treatment, so-called ketosis-prone diabetes (KPD) (Figure 3.1 and Table 3.1).

Table 3.1 AABBCC of diabetes classification.

Autoimmunity	Does this individual have islet **autoantibodies** or a history of **autoimmunity** (i.e. thyroid disease, celiac disease), goiter or vitiligo on exam?
A1c	Is hemoglobin **A1c** worsening on non-insulin therapies?
Body habitus/BMI	Is the **body habitus** or **BMI** inconsistent with type 2 diabetes?
Background	What is the patient's **background**? Is there a family history of autoimmunity and/or type 1 diabetes? Are they from a high-risk ethnic group?
C-peptide	Is the **C-peptide** low or is there clinical evidence that beta cell function is declining?
Co-morbidities	Co-existent cardiac or renal disease and their risk factors could impact the approach to therapy.

Source: Adapted from Leslie, RD, et al. (2021).

Causes of type 1 diabetes

- Type 1 diabetes is an immune-mediated organ-specific disease. The disease is induced by an environmental event or events operating in a genetically susceptible individual (Figure 3.2).
- Many genes are implicated in the genetic susceptibility to type 1 diabetes; the most important are in the histocompatibility leukocyte antigen (HLA) region of chromosome 6.
- The risk of developing childhood-onset type 1 diabetes is about 1:400 in the general population but 1:2 in the identical twin of a young diabetic, 1:10 in the identical twin of an adult diabetic, and 1:17 in a sibling of a subject with type 1 diabetes; the risk is only 1:5 if the sibling is HLA-identical to the affected sibling.

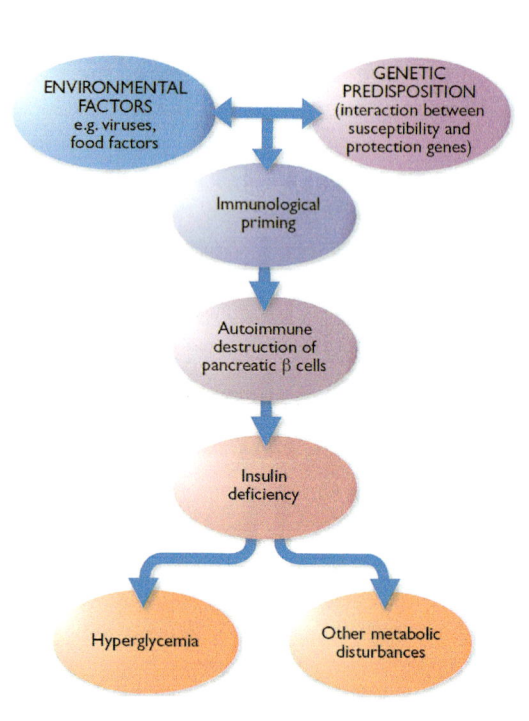

Figure 3.2 Etiological events. Type 1 diabetes is an immune-mediated disease, induced by environmental determinants in a genetically susceptible individual. At every stage in this cascade, a substantial proportion do not progress to the next stage and even destruction of insulin-secreting cells may not progress to total loss.

- The striking discordance between identical twins must be due to nongenetic, probably environmental factors. These environmental factors probably operate in early life, even *in utero*, at least in those cases that present in childhood. Patients presenting in adulthood have a more potent environmental effect, but the nature of the environmental factor or factors is unknown (candidates include the gut microbiome, obesity, viruses, and food).

Five to 10% of patients presenting with adult-onset diabetes have autoimmune diabetes.

- The risk of developing diabetes by age 20 is greater with a father with type 1 diabetes (8%) than with a mother with type 1 diabetes (2%); this discrepancy may be a result of imprinted maternal genes or because fetal exposure to maternal changes may be protective to the offspring. Risk increases as parental age at diagnosis decreases, reflecting greater gene load.
- Whatever the nature of the environmental effect, the interaction of environmental and genetic factors at different stages leads to induction of immune changes, including activation of T lymphocytes and B lymphocytes, with the latter producing autoantibodies to insulin (IAA), zinc transporter8 (ZnT8A), insulinoma-antigen2 (IA-2A), or glutamic acid decarboxylase (GADA).
  ◇ The destructive immune response targets the pancreatic islets, specifically the insulin-secreting cells, with their complete or partial destruction; yet exocrine pancreas is also involved. The immune process in children less than 7 years at diagnosis appears distinct.
  ◇ The destruction can be mediated directly by cellular processes or indirectly through the release of cytokines and chemokines (Figure 3.3).

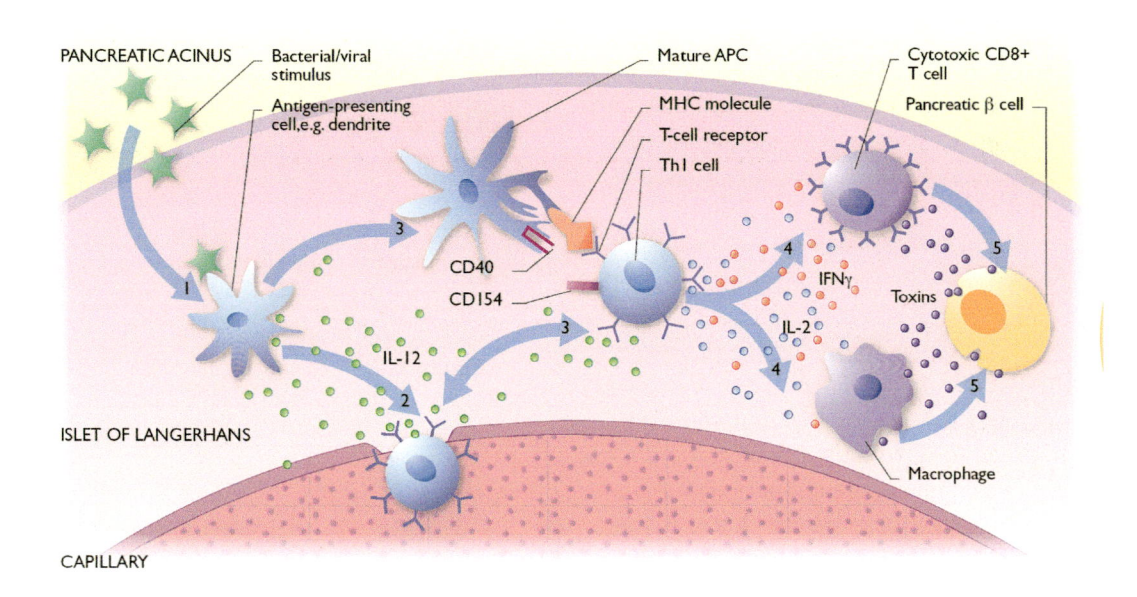

Figure 3.3 Immune-mediated destruction of pancreatic β cells. Upon activation (1), antigen-presenting cells (APCs) such as dendritic cells produce IL-12 cytokines that stimulate the production of Th1 lymphocytes (2). T-cell receptor (TCR) and CD154 molecules on the surface of the Th1 cell bind to the MHC and CD40 molecules on the surface of the APC (3). Th1 lymphocytes also produce large amounts of interferon-gamma (IFN-γ) which, together with IL-2 cytokines, induces macrophages to become cytotoxic, and also stimulates cytotoxic CD8+ cells (4). Both of these release mediators that are toxic to pancreatic islet cells (5).

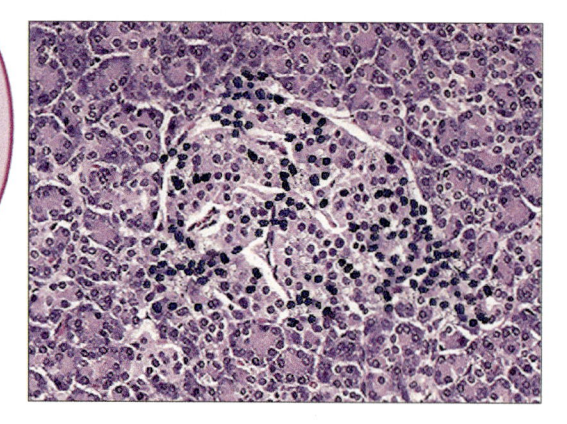

Figure 3.4 Insulitis. Lymphocytic infiltration in a pancreatic islet, suggesting an altered immune response.

Figure 3.5 Islet autoimmunity. The projected cumulative risk for developing diabetes when dysglycemia is present (Stage 2) in those with multiple autoantibodies is close to 100 % so that type 1 diabetes can be designated at that stage and before clinical onset. While progression to diabetes is only 3% in those who had single autoantibodies, at least in childhood. Adult-onset type 1 diabetes and LADA is characterized by a single dominant autoantibody, usually GADA. *From Achenbach et al. (2005).*

At diagnosis, young children show lymphocytes and macrophages surrounding and infiltrating the islets, which is less evident in older cases (Figure 3.4).
- ◇ The younger the onset of the disease, the more severe is this destructive immune process.

Prediction of type 1 diabetes
- ◆ The immune changes associated with type 1 diabetes can be detected months, or even years, before the clinical onset of the disease. These changes, notably the presence of autoantibodies, can predict the disease, with some antibodies and particular combinations of antibodies being more predictive than others allied to metabolic and genetic risk (Figure 3.5).
    - ◇ The ability to predict the disease raises the hope that we may eventually be able to prevent it and clinical trials are now under way with encouraging preliminary data.
- ◆ Autoimmune diseases should show three features:
    - ◇ Defined autoantigens and autoantibodies must be present.
    - ◇ Passive transfer of T lymphocytes (specific or nonspecific) must lead to disease development.
    - ◇ Immunomodulation of subjects with disease must ameliorate symptoms.
- ◆ The first of these is true for type 1 diabetes and the autoantibodies to autoantigens can predict the disease with a degree of certainty. Some immunomodulation therapies can modify, albeit transiently, the disease process, notably anti-CD3 monoclonal antibodies.
- ◆ Type 1 diabetes is associated with other autoimmune diseases, including Hashimoto's thyroiditis, adrenalitis, celiac disease, and pernicious anemia (with vitamin B12 deficiency).

The presence of autoantibodies before clinical onset can predict diabetes.

Genetic factors
- ◆ Type 1 diabetes is genetically determined, as evidenced by family, twin, and genetic studies. Type 1 diabetes is more frequent in siblings of diabetic patients (e.g. in the

UK, 6% by age 30 versus the expected 0.4% by age 30). Higher concordance rates in identical compared with nonidentical twins is consistent with a genetic influence in type 1 diabetes. About 40% of identical twins with type 1 diabetes have a co-twin with the disease (i.e. they are concordant for type 1 diabetes), though that proportion falls as the age at diagnosis of the index twin rises.

- ◇ Remarkably that low twin concordance rate for adult-onset type 1 diabetes implies a limited genetic impact, consistent with disease heterogeneity related to age at diagnosis.

◆ HLA genes are associated with an increased risk of a number of autoimmune diseases. Genes encoding these HLA molecules are found within the major histocompatibility complex (MHC) on the short arm of chromosome 6 (Figure 3.6). HLA genes are highly polymorphic, and this region has been in balanced polymorphism for at least 10 million years. HLA associations with type 1 diabetes probably operate through susceptibility to undefined infections.

- ◇ This MHC complex is a polymorphic gene complex with multiple alleles at each genetic locus. The MHC is divided into class I (HLA -A, -B, and -C), class II (HLA-DR, -DQ, and -DP), and class III (genes for complement components).
- ◇ The class I and class II proteins are transmembrane cell surface glycoproteins involved in both self and foreign antigen presentation to T lymphocytes.

◆ Class II genes are more important than Class I genes, and DQ genes are more important than DR genes.

- ◇ About 95% of European patients have either HLA-DR3 or HLA-DR4, compared with about 60% of the general population, and specific alleles of HLA-DR3 and HLA-DR4 have been identified that are associated with diabetes susceptibility.
- ◇ Other alleles are associated with disease protection, e.g. one haplotype (HLA-DR2, DQB1*0602) is found in about 20% of some populations, but in less than 1% of those that develop the disease.
- ◇ The heterozygous alleles associated with disease susceptibility, HLA-DR3, DQB1*0201, and HLA-DR4, DQB1*0302, decline in frequency with age at diagnosis, as does Class

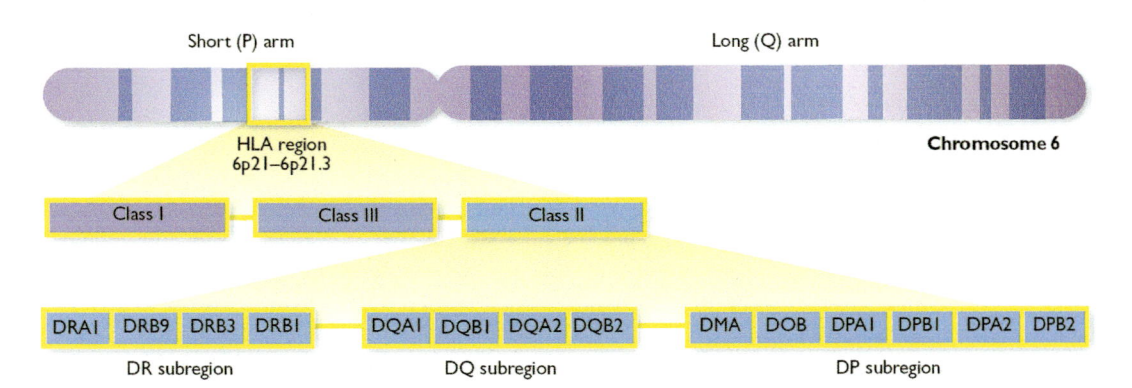

Figure 3.6 Genetic factors. There are numerous regions of the genome associated with type 1 diabetes risk, with IDDM1 on chromosome 6 being the most important. HLA genes within this region account for almost 50% of genetic susceptibility to type 1 diabetes.

1 genetic risk, whereas in adult-onset diabetes, the protective HLA haplotype carries less protection.
- In the HLA molecule, individual residues (i.e. specific amino acids at certain positions) confer a particular susceptibility or protection from disease.

There are over 40 genetic variants associated with type 1 diabetes.

- Other gene polymorphisms are associated with type 1 diabetes, including a gene within the insulin gene upstream promoter region.
  ◊ Of note, the IFIH1 gene plays a role in antiviral defense, clearly implicating viruses in the pathogenesis of the disease; evidence that the type 1 interferon gene response is also altered in islet β-cells implicates that cell in an adverse virus-induced immune dialogue.
- In total, there are some 60 genetic variants associated with type 1 diabetes but only 10 are known to have a function, such as genes involved in T cell immune responses (Figure 3.7).
- Nongenetic factors are important in causing type 1 diabetes, as shown by studies of populations, twins, and migrant populations.
  ◊ Population studies reveal changes in disease incidence within a genetically stable population, both in populations that do not move and those that do.
  ◊ There has been a striking increase in the incidence of type 1 diabetes in children diagnosed under 5 years of age in Europe within a generation, implicating nongenetic factors.
  ◊ An increase has been reported in migrating populations, e.g. Asian children who migrated to Britain from Karachi showed an increased disease risk from 3.1/100,000 per year in 1978–81 to 11.7/100,000 per year in 1988–90, much higher than in their native Karachi (1/100,000 per year) (Figure 3.6).
  ◊ Such increases in disease risk in young children could be due to an accelerated progression to disease, or to an increased disease risk, or both. Current evidence supports both factors being involved.
- A range of environmental factors may cause autoimmune diseases. These factors include:
  ◊ Increased hygiene and decreased rates of infection in childhood.
  ◊ Temperate climate.
  ◊ Viruses, gut microbiome, vaccinations, and antibiotics.
  ◊ Increasing wealth and obesity (possibly relevant for autoimmune and atopic diseases).
- For type 1 diabetes, other factors are:
  ◊ Overcrowding in childhood.

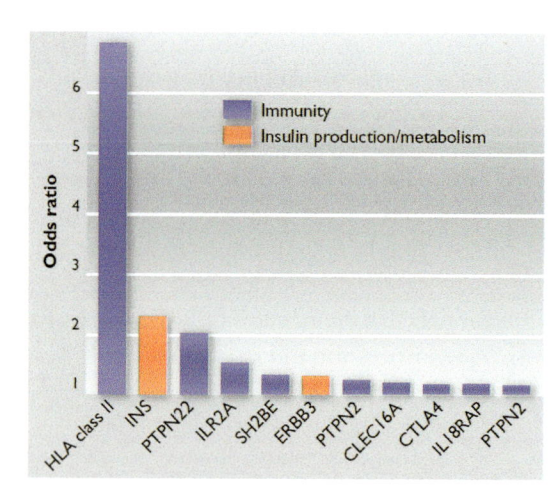

Figure 3.7 Selected genes associated with type 1 diabetes. More than 60 genetic loci that underlie susceptibility to type 1 diabetes have now been identified, with some of the loci associated with a number of candidate genes. While the HLA gene is the most significant, others such as INS, which regulates insulin production and CTLA4, the cytotoxic T-lymphocyte antigen gene, are also of great interest. The graph indicates the estimated odds ratio for risk alleles at each of the indicated loci. *From Todd et al. (2010).*

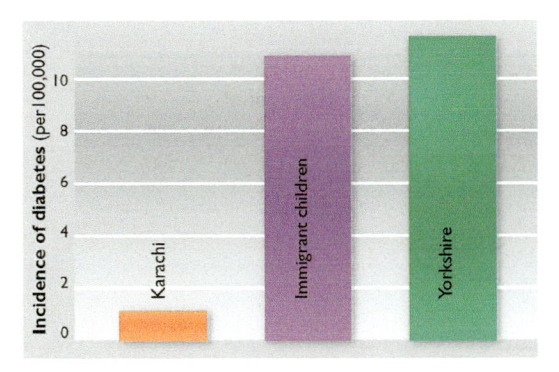

Figure 3.8 Nongenetic factors. *From Swerdlow et al. AJ (2005).*

◇ Reduced rates or duration of breast feeding.
◆ Several or one of these factors could account for the disease in any given individual (Figure 3.8).

Development of type 1 diabetes

Pancreatic β-cell dysfunction

- There is a continuous spectrum of loss of insulin secretory capacity associated with autoimmune diabetes. The severity of the destructive immune effect is age related, being more severe in children than in adults and more severe in adults with type 1 diabetes initially requiring insulin or not (as with LADA).
- Some individuals, before they develop type 1 diabetes, pass through a 'prediabetic' stage of impaired glucose tolerance or even noninsulin-requiring diabetes, before becoming frankly insulin-dependent (Figure 3.9). In that sense, LADA does no more than reflect delayed progression of type 1 diabetes.
- The rate of progression to clinical diabetes is more rapid in those patients presenting at less than 5 years of age than in patients presenting with diabetes much later in life.

Insulin resistance

- The normal relationship between insulin sensitivity relative to insulin secretion is disrupted in the 'prediabetic' phase, just as it is in type 2 diabetes.

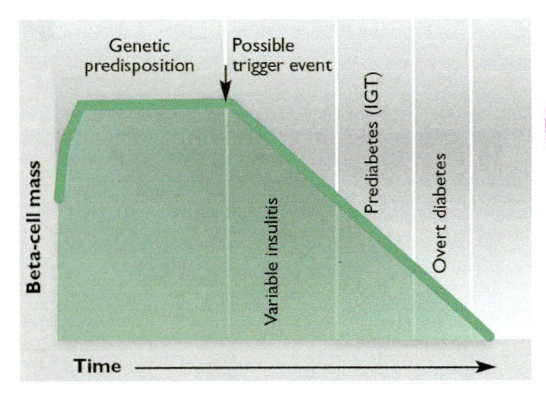

Figure 3.9 Disease progression. Time-related decline in β-cell mass, showing critical transitions from genetic susceptibility to frank diabetes. *From Gianani R and Eisenbarth GS (2005).* Stage 1 is the induction of autoantibodies; Stage 2 represents autoantibodies and dysglyaemia, and when multiple autoantibodies are present the clinical diagnosis of type 1 diabetes can be made; Stage 3 is overt clinical diabetes.

- Those autoantibody-positive individuals who develop type 1 diabetes show changes in insulin sensitivity during this period. It follows that metabolic decompensation, which leads to frank diabetes, can result from any cause of reduced insulin sensitivity, as is seen with increased linear growth and increased childhood obesity, both of which are related to age at presentation.

Mortality

- Studies have demonstrated that the pattern of causes of death changes, depends on the duration of type 1 diabetes, and is particularly high in those with chronic kidney disease (Figure 3.10).
  ◇ Cardiovascular disease was the principal cause of death among people who had had type 1 diabetes for more than 30 years.
  ◇ Renal disease formed the largest proportion of causes of death among people whose disease duration was between 10 and 19 years.

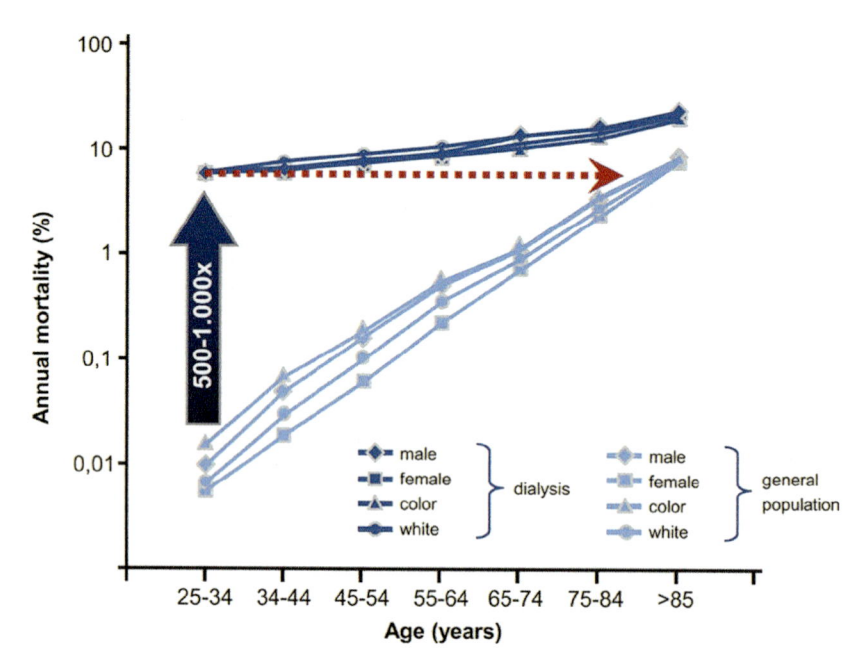

Figure 3.10 Diabetes complications. Excess mortality is particularly striking in those diagnosed at a younger age and strongly dependent on diabetes duration. Cases with chronic kidney disease, irrespective of gender or race, show the highest excess mortality (500–1000-fold greater) which approximates to the normal population in the elderly, yet remains excessive. *From Cardiovascular Disease in Chronic Kidney Disease. Pathophysiological Insights and Therapeutic Options. Joachim Jankowski et al, Originally published 15 Mar 2021. https://doi.org/10.1611/CIRCULATIONAHA.120.050686 Circulation. 2021;143:1157–1172.*

- ◇ In contrast, for those who died less than 10 years after diagnosis, the major causes of death were other diabetes-related complications such as hypoglycemia and diabetic ketoacidosis.
- ◆ Recent studies also identify acute complications of diabetes as the major cause of death in teenagers and cardiovascular disease as the major cause of death in people over 30 years of age. It has also been noted that South Asian patients with insulin-treated diabetes suffer an exceptionally high mortality, which may be related to a higher risk of cardiovascular disease.
- ◆ Cancer mortality among people with type 1 diabetes is thought to be generally similar to that of the general population.
  - ◇ There may be greater incidence of ovarian cancer and mortality, as implied by at least one study (Figure 3.10).

Cardiovascular disease is the major cause of death in patients who have had type 1 diabetes for over 30 years.

Screening for potential type 1 diabetes

- ◆ Autoimmune diseases are the third leading cause of morbidity and mortality in the developed world, surpassed only by cancer and heart disease.
- ◆ Autoimmune diseases are complex, chronic disorders that develop over the course of years and are characterized by autoantibodies, which appear in the peripheral blood months, even years, before the onset of clinical symptoms. Since the genes associated with autoimmune diseases are susceptibility genes

and therefore carry a limited predictive value, attention has turned to the immune response, and specifically disease-associated autoantibodies, as potential predictors.

- Screening for autoantibodies as predictors of disease has been convincingly demonstrated for a number of autoimmune diseases, including type 1 diabetes. These studies, involving thousands of subjects, showed that autoantibodies:
  - Can appear at an early age, even around the time of birth.
  - Can precede the clinical onset of diabetes by some years.
  - Recognize different autoantigens and some antigen-specific autoantibodies are more predictive of type 1 diabetes than others.
  - Have a positive predictive value that increases for one, two, or three autoantibodies from approximately 10% to 50% and 80%, respectively, within 5 years and even higher thereafter.
  - Combination of autoantibodies with genetic risk, including gene risk scores calculated by summing odds ratio of risk for selected single-nucleotide polymorphisms, plus the assessment of insulin secretion using C-peptide as a proxy for insulin.
- The success of screening with autoantibodies for type 1 diabetes suggests that autoantibody screening will be useful in predicting other chronic autoimmune diseases. Such screening is being used in research settings to identify subjects at risk in the immediate family or the general population, in order to identify those suitable for prevention therapy when it becomes available and in an informed setting with counseling to reduce the risk of diabetic ketoacidosis by alerting patients at risk. Biomarkers can also be used to classify disease, notably when patients present with initially noninsulin-dependent diabetes as adults, of whom some 5–10% have autoimmune type 1 diabetes.

CHAPTER 4

Type 2 diabetes

Epidemiology

- Type 2 diabetes is a common chronic disease of global importance (see Figure 1.2). Most patients (>85%) with diabetes have type 2 diabetes.
- The rate of increase of type 2 diabetes is such that there is effectively a global epidemic. The WHO estimated that 30 million people had diabetes in 1985; in 2019, the estimate was 463 million, and projections are that numbers will reach 578 million by 2030.
- Diabetes has traditionally been viewed as a disease of rich countries. However, recent estimates of diabetes prevalence show that 80% of people with diabetes live in countries classified by the World Bank as low- and middle-income countries, and this proportion is increasing.
- The prevalence of type 2 diabetes is related to increasing age, increasing calorie intake, increasing obesity (Figure 4.1), and reduced physical activity. Pregnancy, drug therapy (such as corticosteroids), and intercurrent illness are associated with precipitating diabetes.
- Type 2 diabetes can remain undiagnosed for many years.
- Worldwide, around 8.5% of the population over the age of 18 has diabetes.
  ◇ In some previously undeveloped societies, however, such as Pima Indians in the United States and the Naruans

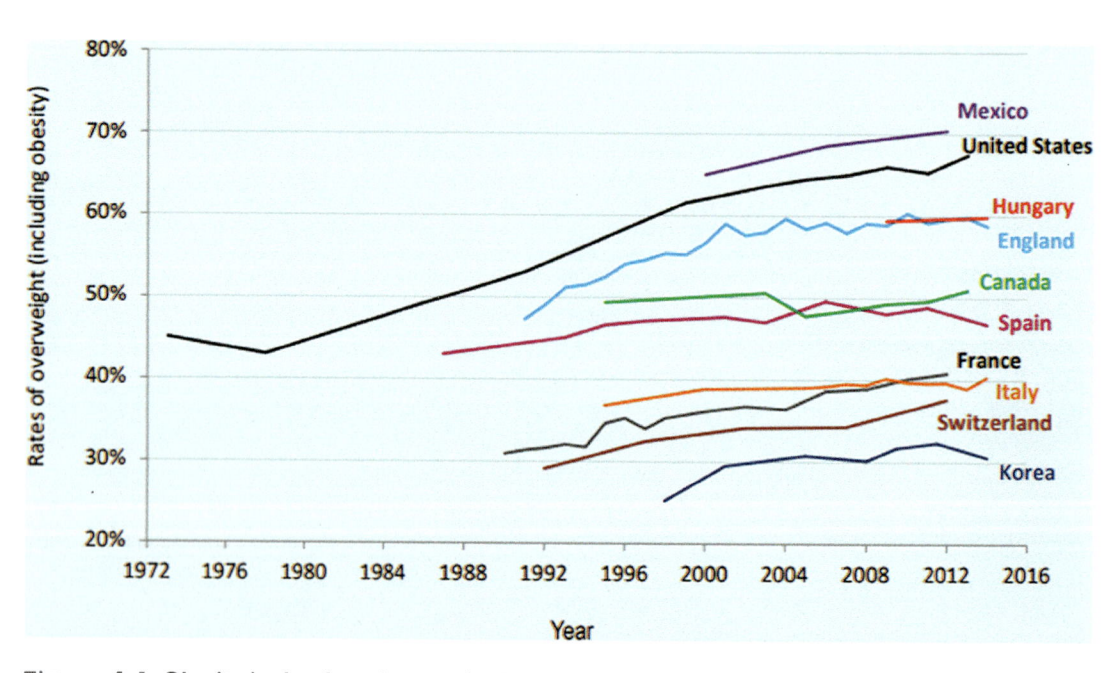

Figure 4.1 Obesity in developed countries. Levels of obesity have been increasing consistently over the past three decades.

from Micronesia, the prevalence is up to 50%.
- Recognized morphological associations of type 2 diabetes include shorter stature (by 1–4 cm compared to nondiabetic subjects) with obesity of the 'android' (also known as 'apple', 'upper body', 'central' or 'visceral') type, marked by a high waist:hip ratio, low capillary density in skeletal muscle, and high ratios of slow twitch: fast twitch muscle fibers.

Causes of type 2 diabetes

- Type 2 diabetes is unlikely to be a single condition. Some late-onset diabetes, initially presumed to be type 2, may turn out to be latent autoimmune diabetes in adults (LADA), while other patients thought to have type 2 diabetes may upon investigation be shown to have secondary types such as pancreatic, or monogenic diabetes.
- In all patients with type 2 diabetes, there is a variable degree of insulin resistance and relative insulin deficiency.
- With time (typically 5–15 years from diagnosis), glycemic control in people with type 2 diabetes usually becomes more difficult, insulin deficiency more apparent and a subgroup of patients may become ketosis-prone. Data from the UKPDS trial suggested that the average time to insulin use was approximately 8 years after diagnosis of type 2 diabetes and confirmed the clinical impression of a progressive rather than static disease process. The advent of newer therapies for type 2 diabetes, however, may extend the period to insulin requirement considerably.

Type 2 diabetes is associated with both insulin resistance and relative insulin deficiency.

Environmental risk factors

- The typical patient with type 2 diabetes is overweight (average body mass index [BMI] at presentation, >27 kg/m^2), with a central distribution of obesity (most conveniently assessed by waist circumference, or waist:hip ratio) conferring risk which is independent of, and additional to, that of elevated BMI (Table 4.1).

Table 4.1 Risk factors. The main determinants for type 2 diabetes are linked to social factors, such as socioeconomic status. Age, family history, poor diet, and physical inactivity are the main risk factors.

Determinants and risk factors for type 2 diabetes	
Lifestyle and behavior related	'Westernization, urbanization, modernization' Obesity (including distribution of obesity and duration) Physical inactivity Diet Stress
Genetic	Genetic markers 'Thrifty gene(s)' Family history
Demographic	Sex, age, ethnicity Other demographic characteristics
Metabolic determinants and intermediate risk categories	Impaired glucose tolerance Insulin resistance Pregnancy-related determinants (parity, gestational diabetes, diabetes in offspring of women with diabetes during pregnancy, intrauterine mal- or overnutrition)

- Other independent risk factors for type 2 diabetes include lack of exercise, being born to a mother with gestational diabetes, or being of exceptionally high or low birth weight.
    - Low birth weight is postulated by the Barker hypothesis to predispose to diabetes and obesity by various mechanisms, including switching on 'thrifty' genes to counter the effects of intrauterine malnutrition.
- Leaner patients with type 2 diabetes tend to show more severe insulin deficiency (and within this subgroup one typically finds LADA patients).
- Greater degrees of obesity are associated with more insulin resistance.
- There is longstanding controversy as to whether, for the type 2 diabetes typical of patients of European origin, the prime defect in glucose homoeostasis is insulin deficiency, insulin resistance, or both. Given that many individuals with severe insulin resistance do not have diabetes and that some patients with type 2 diabetes have little insulin resistance, it is probable that insulin resistance alone is not the cause; rather, some degree of β-cell dysfunction (either as an inherited tendency or a result of reduced β-cell function as part of a degenerative process) is the *sine qua non* of type 2 diabetes.
    - Such β-cell dysfunction may take the form of a relative lack of insulin secretion and/or of abnormal patterns of insulin secretion.
    - Such abnormalities have been described in patients who later developed type 2 diabetes and include changes in the amplitude and frequency of insulin secretory pulses, and in the loss of first-phase insulin secretion with prolongation and augmentation of second-phase secretion.
    - These abnormalities of insulin secretion have been shown to be largely reversible with weight loss, or after certain forms of bariatric surgery for morbid obesity in patients with type 2 diabetes.
- Population studies indicate that the concurrent existence in an individual of both a cause for insulin resistance (usually obesity) and of a relatively low insulin secretory reserve predicts the onset of type 2 diabetes.
- The differentiation of type 2 diabetes and 'secondary' diabetes can be difficult.
    - Secondary diabetes implies that another disease process has caused or substantially contributed to the diabetes (see Table 1.3). While there is good understanding of the natural history and treatment approach for type 2 diabetes, this is less so for secondary diabetes. Occasionally, the secondary diabetes may be significantly improved by treating the primary condition.

Genetic factors

- Family studies suggest that type 2 diabetes is strongly inheritable:
    - Concordance rates for identical twins exceed 70%.
    - Some racial groups have a very high incidence of type 2 diabetes; notable examples of this include the Pima Indians of Arizona (Figure 4.2) and South Sea Islanders, with prevalence rates of up to 50%.
    - In the UK, the prevalence of type 2 diabetes among people of South Asian extraction is approximately three times that among those of European origin. African-Caribbeans show an intermediate prevalence (Figure 4.3). In the USA, Hispanic and African Americans have higher rates of diabetes than those of European origin.
    - The natural history of type 2 diabetes and its propensity to give rise to

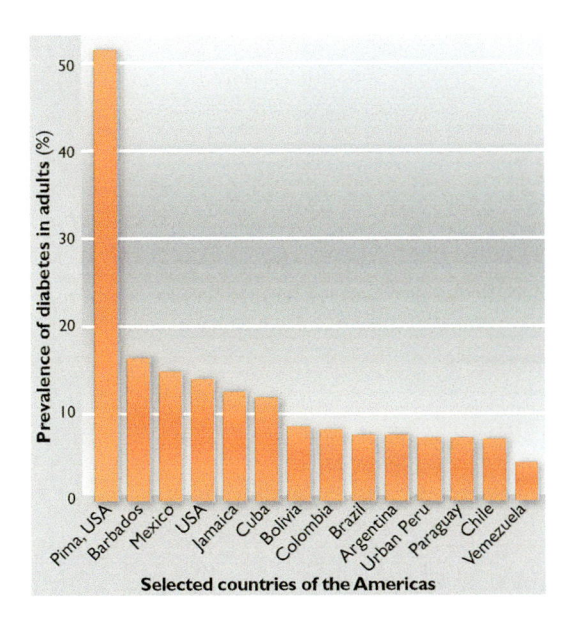

Figure 4.2 Genetic versus environmental factors. The Pima Indians of Arizona have the highest prevalence of type 2 diabetes in the world, far higher than other American populations. A homogeneous group, they have been extensively studied. There is an increased prevalence among Native Americans in general, possibly due to the interaction of genetic predisposition and a change from traditional diets. Genetically similar Pimas in Mexico, among whom the prevalence of obesity is less, are much less susceptible to diabetes.

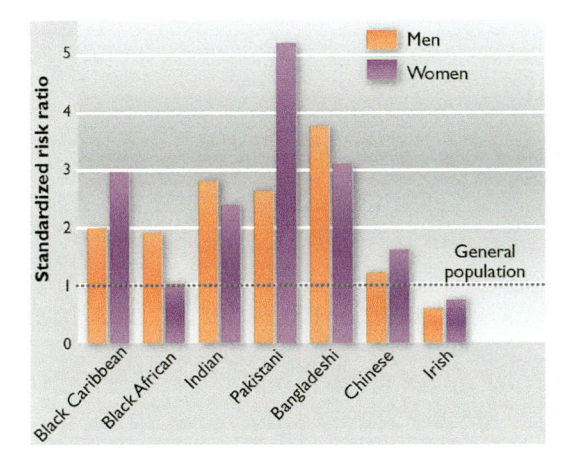

Figure 4.3 Ethnic minorities in England (2004). All minority ethnic groups, except Irish, have a higher standardized risk of (doctor-diagnosed) diabetes compared to the general population, with Pakistani women being particularly vulnerable.

long-term complications also vary between races (examples being the relative lack of diabetic foot disease in British Asians and the high prevalence of diabetic nephropathy among those of African-Caribbean descent).

◆ In most patients with type 2 diabetes, the pattern of inheritance suggests a polygenic disorder, with an important role for environmental factors (Figure 4.4) such as obesity and a low level of exercise. The specific genes already associated with the disease are, by and large, genes associated with reduced insulin secretion. A few genes, such as the fat mass and obesity associated (FTO) gene, have a modest effect leading to obesity; in the case of FTO probably due to increased food intake.

◆ Most recognized genes increase type 2 diabetes risk by 10–20% (OR 1.1–1.2), compared to obesity 510% (OR 5.1).

◆ Molecular biological techniques have not yet shown type 2 diabetes to be consistently associated with any abnormalities of the DNA coding for insulin, the insulin receptor or glucose transporter peptides (except in a small percentage [<5%] of cases). Abnormalities of the glucokinase gene and of certain hepatic nuclear factor genes cause some cases of MODY (see Table 1.3), but not typical type 2 diabetes.

Associated conditions

◆ In Western populations, type 2 diabetes usually forms part of a syndrome of morphological and metabolic abnormalities. Some of these associations are referred to as 'metabolic syndrome' (see p. 43).

◆ The metabolic features of type 2 diabetes include fasting hyperinsulinemia, hyperglycemia, dyslipidemia, and high circulating concentrations of lactate, pyruvate, and glucogenic amino acids.

◆ Other associated conditions include hypertension, hyperuricemia, high plasma

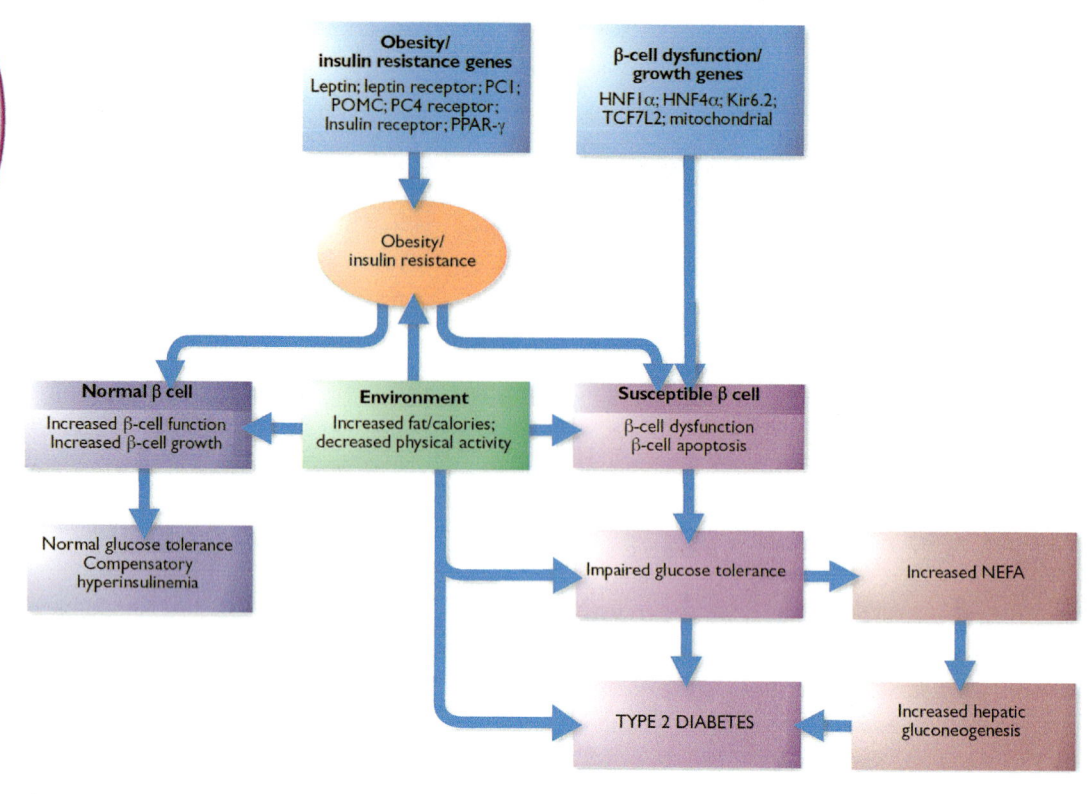

Figure 4.4 The etiology of type 2 diabetes. Interaction between genes and the environment can lead to obesity/insulin resistance. Genetically susceptible β cells are unable to compensate for the increased secretory demand, resulting in dysfunction and cell death. *From Kahn, Hull, et al, 2006.*

androgen:estrogen ratios, hypercoagulability of blood, endothelial dysfunction, and accelerated atherosclerosis.
  ◊ A higher prevalence of and mortality from cancers, such as pancreatic, colorectal and liver cancers, have been observed in type 2 diabetes.

Hyperinsulinemia and hyperglycemia
◆ The typical natural history of type 2 diabetes is reflected in a progressive decline in insulin secretory capacity, so that the metabolic picture changes over a period of years (Figure 4.5).
  ◊ Patients become insulin resistant, almost always because of obesity and physical inactivity.
  ◊ Insulin resistance causes the patient to progress over the years through a phase of hyperinsulinemia ('metabolic syndrome').

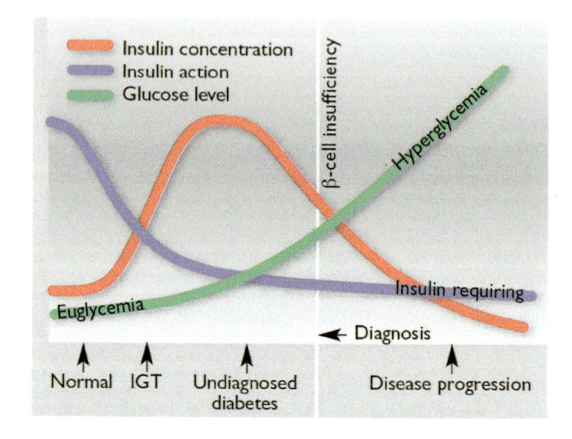

Figure 4.5 Natural history of type 2 diabetes. This model (the De Fronzo hypothesis) shows that patients progress from normal glucose tolerance to IGT to diabetes. Though decreased insulin action is a contributor, it is the decline in β-cell production of insulin that heralds the onset of diabetes.

- ◇ The hyperinsulinemia puts a strain on the β cells and progressive pancreatic failure is added to the pathophysiology.
- ◇ Thereafter, the patient proceeds through phases of increasingly severe hyperglycemia. At first, the glycemic defect will be subtle, such as IGT or IFG, but will then progress to become type 2 diabetes.
- ◆ Initially, therapy for type 2 diabetes may involve just lifestyle interventions, but typically, oral hypoglycemic agents and later, exogenous insulin, may be needed as worsening β-cell failure supervenes.

Hypertension

- ◆ The association between diabetes and hypertension is strong and long recognized. The incidence of hypertension in obese patients with type 2 diabetes is about 50% in some series.
- ◆ Hypertension is associated with obesity and short stature in nondiabetic as well as diabetic groups.
- ◆ People with diabetes are liable to develop the same secondary forms of hypertension as the nondiabetic population (renal artery stenosis is commoner in diabetes).
- ◆ In type 1 diabetes, hypertension is strongly linked with diabetic nephropathy. Although it is often uncertain whether this is initially cause or effect, it becomes a vicious cycle.
  - ◇ There appear to be familial effects, with nondiabetic relatives of diabetic nephropathic hypertensive patients showing an increased propensity to develop essential hypertension.
- ◆ Sodium retention and impaired natriuresis are characteristically found both in patients with type 1 and type 2 diabetes with hypertension; exchangeable body sodium is increased by an average of 10%. This may be seen even before the development of any clinically detectable complications of diabetes.
  - ◇ Possible mechanisms include increased glomerular filtration of glucose leading to enhanced proximal tubule sodium-glucose co-transport, hyperinsulinemia-induced overactivity of tubular sodium transporters, an extravascular shift of fluid with sodium and, in later stages, renal impairment.

Hypertension is common in type 2 diabetes patients and is often needs multiple therapies.

- ◇ In glycemically controlled patients with type 1 and type 2 diabetes, plasma renin activity, angiotensin II, aldosterone, and catecholamine concentrations are usually normal.
- ◇ Conversely, plasma atrial natriuretic peptide concentrations tend to be increased, and an exaggerated vascular reactivity to norepinephrine and angiotensin II is common, even in uncomplicated types 1 and 2 diabetes.
- ◆ Data from the UKPDS confirm that hypertension in type 2 diabetes is often refractory to treatment and a combination of antihypertensive agents is typically required to maintain tight blood pressure (BP) control. This study also made clear the relationship between BP and diabetic nephropathy, showing that a modest reduction in BP reduced the incidence of nephropathy and death.

Abnormalities of lipid metabolism

- ◆ Diabetes is associated with abnormalities of lipid metabolism. Several mechanisms have been suggested for these associations.
  - ◇ The obesity and body fat distribution common in type 2 diabetes are linked with dyslipidemias in nondiabetic subjects.
  - ◇ Nonenzymatic glycation of apolipoproteins impairs lipoprotein clearance.

- ◇ Insulin is the principal regulator of lipolysis and, without its action, NEFA release from adipose tissue may be increased.
- ◇ Much of this extra NEFA will be re-esterified by the liver to VLDL-triglyceride.
- ◇ Peripheral VLDL-triglyceride clearance may be impaired because insulin is needed to synthesize and secrete lipoprotein lipase, the principal enzyme responsible for clearing VLDL-triglyceride in some tissues.
- ◇ Insulin also promotes LDL receptor function.
- ◆ Poor glycemic control in type 1 diabetes is associated with high concentrations of VLDL-cholesterol, LDL-cholesterol and total triglycerides, and sometimes with low HDL-cholesterol. Adequate insulin therapy usually leads to a fall in total triglyceride, and abnormalities of VLDL and LDL also improve. Patients with well-controlled type 1 diabetes can achieve plasma lipid concentrations similar to those of nondiabetic subjects; HDL may even be elevated.

Abnormalities of lipid metabolism are frequently present in patients with diabetes.

- ◆ Type 2 diabetes is strongly associated with low HDL-cholesterol, yet high VLDL-cholesterol and elevated triglyceride concentrations. Total cholesterol is often normal, but HDL:LDL or HDL:total cholesterol ratios are low.
  - ◇ In type 2 diabetes, the composition of VLDL particles changes, with more triglyceride and cholesterol ester relative to the apoprotein content.
  - ◇ LDL particles are typically small and dense.
  - ◇ These abnormalities are particularly atherogenic and there is a need to consider the HDL and triglycerides, rather than just total or LDL cholesterol, in the treatment of dyslipidemia in type 2 diabetes.
  - ◇ Improved glycemic control only partially improves the dyslipidemia of type 2 diabetes.

Metabolic syndrome and obesity

- ◆ Many of the associated features of type 2 diabetes co-segregate in members of a population even in nondiabetic subjects. Various overlapping syndromes have been introduced to reflect this fact, e.g. syndrome X, insulin resistance syndrome, metabolic syndrome.
- ◆ Subjects with glucose intolerance (type 2 diabetes or IGT), fasting hyperinsulinemia, hypertriglyceridemia (mainly VLDL-triglyceride), low HDL cholesterol, and hypertension have an increased predisposition to atherosclerosis and were said to have syndrome X.
- ◆ Metabolic syndrome is the more frequently discussed syndrome and includes abdominal obesity, but no formal requirement for insulin resistance. There has been debate on the cutoff points for the presence or absence of these features, and on the number of features required before an individual is labeled as having these related syndromes (Table 4.2).
  - ◇ Not all components are measured in routine clinical practice and the labels have no especial management implications. Some workers specifically exclude obese subjects from syndrome X but there are many features in common between slim subjects with syndrome X and those who are obese with metabolic syndrome.
- ◆ Insulin resistance is a prominent feature of obesity, especially of the android type. Obesity provokes compensatory hyperinsulinemia and the dyslipidemia and hypertension associated with obesity may

Table 4.2 Metabolic syndrome. People with metabolic syndrome have a five-fold greater risk of developing type 2 diabetes. The International Diabetes Federation (IDF) and the National Cholesterol Education Program (NCEP) have both recently issued updated diagnosis guidelines.

Definitions of metabolic syndrome

	IDF (2006)	WHO (1999)	EGIR (1999)	AHA/NCEP (2004)
Qualifying criteria	Central obesity (defined as waist circumference with ethnicity-specific values) AND any two of the other factors below	Presence of either: diabetes; impaired glucose tolerance; impaired fasting glucose; OR insulin resistance AND any two of the other factors below.	Insulin resistance (defined as the top 25% of the fasting insulin values among nondiabetic individuals) AND any two of the other factors below	Any three of the factors below
Central obesity	As above. NB: If BMI is >30 kg/m², central obesity can be assumed and waist circumference does not need to be measured	Waist:hip ratio of males: >0.90; females: >0.85 AND/OR BMI >30 kg/m²	Waist circumference of males: ≥94 cm; females: ≥80 cm	Waist circumference of males: ≥102 cm; females: ≥88 cm
Triglycerides	Levels of >1.7 mmol/L (150.5 mg/dL) OR specific treatment for this lipid abnormality	Dyslipidemia counts as one criterion; triglyceride levels of ≥1.695 mmol/L (150 mg/dL)	Dyslipidemia counts as one criterion; triglyceride levels of ≥2.0 mmol/L (177 mg/dL)	Levels of ≥1.7 mmol/L (150.5 mg/dL)
High-density lipo-protein cholesterol (HDL)	Levels of <1.03 mmol/L (39.8 mg/dL) (males); <1.29 mmol/L (49.8 mg/dL) (females) OR specific treatment for this lipid abnormality	AND HDL levels of 0.9 mmol/L (34.7 mg/dL) (males); 1.0 mmol/L (38.6 mg/dL) (females)	AND/OR HDL levels of <1.0 mmol/L (38.6 mg/dL) OR treated for dyslipidemia	Levels of males: <1.03 mmol/L; females: <1.29 mmol/L
Blood pressure (BP)	Systolic BP of >130 mmHg OR diastolic BP of >85 mmHg OR treatment of previously diagnosed hypertension	Levels of ≥140/90 mmHg	Levels of ≥140/90 mmHg OR treatment of previously diagnosed hypertension	Levels of ≥130/85 mmHg OR treatment of previously diagnosed hypertension
Fasting plasma glucose (FPG)	Levels of >5.6 mmol/L (100 mg/dL) OR previously diagnosed type 2 diabetes	As above	Levels of ≥6.1 mmol/L (110 mg/dL)	Levels of ≥5.6 mmol/L (100 mg/dL) OR use of medication for hyperglycemia
Microalbuminuria		Urinary albumin excretion ratio of ≥20 mg/min OR albumin:creatinine ratio of ≥30 mg/g		

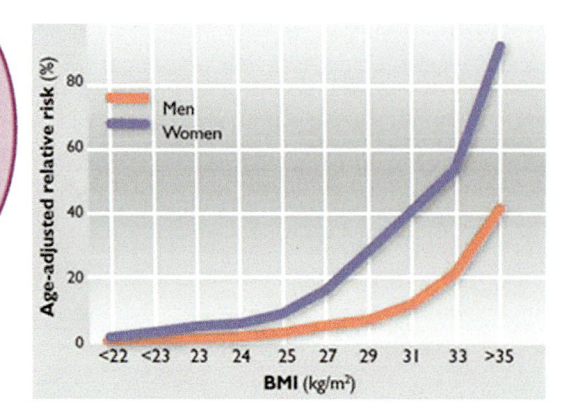

Figure 4.6 Obesity and diabetes. The link between obesity and type 2 diabetes is firmly established.

follow from the insulin abnormalities. Obesity is a powerful indicator of type 2 diabetes risk (Figure 4.6).

Development of type 2 diabetes

Glucoregulatory defects in type 2 diabetes

- The causes of type 2 diabetes are partially understood.
  - ◇ Reduced insulin secretion plays a major role, together with reduced insulin sensitivity.
  - ◇ Hyperglycemia is due to elevated hepatic glucose output and (to a lesser extent) failure of skeletal muscle to take up glucose and store it as glycogen.
  - ◇ There are also abnormalities in metabolic fluxes (Table 4.3).

Pancreatic β-cell deficiency

- The importance of β-cell deficiency varies in different groups and individual cases of type 2 diabetes. In general, the β-cell deficiency becomes more severe with time. There are abnormalities of insulin secretion in all these patients, but the causes of these defects are not yet established.
  - ◇ In individual patients it is often difficult to define the severity of the insulin secretory defect. Although β-cell dysfunction may be the prime abnormality in some cases of type 2 diabetes, usually the β-cell dysfunction is more subtle than in type 1 diabetes and is secondary to the preceding insulin resistance.
- The finding of marked insulin deficiency in an apparent type 2 patient should provoke a consideration of LADA.
- Some patients with type 2 diabetes, especially obese subjects with mild glucose

Table 4.3 Alterations in metabolic fluxes. Insulin resistance causes increased flux of free fatty acids, leading to increased VLDL synthesis in the liver.

Metabolic fluxes in insulin resistance syndrome/early type 2 diabetes		
	CONCENTRATION	FLUX
Glucose	Increased fasting concentration	Normal whole body disposal rate; normal whole body glucose production and clearance
NEFA	Variable	Usually normal fasting total body production; impaired responsiveness to meal
VLDL	Increased concentration	Increased production, increased plasma half-life and increased whole body clearance
Oxidized fuel	Whole body respiratory quotient* reflects diet	Whole body respiratory quotient reflects diet, but seems to be higher in diabetes

*Respiratory quotient is the ratio of oxygen consumption to carbon dioxide production during biological oxidation at tissue level.

intolerance, may have hyperinsulinemia throughout the whole 24 hours.
- ◇ Some patients can exhibit both insulinopenia and hyperinsulinemia (relative to normal weight controls) at different times during a single day.
- ◇ It is fairly common to have fasting hyperinsulinemia combined with reduced β-cell reserve, relative to healthy subjects.

◆ The time course of insulin secretion in type 2 diabetes is abnormal, with patients typically exhibiting relative insulin deficiency during both the early phase of insulin secretion after an oral glucose load or meal and the first-phase insulin response to an intravenous glucose load. This loss of early insulin response to glucose is paralleled by defects in the pulsatility of insulin secretion.

◆ Insulin clearance is thought to be normal in type 2 diabetes, so hyperinsulinemia is a reflection of true hypersecretion. This hypersecretion represents a load on the pancreas and explains why increased concentrations of insulin precursors (such as pro-insulins) are seen in type 2 patients.

◆ However, over time, even patients who were hyperinsulinemic at diagnosis become progressively more insulin deficient. Such patients, together with those who are insulin deficient from diagnosis, often need exogenous insulin treatment to maintain near-normal glycemia. These patients may then be termed 'insulin-treated' or 'insulin-requiring', but it should be recognized that such insulin-*treated* patients form a heterogeneous group, very different in character from type 1, insulin-*dependent* patients.

All patients with type 2 diabetes have some beta-cell deficiency, which often gets more severe with time.

Insulin resistance

◆ In 1970, Berson and Yalow defined insulin resistance as 'a state in which greater than normal amounts of insulin are required to elicit a quantitatively normal response.'

◆ Following the discovery of insulin in 1922, it was widely assumed that diabetes was due exclusively to a deficiency in insulin secretion. The concept of insulin resistance arose in the 1930s when Himsworth noted that the same amount of exogenous insulin injected into different subjects with diabetes had different antihyperglycemic effects. Those with lesser antihyperglycemic responses were termed insulin insensitive (or insulin resistant). When the development of radioimmunoassay showed that many patients with type 2 diabetes had high levels of circulating insulin, the concept of insulin resistance was reinforced. Such patients are hyperglycemic, and hence by definition relatively insulin deficient, yet they actually have more immunoreactive insulin than other people, such that their true 'insulin requirement' was believed to be larger still.

◆ Hyperinsulinemia with eu- or hyperglycemia is taken to indicate insulin resistance, since hyperinsulinemia produces hypoglycemia in subjects with normal insulin sensitivity.

◆ As insulin has several actions, resistance to insulin action may take several forms:
- ◇ Some subjects show resistance to hepatic effects.
- ◇ Some show resistance to skeletal muscle effects. (Activation of muscle glycogen synthase by insulin is often defective.)
- ◇ Some show resistance to liporegulatory effects.
- ◇ The degree of resistance may be different for different actions of insulin so that some subjects may have marked liver insulin resistance but relatively normal lipids (or other combinations).

Insulin resistance means that more insulin than normal is needed to exert the glucoregulatory effects.

- There is incomplete consensus as to the cellular mechanisms underlying insulin resistance in most patients with type 2 diabetes, though multiple mechanisms have been suggested:
  ◇ Competition between carbohydrate and lipid fuels (Randle cycle hypothesis). High circulating concentrations of alternative fuels, such as triglycerides, NEFA, lactate, and ketone bodies, compete with glucose for metabolism and, in their presence, glucose clearance will be reduced.
  ◇ Some insulin resistance can be interpreted as a result of 'cellular satiety', seen whenever intracellular sensors, such as UDP glucosamine, detect overabundant energy supply.
  ◇ Some insulin resistance is attributable to specific cellular abnormalities, such as reduced numbers of insulin receptors, reduced receptor function, dysfunction of second messenger systems, and intracellular antagonists of insulin effects.
- These different hypotheses are not necessarily mutually exclusive. Lipid fuel competition may contribute to cellular satiety and provoke specific second messenger changes.
- Most glucose clearance occurs independently of insulin. This insulin-independent glucose clearance is defective in type 2 diabetes and contributes to hyperglycemia. Reduced tissue blood flow, particularly within skeletal muscle, may also reduce clearance of plasma glucose in diabetes.

Incretin hormones

- The incretin effect describes the physiological phenomenon whereby oral glucose elicits a much greater insulin stimulatory effect than that of intravenously administered glucose.
- Incretin hormones (glucagon-like peptide-1 [GLP-1] and gastric inhibitory peptide [GIP] – also known as glucose-dependent insulinotropic polypeptide) are responsible for the incretin effect. These are hormones produced by the L-cells of the small intestine in response to nutrient.
- Incretin hormones stimulate insulin release from the pancreatic beta cells in a glucose-dependent manner. GLP-1 also inhibits glucagon secretion from the pancreatic alpha cells.
- In addition, they reduce appetite by reducing gastric emptying.
- Incretin hormones are rapidly degraded by the enzyme dipeptidyl peptidase-4 [DPP-4], and inhibition of this enzyme with DPP-4 inhibitors can lead to increased endogenous incretin hormone levels.
- In people with type 2 diabetes, the incretin effect (the ability of glucose to stimulate insulin release) is considerably diminished (Figure 4.7). In addition, the glucagon suppression effect of nutrient administration in people with type 2 diabetes is also diminished.
- This has formed the basis for therapeutic intervention in type 2 diabetes with incretin analogues (see p. 187) (Figure 4.7).

The role of amylin

- Amylin (also known as islet amyloid polypeptide, IAPP) is a 37-amino-acid peptide co-secreted with insulin by β cells in all subjects with intact insulin secretion (and so not those with type 1 diabetes or those type 2 patients with severe insulin deficiency). The amino acid structure has some homology with calcitonin gene-related peptide.
- It is suggested that amylin may have a physiological role in the regulation of insulin secretion within the islet.
- Amylin may induce insulin resistance in skeletal muscle.

Diabetes & The "Incretin Effect"

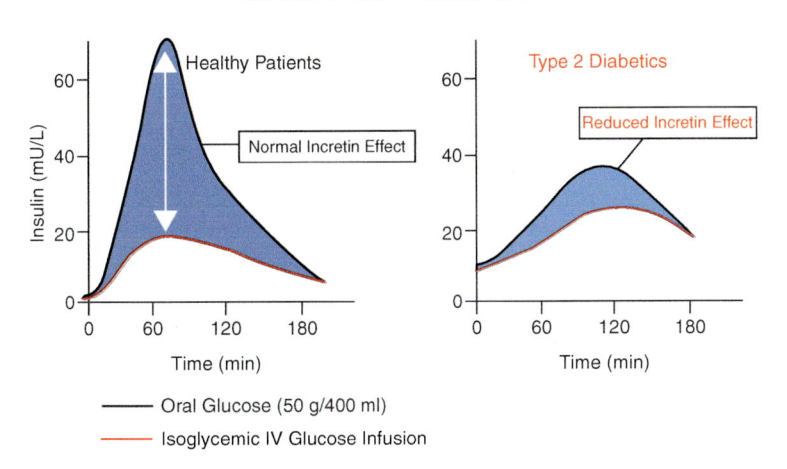

Figure 4.7 Insulin response to oral glucose and intravenous glucose in healthy patients and people with Type 2 diabetes. Healthy patients show a much greater rise in insulin levels in response to oral glucose compared to intravenous glucose. This difference is called the "incretin effect", and is mediated by incretin hormones produced by the small intestinal L cells. In people with Type 2 diabetes, the incretin effect is diminished.

- Amylin fibrils (with typical amyloid features of secondary protein structure and insolubility) are deposited in islet cells in conditions of excess insulin secretion (such as insulinoma) and in situations where insulin secretion may have initially been increased but has subsequently declined (such as old age and type 2 diabetes). The possible role of amylin in the islet damage of type 2 diabetes is unclear.

Glucotoxicity and lipotoxicity

Glucotoxicity
- Acute elevation of plasma glucose concentrations is able to induce a state of insulin resistance, coupled with impairment of insulin secretion in response to glucose (Figure 4.8).
- In the presence of normal β-cell mass, transient elevation of plasma glucose to levels just above the physiological range potentiates insulin secretion in both humans and animals, but chronic hyperglycemia reduces insulin secretion.
- Conversely, strict metabolic control is able to induce improvements in both insulin secretion and sensitivity, although not usually to normality. It is likely that

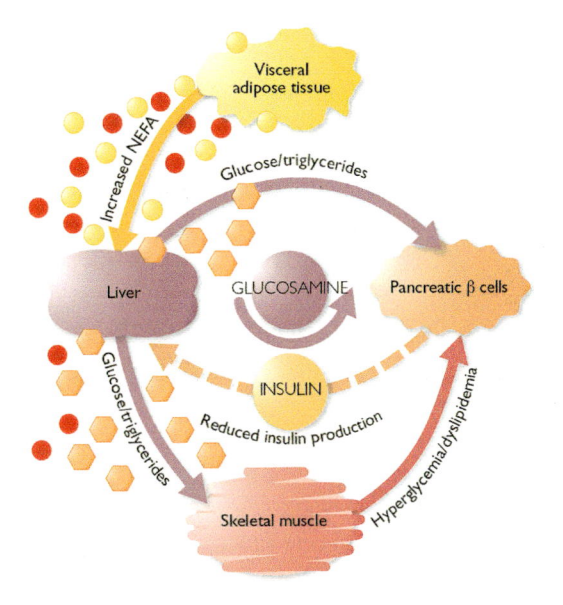

Figure 4.8 Glucotoxicity and lipotoxicity. Insulin resistance is related to elevated levels in the blood of both glucose and free fatty acids (NEFA). The metabolism of glucose to glucosamine is a possible unifying mechanism for both glucotoxicity and lipotoxicity whereby the glucosamine pathway inhibits a number of steps in the insulin-signaling cascade.

multiple mechanisms contribute to this effect, including:
- ◇ Changes in the K_m of glucose sensing systems, such as glucokinase/hexokinase, which may lead to alteration of

the dose-response curve of the islet cell to blood glucose concentrations.
- ◇ Changes in the ratio of proinsulin to insulin secretion.
- ◇ Alteration in the functional activity of the membrane sulfonylurea-sensitive K+ channel.
- ◆ It is likely that the 'honeymoon period' often observed in new-onset type 1 diabetes is at least partly attributable to a reduction in glucotoxicity.

Lipotoxicity
- ◆ Although adipose tissue has a large number of functions related to thermal insulation, immunity, fertility, and protection of structures such as the eye, its main function is the uptake of energy during the postprandial state, energy storage in the form of triglycerides, and the release of lipids in the form of NEFA in the fasting state (Figure 4.8).
- ◆ The consequences of an accumulation of lipids in non-adipose tissues include hepatic steatosis, lipid-induced cardiomyopathy, insulin resistance, and type 2 diabetes. This process is termed lipotoxicity.
- ◆ In fatless rodents and humans with generalized lipodystrophy there can be an especially severe form of lipotoxicity (including lipoapoptosis where programmed cell death occurs). This severe form is reversible in rodents by the transplantation of small amounts of normal adipose tissue into fatless rodents, but not by the transplantation of adipose tissue from *ob/ob* mice, which lack the ability to secrete leptin.
  - ◇ In humans with generalized lipodystrophy, long-term treatment with leptin improves insulin resistance, hyperlipidemia, and hepatic steatosis dramatically.
- ◆ NEFA can induce insulin resistance in muscle via at least three putative mechanisms:
  - ◇ The Randle cycle, mentioned earlier.
  - ◇ Increased activity of protein kinase C via intermediates of fatty acid metabolism, such as diacyl glycerol, which promotes inactivating phosphorylation of the insulin receptor.
  - ◇ NFκB activation, which has supposed vascular effects that might contribute to the observed increase in vascular damage preceding hyperglycemia.
- ◆ In the liver, NEFAs inhibit the suppression of glycogenolysis by insulin.
- ◆ Other mechanisms of lipotoxicity include modulation of adipocytokines, such as adiponectin, that could promote insulin resistance.
- ◆ Not all individuals with obesity and elevated NEFA rapidly develop diabetes. One explanation for this may lie in the fact that NEFAs are potent stimulators of insulin in normal individuals, an effect that might mitigate the tendency for NEFAs to induce insulin resistance. However, in subjects with type 2 diabetes and in their normoglycemic first-degree relatives, NEFAs do not induce a sufficient compensatory rise in insulin secretion to overcome the induced insulin resistance. Thus NEFAs may be able to cause diabetes in those with a genetic predisposition to β-cell dysfunction, but not in those with full β-cell reserve.
- ◆ PPARγ activators may alleviate several of these NEFA-induced abnormalities by reducing plasma NEFA levels, increasing adiponectin and redistributing fat from visceral to subcutaneous deposits, thus reducing the direct effects on the liver and elsewhere.

Very high plasma glucose concentrations can induce a state of insulin resistance.

Screening and prevention

- ◆ Screening for diabetes can be undertaken using glucose tests or, more conveniently, HbA1c (see Table 1.2).

- IGT, IFG, and prediabetes are recognized as high-risk states for the development of type 2 diabetes. The standard definition has been updated on several occasions, but the evidence remains that IGT is a powerful predictor of diabetes progression, with a concomitant increased risk for cardiovascular disease.
- IGT, IFG and prediabetes are common, affecting up to a third of adults in the UK and USA.
- Several additional factors determine the risk of progression from prediabetes, IGT, or IFG to type 2 diabetes: family history of diabetes, age, central and total obesity, physical inactivity, fetal maturation, and ethnic origin. The risk of progression to diabetes is greater for those with IGT than for those with IFG (Figure 4.9).
- As with type 2 diabetes, IGT is an insulin-resistant state and subjects have a reduced early-phase insulin response to intravenous or oral glucose challenge. It follows that glucose tolerance, as with diabetes, can be improved by improving insulin sensitivity and insulin secretion.

◇ Following intervention to reduce weight, reduce calorie intake, and increase exercise, middle-aged subjects with IGT have been successfully treated with these lifestyle changes with or without metformin, acarbose, and orlistat. For example, lifestyle changes (diet and exercise) reduced the 4-year incidence of diabetes by 58% in middle-aged, obese, IGT subjects in one study; by 58% in similar subjects by 3 years in another study; and by 31% by 3 years with metformin.
◇ Intervention with very low-calorie diets in people with recent onset type 2 diabetes can lead to successful remission in over 50% of patients at one year.

IGT is a powerful predictor of diabetes progression.

- Type 2 diabetes can be predicted using diabetes-associated conditions such as

Early identification of risk

RISK FACTORS (AGE ≥30 IF HIGH RISK)
Family history of diabetes
Overweight
Sedentary lifestyle
Higher-risk ethnic origin
Previously identified IGT or IFG
Hypertension
Elevated triglycerides, low HDL, or both
History of gestational diabetes
Delivery of a baby of >4 kg (9 lb)
Severe psychiatric illness

Lifestyle modification

INTERVENTION
Medical nutrition therapy (MNT)
Physical fitness program (30 min exercise, equivalent to brisk walking, 5 times a week)
Weight loss (5–7% reduction in body weight, if overweight)

Pharmacologic therapy

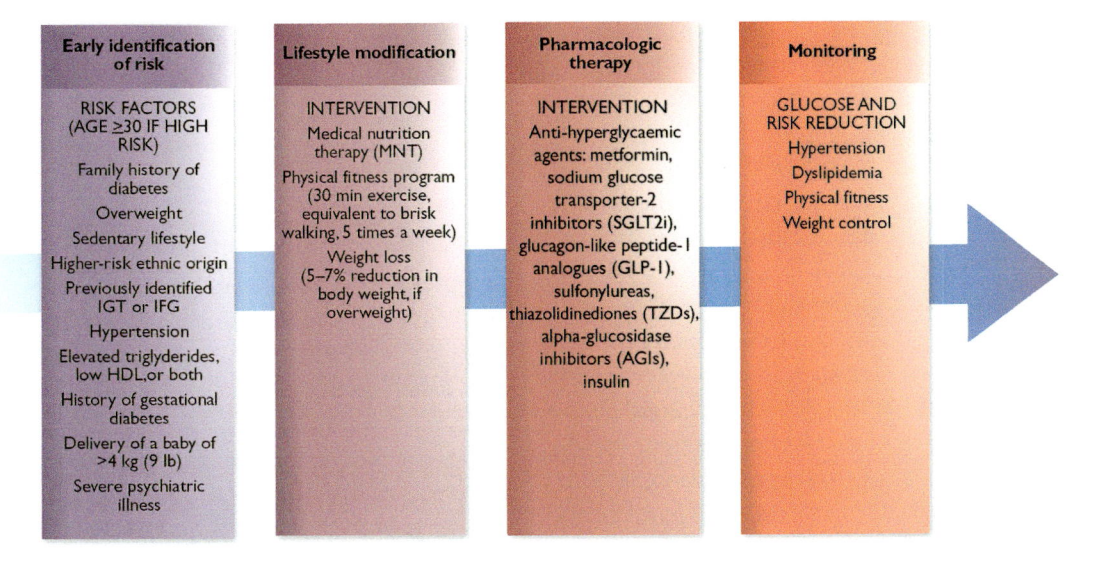

INTERVENTION
Anti-hyperglycaemic agents: metformin, sodium glucose transporter-2 inhibitors (SGLT2i), glucagon-like peptide-1 analogues (GLP-1), sulfonylureas, thiazolidinediones (TZDs), alpha-glucosidase inhibitors (AGIs), insulin

Monitoring

GLUCOSE AND RISK REDUCTION
Hypertension
Dyslipidemia
Physical fitness
Weight control

Figure 4.9 Prevention of type 2 diabetes. Screening and identification of those most at risk is the first step in preventing type 2 diabetes. There is convincing evidence that lifestyle modification is the most effective tool in preventing or delaying its onset, with moderate weight loss and physical activity substantially reducing the risk. However some patients will also require pharmacologic intervention.

obesity; presence of IGT, IFG, or prediabetes; and metabolic syndrome.
- ◇ Evidence from long-term trials suggests that lifestyle interventions are more effective in the prevention of type 2 diabetes than drug therapy. This may be expected since lifestyle intervention focuses on the pathogenetic mechanisms underlying the development of type 2 diabetes, in particular factors causing insulin resistance.
- ◇ Theoretically, it would be possible to delay over 70% of cases of type 2 diabetes in persons at increased risk, if they were able to maintain normal body weight and engage in physical activity throughout their lives.
- ◇ More than preventing diabetes, a healthy diet and lifestyle could prevent or delay heart disease.

Type 2 diabetes prevention studies

- ◆ Type 2 diabetes may be prevented or at least delayed by relatively modest degrees of weight loss and exercise. The interventions have involved individual counseling regarding weight loss, total fat intake, saturated fat intake, fiber intake, and physical exercise.
    - ◇ Lifestyle interventions resulting in average weight loss of <7 kg over 6 months with some later regain resulted in a 58% reduction in cumulative diabetes incidence in the intervention groups during the period of the studies.
- ◆ There is evidence that medications may reduce progression to diabetes, especially in younger subjects.
- ◆ For patients unable to lose weight after appropriate lifestyle interventions, treatment with metformin may bring about a modest reduction in the incidence of type 2 diabetes.
- ◆ Other studies have shown that adopting a more physically active lifestyle appears to confer useful protection independently of body weight. Several trials have shown

Table 4.4 Type 2 diabetes prevention studies. Several long-term trials have studied the effectiveness of a range of medications as well as lifestyle changes: lifestyle change and glitazones have proved the most successful, although both troglitazone and rosiglitazone have since been withdrawn due to concerns over side effects.

Trials determining prevention/delay of progression from IGT to type 2 diabetes

Lifestyle change trials	Risk reduction vs placebo (%)
Malmö study	63
Da Qing study	42
Finnish Diabetes Prevention Study (DPS)	58
Diabetes Prevention Program (DPP)	58

Medication trials	
TRIPOD: troglitazone	55
STOP-NIDDM: acarbose	25
XENDOS: orlistat	37
DPP: metformin	75
DREAM: rosiglitazone and ramipril	60
NAVIGATOR: nateglinide/valsartan	0/14

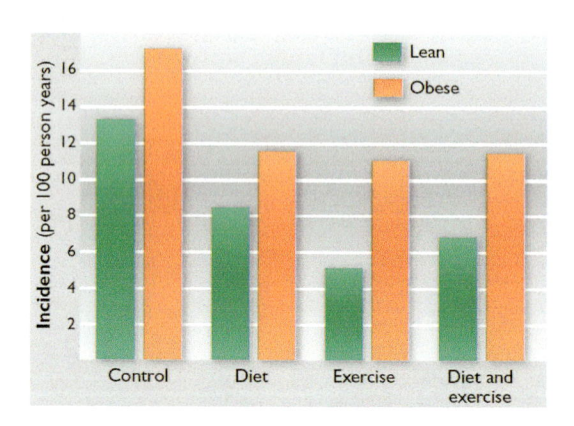

Figure 4.10 Lifestyle interventions. The Da Qing study examined the effect over 6 years of diet and exercise intervention in Chinese subjects with IGT and a mean age of 45. The diet intervention saw a 31% reduction in the risk of developing type 2 diabetes, while exercise or exercise combined with diet showed a 46% reduction and a 42% reduction, respectively.

successful prevention or delay of progression from a state of IGT to type 2 diabetes by adopting different interventions (Table 4.4 and Figure 4.10).

CHAPTER 5

Diabetes screening and patient care

Management overview

- The goals of diabetes management are, at first glance, easily established. We know that the excess mortality associated with diabetes is predominantly due to macrovascular disease, although more recently there is growing data to suggest that cancer is a growing cause of mortality in people with diabetes. The morbidity due to diabetes results from both macrovascular and microvascular disease. The aim of therapy is to normalize excess mortality and morbidity, so therapy should be aimed at risk factors for both macrovascular and microvascular diseases.
  - ◇ Modifiable risk factors for macrovascular disease are hypertension, hypercholesterolemia, obesity, smoking, and hyperglycemia.
  - ◇ Risk factors for microvascular disease are largely the same, but predominantly hyperglycemia and hypertension.
  - ◇ Since many patients with type 2 diabetes have a combination of these risk factors, many patients will require a combination of drugs to manage their diabetes.
  - ◇ In type 1 diabetes, insulin therapy is mandatory once insulin dependence is established, and in these patients the focus is much more on management of glycemia, as these patients are generally younger and have fewer modifiable risk factors than patients with type 2 diabetes.
- The management of type 2 diabetes is complex and the physician will have to consider the interplay between the psychosocial background, various risk factors, and several therapeutic agents before deciding on a regimen appropriate to the patient. In practical terms the therapy of type 2 diabetes involves a trade-off between what is desirable and what is practically possible.
- There is strong evidence that patient-focused education early in the diagnosis of diabetes can considerably improve outcomes.
- Different studies of treatment, including the UKPDS and DCCT, illustrate the significant benefits that may be achieved by appropriate treatment. Cost/benefit assessments indicate that improved diabetes care compares favorably with other established healthcare programs, such as breast cancer screening.
- Newer therapeutic agents have shown significant benefits in terms of cardiovascular and renal outcomes, and their place in treatment of type 2 diabetes is expanding.

Risk factors

- Patients with type 2 diabetes have an increased mortality (up to four times that of the nondiabetic population) attributed mainly to macrovascular disease, notably cardiovascular disease.
- In high-income countries, diabetes is the commonest single cause of limb

amputations, the commonest cause of blindness in working life, and the commonest cause of end-stage renal failure.
- The macrovascular disease risk is associated with smoking, lack of exercise, hypertension, obesity, dyslipidemia, and hyperglycemia. This network of risk factors, when it occurs concurrently, is called metabolic or insulin-resistance syndrome, since all these factors are associated with insulin resistance and can precede type 2 diabetes (see p. 43).
  - Metabolic syndrome may be present in up to 25% of the non-diabetic population and, in adult life, about 2–12% per year of these individuals progress to diabetes.

Annual examination

- Diabetes patients should be reviewed, at the very least once per year, by one of the following:
  - Their appropriately trained primary health care provider.
  - A specialist diabetes clinic.
  - OR a combination of these.
- All diabetes patients should have access to advice outside the routine primary care clinic.
- The purposes of a diabetes review are to:
  - Optimize therapy (e.g. targets set for risk factors).
  - Provide patient education.
  - Screen for diabetes complications.
  - Treat established or developing complications.
- Monitoring of therapy includes assessment of:
  - Weight.
  - Height (using centile charts for children).
  - Urine (microalbuminuria).
  - HbA1c, blood glucose, lipid profile, creatinine.
  - Blood pressure.
  - Smoking status

- There are key areas to be considered when examining a patient with diabetes outlined below.

Diabetes patients should be reviewed at least once per year.
Since prevention of complications is better and easier than cure, early referral is preferable.

Screening for complications

Eyes

- Most retinal screening should be undertaken annually using digital photography by trained screeners (Figure 5.1). This involves:
  - Determine visual acuity. This can be done using the commonly used Snellen's chart.
  - Extraocular eye movements can also be checked at this time.
  - Dilate pupils 30 minutes before the eye is examined with a mydriatic, such as tropicamide 0.5%.
    - Dilating drugs should not be used in patients with a history of glaucoma, except with the advice of an ophthalmologist.
- Ophthalmoscopy may be used to carry out a systematic examination of the eyes, but is inadequate for an annual retinal screen (Figure 5.1).
- Patients with retinopathy should be examined regularly by an ophthalmologist. The following circumstances dictate immediate referral to an ophthalmologist:
  - Deteriorating visual acuity.
  - Hard exudates encroaching on the macula.
  - Pre-proliferative changes (cotton-wool spots or venous beading).
  - New vessel formation.

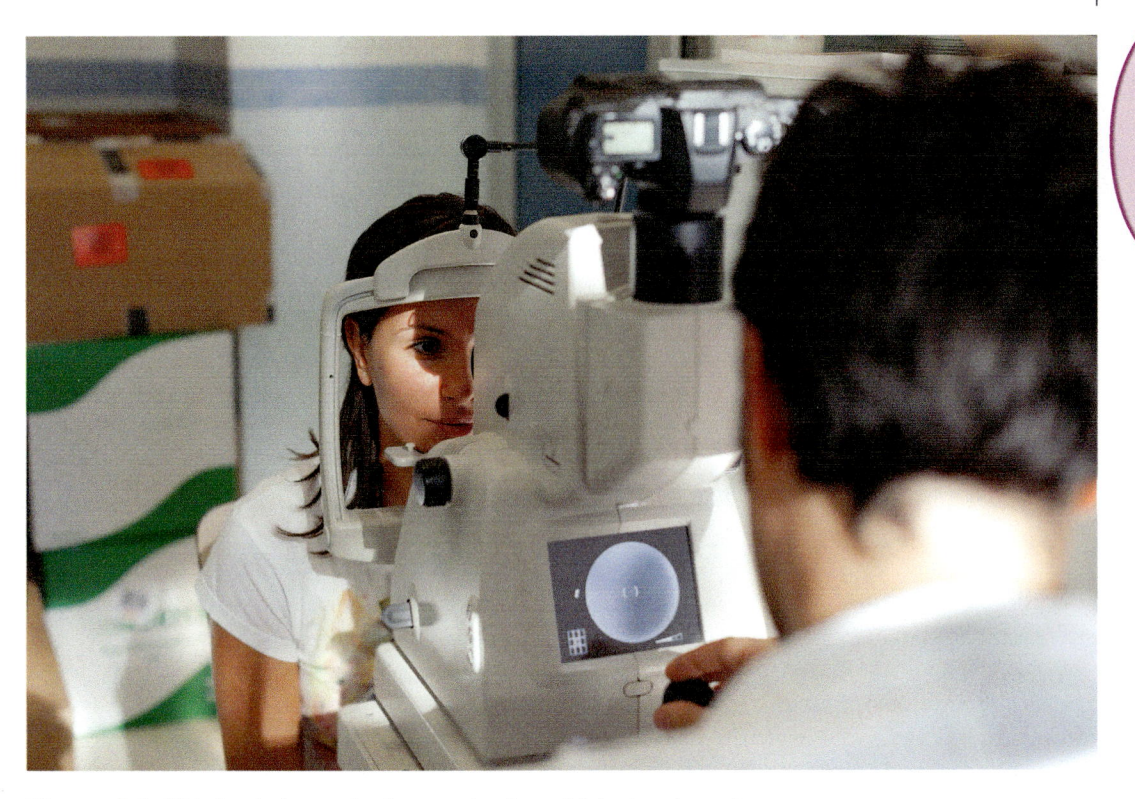

Figure 5.1 Digital retinal screening for annual review of diabetic retinopathy.

Table 5.1 Values for urine albumin screening.

	Urine albumin creatinine ratio (ACR) (mg/mmol)	Urine albumin creatinine ratio (ACR) (mg/g)	24 hour urine (mg/24hrs)	Timed urine collection (mcg/min)
Normal	<3	<30	<30	20
Microalbuminuria	3-30	30-300	30-300	20-200
Macroalbuminuria	>30	>300	>300	>200

Kidneys
- Urine is screened for microalbuminuria using a first voided specimen to determine the urinary albumin creatinine ratio (Table 5.1).
  ◇ This is valid as a marker of early kidney disease in children and young adults only when present on at least two separate occasions in an early morning urine sample.
  ◇ If microalbuminuria is confirmed, treatment with an angiotensin-receptor blocker (ARB) or angiotensin-converting enzyme (ACE) inhibitor should be started. More recently in patients with type 2 diabetes, sodium glucose transporter-2 inhibitors (SGLT-2i) have been shown to reduce progression of diabetic nephropathy and should be consider early.
- Serum creatinine should be analyzed annually.
- Referral to a renal specialist is advised once the estimated glomerular filtration rate (eGFR) reaches 30 mL/min/1.73 m^2, or there is rapid progression of renal dysfunction or albuminuria.

Feet

- Inspection of the feet is performed to identify anatomical distortions, pressure points, ulcers, injuries, or problems with footwear.
- Examination is carried out for blood supply (by checking peripheral pulses) and nerve supply (by checking vibration and fine touch peripheral sensation, using a 10 g monofilament (Figure 5.2).
- Refer to a chiropodist for education on self-management if foot problems are identified. Since prevention is better and easier than cure, early referral is preferable.

Erectile dysfunction

- History should assess whether the patient can get an erection, penetration, or emission. Questions should be direct and unequivocal, as otherwise the response may not be informative.
- Examination should exclude hypogonadal features, small testes, and penile changes, such as Peyronie's disease.

Vascular disease

- History should be assessed, e.g. pain in chest or legs, erectile dysfunction.
- Examination includes checking for bruit in carotids, palpating peripheral foot pulses.
- Special investigations may be necessary, e.g. an electrocardiogram (ECG), or CT coronary angiography.
- Refer to a cardiologist if there is either angina or cardiac dysfunction.

Treating children

Types of childhood diabetes

- Most children (under 18 years) with diabetes have type 1 diabetes (Table 5.2)
    ◇ As childhood obesity increases throughout the world an increasing proportion have type 2 diabetes (Figure 5.3).
    ◇ A small proportion will have maturity onset diabetes of the young (MODY) (see p. 7).

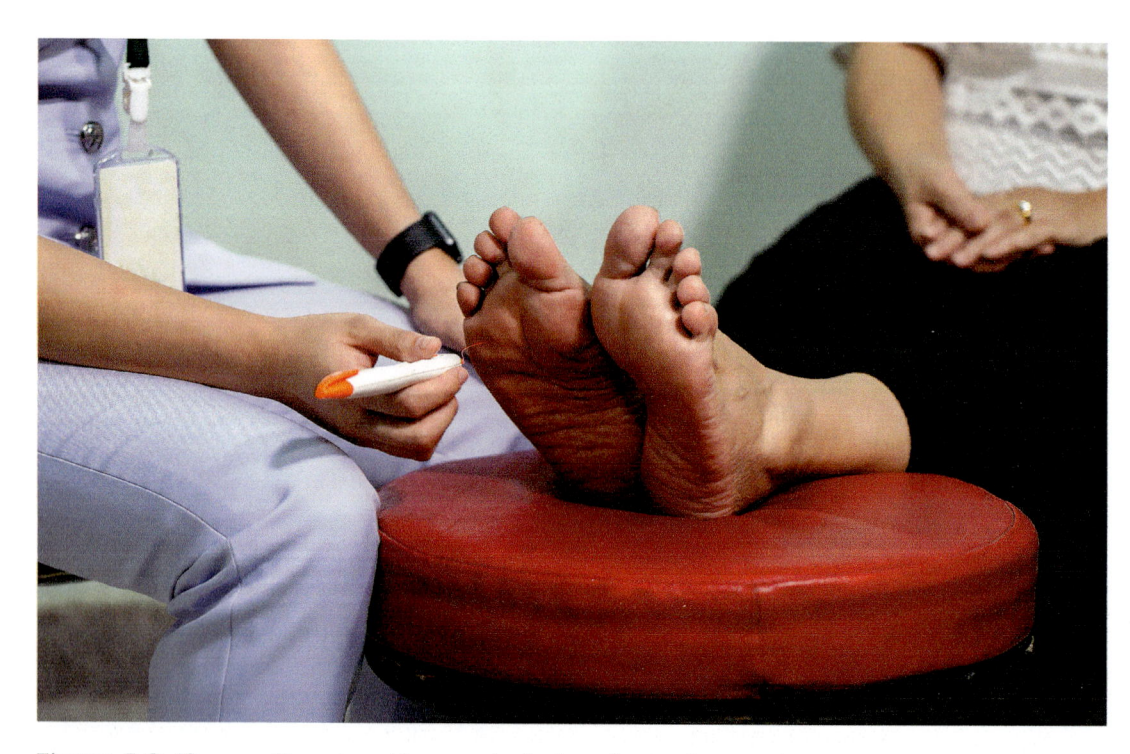

Figure 5.2 10 g monofilament used for screening for loss of protective sensation.

Table 5.2 Childhood diabetes. While type 1 diabetes accounts for most cases in children, in industrialized societies, type 2 is increasingly prevalent. MODY accounts for only 1% of cases.

Diabetes in childhood	
TYPE OF DIABETES	**PRINCIPAL CAUSES**
Type 1 diabetes	Autoimmune (see Chapter 3)
Type 2 diabetes	Decreased insulin secretion and obesity (see Chapter 4)
Maturity-onset diabetes of the young (MODY)	Dominantly inherited variant of type 2 diabetes mellitus (see Chapter 1)
Secondary diabetes	
Chromosomal abnormalities:	Down syndrome; Turner syndrome; Klinefelter syndrome
Inherited disorders:	Prader–Willi syndrome; Laurence–Moon–Biedl syndrome; DIDMOAD syndrome; Leprechaunism; Lipodystrophy; Ataxia–telangiectasia; (Rabson) Mendenhall syndrome
Inherited disorder with pancreatic disease:	Cystic fibrosis; Cystinosis; Thalassemia
Acquired pancreatic disorders:	Postpancreatectomy

- ◇ An even smaller proportion have neonatal diabetes, which may be permanent or transient, and predominates when diabetes is diagnosed before 2 years of age and especially within 6 months of birth.
- ◆ Type 1 diabetes is invariably treated with insulin.
- ◆ The optimal treatment of type 2 diabetes in children and adolescents remains to be determined. Common sense suggests that treatment regimens similar to those for adults with type 2 diabetes would be appropriate. However, many of these patients will be started on insulin initially on the assumption that they have type 1 diabetes, before the correct diagnosis is established.

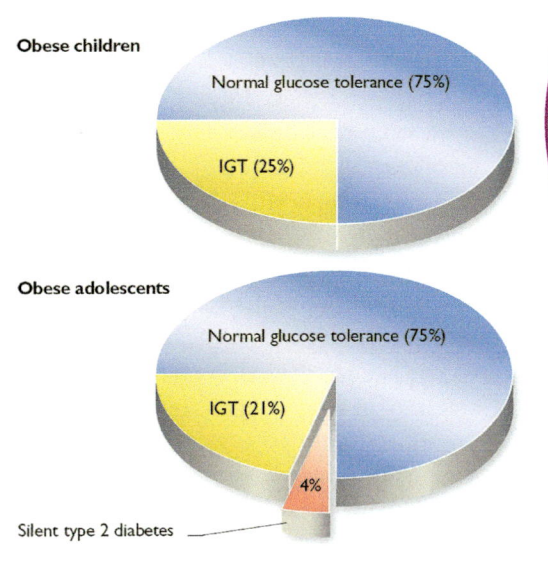

Figure 5.3 Childhood obesity and IGT. The prevalence of impaired glucose tolerance and type 2 diabetes in obese children and adolescents has been found to be high.

Obese children: Normal glucose tolerance (75%); IGT (25%)

Obese adolescents: Normal glucose tolerance (75%); IGT (21%); Silent type 2 diabetes 4%

Diabetes screening and patient care

- ◆ Treatment of certain types of MODY with sulfonylureas often achieves excellent glycemic control, and the use of these agents in this context has been useful in confirming their long-term safety in younger patients. The physician should be alerted to MODY when there is a strong family history of early onset diabetes.
- ◆ The causes of neonatal diabetes are predominantly genetic mutations in the sulfonylurea or potassium channels, so these children respond to sulfonylurea therapy.

Good glycemic control in the early years of diabetes may have a lasting effect on prevention of complications.

Management of young patients
- ◆ Management of children is not unlike management of the adult. However, it often requires particular sensitivity to the balance between the child's social independence and dependence on others. Younger children will be much

more dependent on family and friends for supervision of their care. Developing independence as children get older is important for their ability to manage diabetes throughout their lifetime. Understanding and dealing in a sympathetic way with parents' understandable reluctance to cede too much independence is crucial to the management of teenage diabetes.

- ◆ Hypoglycemia is a particular problem in children, in whom the warning symptoms can differ from hypoglycemia in adults.
- ◆ Symptoms of note due to hypoglycemia in young children include:
  - ◇ Bedwetting.
  - ◇ Naughtiness.
  - ◇ Tearfulness.
  - ◇ Bad temper.
  - ◇ Poor performance in school.
- ◆ Glycemic targets should be essentially the same as in adult patients.
- ◆ Long-term follow-up of the young adults who constituted the DCCT cohort has suggested that good glycemic control in the early years of diabetes may have a lasting effect on prevention of complications, even when there is a subsequent modest decline in glycemic control. This study also showed for the first time that early glycemic control protects against cardiovascular disease later in life as well as microvascular disease. The DCCT did not specifically enroll patients who had developed diabetes in early childhood, but there is no reason to believe that the lessons from the study would not apply.
  - ◇ It makes sense, therefore, to try to apply the same standards of care in childhood diabetes that we would strive for in more mature patients.
- ◆ Even when there is reason to question the level of competence for self-management among children with diabetes and their families, instruction on intensive insulin treatment can be very beneficial (Figure 5.4).

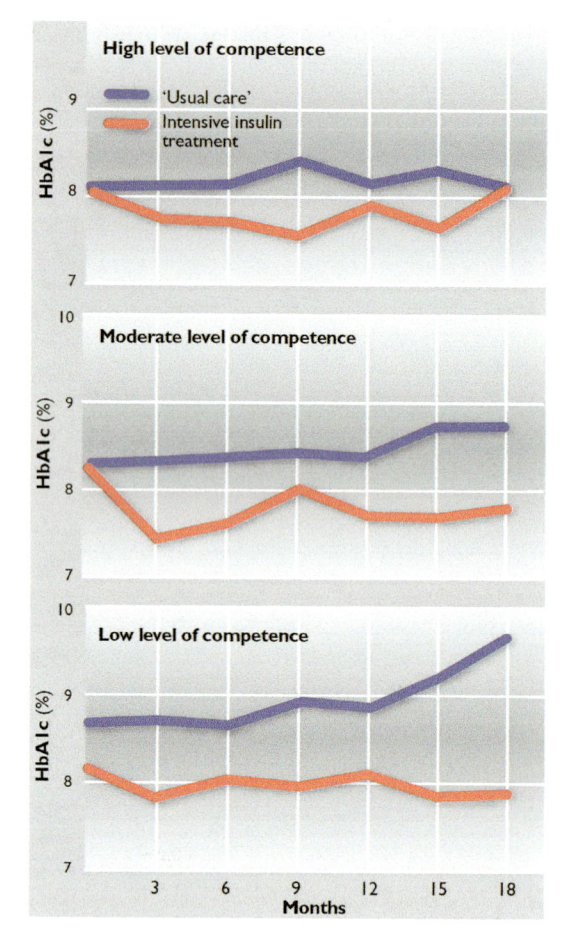

Figure 5.4 Diabetes self-management. In a study of 142 young people, intensive therapy gave improved glycemic control irrespective of self-management competence, but competence level was more significant with 'usual care'. *From Wysocki T, et al. Diabetes Care, 2003.*

- ◆ Sometimes the fear of hypoglycemia limits attempts to obtain optimum diabetes control, and this is understandable.
- ◆ Optimal use of newer insulin analogs in 'basal and bolus' regimens, or of continuous subcutaneous insulin infusion pumps (see p. 198), should enable most young people with diabetes to achieve reasonably good control with less risk of hypoglycemia. Adolescents and many young children embrace the technologies of newer delivery devices and monitoring systems much more readily than older patients.

- Newer continuous glucose monitoring devices (real-time or intermittently scanned) offer a method of improving glucose control in such patients with minimal finger-prick testing which can be a significant barrier.
  ◇ In light of the potential long-term benefit of excellent glycemic control achieved early in the course of diabetes, every effort should be made to facilitate access to these newer technologies to as many children and adolescents with diabetes as possible.
  ◇ However, if optimum control is difficult, any reduction in HbA1c is associated with a marked decrease in complication risk. Thus, never abandon trying to get better control.

- Common issues regarding children with diabetes:
  ◇ Immunization programs in diabetic children are unaltered.
  ◇ Illness is no more prevalent in diabetic children, though urinary tract infection is more common.
  ◇ Bedwetting is no more prevalent in diabetic children but might be due to nocturnal hyperglycemia or hypoglycemia.
  ◇ Reluctance to take injections should be sympathetically handled and expert advice sought on needleless pens and injection technique.
  ◇ Hypoglycemia may present differently. Measure blood glucose if in doubt.
  ◇ Diet should be similar as for the rest of the family, and low in refined sugar. Try to keep mealtimes to a routine, but avoid being obsessive about it.
  ◇ Diabetic children should be encouraged to participate in all aspects of sport and play at school. Teachers may need to be advised.
  ◇ People around the child should be aware that the child has diabetes and what to do in case they develop hypoglycemic coma.
  ◇ Diabetes is an excellent opportunity for manipulative behavior.
  ◇ Linear growth is, on average, only slightly reduced in diabetes, especially in very young children with poor control. Puberty may also be delayed by 2 years or arrested. Both should be monitored (Figure 5.5) and

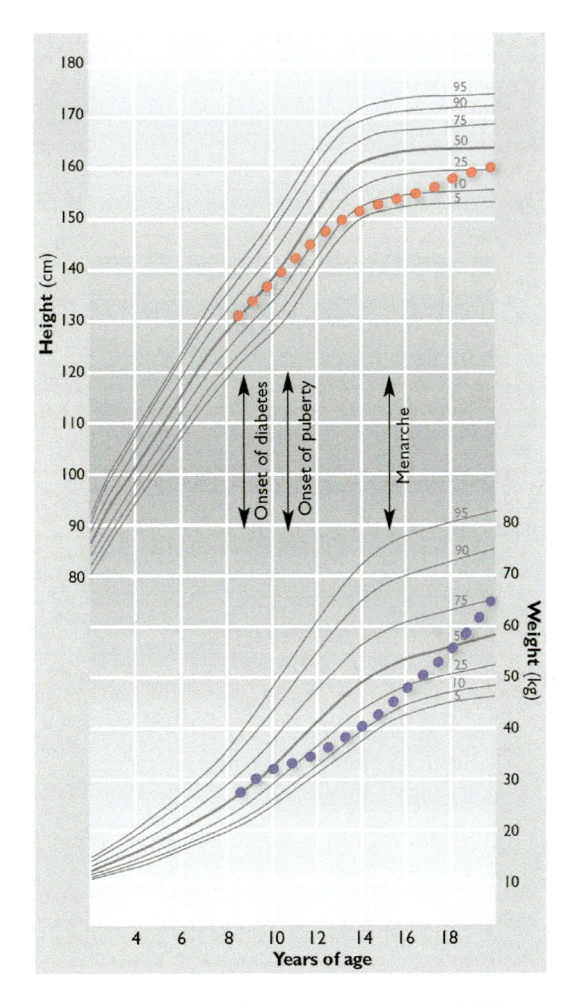

Figure 5.5 Growth and development. Height and weight increase with age in a child developing type 1 diabetes. This girl had poor glucose control postdiagnosis. Note the fall in both height and weight from the 60th centile to lower centiles after diagnosis, with a delay in both puberty and the onset of menarche. Note also the start of catch-up growth after menarche and the mismatch between weight and height associated with relative overweight thereafter.

if changes are noted then referral to a specialist may be required to exclude other causes (e.g. hypothyroidism, gluten enteropathy) and for therapy as required.

Developing independence is important to enable children to manage diabetes throughout their lifetime.

The elderly person with diabetes

- The number of elderly people with diabetes has been increasing steadily.
    - Approximately 10% of people over 65 years of age have diagnosed diabetes and another 10% have undiagnosed hyperglycemia. In the US, total prevalence of DM (i.e. diagnosed plus undiagnosed) is 20.9% in those above 60 years.
    - In the UK, half of all people with type 2 diabetes are over 65 years old.
- In part, the increase in diabetes prevalence is due to age-related changes in glucose metabolism, including decreased insulin secretion and decreased insulin sensitivity (Figure 5.6).
- Hyperglycemia in an elderly person is usually due to type 2 diabetes, but type 1 diabetes may also present late in life.
- Diabetes as a feature of underlying pancreatic cancer is more likely in the elderly, but accounts for only a small proportion of all cases of diabetes.
- Clinical presentation in older people may be 'atypical' and not as clear cut as in children or younger adults – for example, unexplained weight loss without other 'classic' symptoms of hyperglycemia.
- Hyperosmolar, hyperglycemic syndrome (HHS) with extreme hyperglycemia, but no antecedent history of thirst or polyuria, may be a presenting feature of diabetes in the elderly, particularly in patients treated with diuretic drugs or steroids.
- As with children and adolescents, attention must be paid to achieving a balance between social autonomy and dependence. In principle, the aims of treatment are no different than in younger patients – relief of symptoms and prevention of complications.
- Macrovascular disease, hypertension, renal impairment, and failing vision due to macular degeneration or cataracts are all increasingly prevalent with advancing age regardless of diabetes, so efforts to combat the additional risk that diabetes presents in respect of these disabilities should be just as strenuous in the elderly as in younger people.

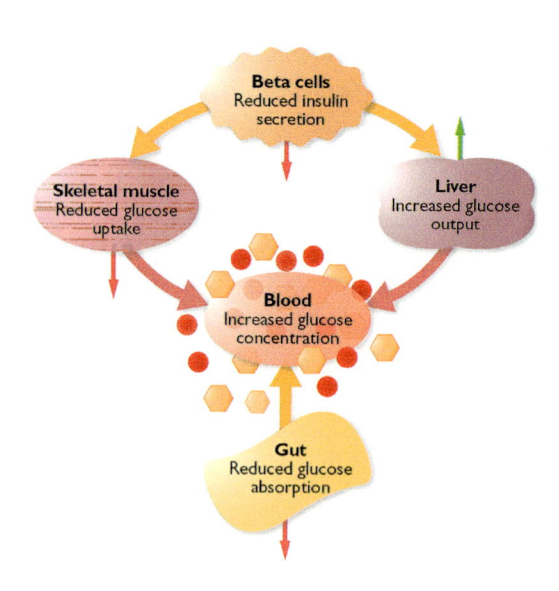

Figure 5.6 Glucose metabolism in the elderly. Decreased insulin secretion and sensitivity lead to raised glucose levels, despite reduced glucose absorption.

By 2025 about a third of diabetes patients will be 75 years or older.

Management of elderly patients
- A number of factors in the elderly may interfere with concordance and complicate the management of patients:

- ◇ Multiple pathologies and drug therapies can result in drug interactions and poor concordance. Concordance is related inversely to the number of drugs.
- ◇ Drugs in the elderly are not metabolized so efficiently as in the young, and dosages may need to be lower.
- ◆ It may be considered necessary or prudent to identify the most important areas for intervention rather than identify all therapies required. There may be circumstances where intensifying treatment would not be expected to have a significant impact – or, worse, may have an adverse one – on a patient's overall sense of well-being or eventual outcome.

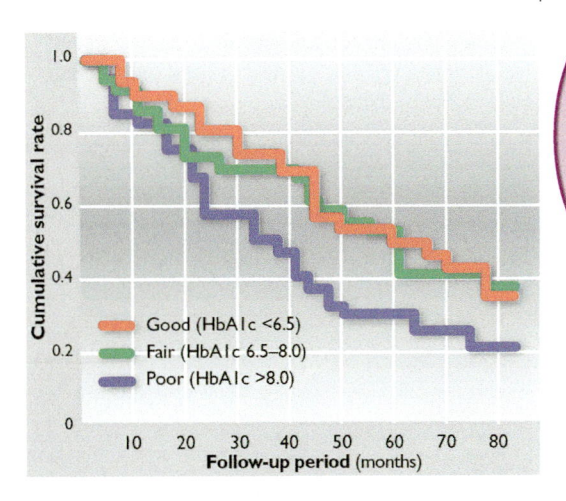

Figure 5.7 Glycemic control and survival rates. Survival rates in groups of diabetic patients on chronic hemodialysis over a 7-year period, indicating a better survival in patients with fair to good HbA1c levels. The average age of entry was over 60 years. From Oomichi T, et al, Diabetes Care, 2006.

Avoidance of hypoglycemia

- ◆ There is, however, the danger of acquiescing in the face of poor glycemic control or inadequate management of hypertension or hyperlipidemia in the mistaken belief that control of these risk factors for vascular disease is less worthwhile or effective in the elderly.
  - ◇ A recent study from the Veterans Administration in the US confirmed that older patients and those with comorbid illnesses were least likely to have their therapy stepped up at outpatient clinic visits when glycemic control was clearly inadequate.
  - ◇ It has been shown that poor glycemic control is an independent predictor of decreased survival in diabetic patients – many elderly – on hemodialysis (Figure 5.7), so it seems reasonable to assume a similar potential benefit in other situations of chronic ill health. (Tables 5.3, 5.4).
- ◆ Strenuous efforts should be made to avoid hypoglycemia.
  - ◇ Severe hypoglycemia is a hazard with sulfonylureas in the elderly, especially when there is impairment of renal function; short-acting insulin secretagogues such as glipizide, gliclazide, repaglinide, or nateglinide are preferable.
  - ◇ Non-insulinotropic agents, such as metformin, DPP-4 inhibitors, SGLT-2 inhibitors, or GLP-1 analogues, are unlikely to cause hypoglycemia.
  - ◇ Metformin should be used with caution in patients with impaired renal or cardiac function because of the rare occurrence of lactic acidosis. Serum

Table 5.3 Management problems. Social, economic, and other health problems may lead to poor compliance with diabetes management among the elderly.

Management problems in the elderly
Living alone, poverty, poor diet – poor compliance
Intellectual impairment, depression, and dementia – poor compliance
Poor vision and dexterity – difficulty with blood test and injections
Coexisting diseases and drugs – potential for confusion and drug interaction
Multiple drug therapy – poor compliance
Decreased mobility and exercise – poor lifestyle

Table 5.4 Therapy key points. Therapy should be chosen based on the individual needs, wishes, and abilities of each patient.

Therapy for diabetes in the elderly
Determine current quality of life and prognosis
Assess priorities in treating diabetes and other diseases
Avoid hypoglycemia
Treat diabetes according to individual targets
Screen for complications and treat to maintain quality of life
Be cautious with drug dosages and insulin use

creatinine will often underestimate the degree of renal impairment in older, frail patients.
- ◇ The glucose-dependent action of GLP-1 means that DPP-4 (dipeptidyl peptidase-4) inhibitors have little inherent hypoglycemic risk; this makes these oral agents an attractive option in the elderly, although they do not provide cardiovascular protection. Dose adjustment may be required with impaired renal function.
♦ Similar care to avoid hypoglycemia is required with insulin treatment in the elderly, but fear of hypoglycemia should not lead to avoidance of insulin treatment when it is clearly the most appropriate option.
  - ◇ Failing eyesight, decreased manual dexterity, and problems with memory may all be cited as barriers to insulin treatment; however, ways should be found to overcome such barriers when insulin treatment is essential or clearly better than other options.
  - ◇ Use of long-acting insulin analogues once a day may be sufficient to protect against hyperglycemic emergencies, if additional mealtime insulin is just not practical due to social circumstances.
  - ◇ When mealtime insulin is used, rapid-acting insulin analogs are preferred; timing of the injection is vitally important, either immediately before or after the meal, with dosage adjustment if there is concern about ability to complete the meal, in order to avoid hypoglycemia.
  - ◇ Biphasic insulins are an option, but mealtime regularity is required with these insulins.
♦ It is worth considering that, for the person with limited social independence who nevertheless lives alone, the employment of a carer to give insulin will help prevent social isolation.

Ethnic minorities

♦ Patients with diabetes should be treated in the same manner, irrespective of their race, and according to the type of diabetes and risk factors.
♦ The following points are of particular note:
  - ◇ There is wide variation in diabetes incidence according to race, both for type 1 and type 2.
  - ◇ Macrovascular disease is particularly prevalent in some ethnic groups such as Asian Indians.
  - ◇ HHS is more common in African Americans than in people of European origin.
  - ◇ Hypertension in patients of African origin is often low-renin, which may explain why response to angiotensin-converting enzyme inhibitors is poor. Nevertheless, these agents, and calcium channel blockers are the first choice (though evidence for the success of this strategy is lacking).

Ramadan and dietary preferences
♦ Fasting during the month of Ramadan can prove challenging for Muslim patients with diabetes. Fasting involves complete abstinence from food and water from dawn to dusk. As a result, hypoglycemia

can be a risk, although hyperglycemia due to feasting at the break of fast can also be problematic. The person with diabetes should be carefully assessed for their risk of fasting and advised whether it is safe for them to do so. If deemed safe, the person should have adjustments to therapy undertaken to reduce risk of hypo- or hyperglycemia. There is good evidence that Ramadan-focused education can improve the safety of Ramadan fasting in people with diabetes, and ideally such a service should be offered for this group of patients.

◆ Patients of differing ethnicities have diverse dietary preferences, and one of the features of the ethnic heterogeneity of modern western society is the much greater variety of cuisine available to, and enjoyed by, all. It is important, therefore, that the nutritional advice offered takes into account the fact that many patients will not be following a traditional western-type diet.

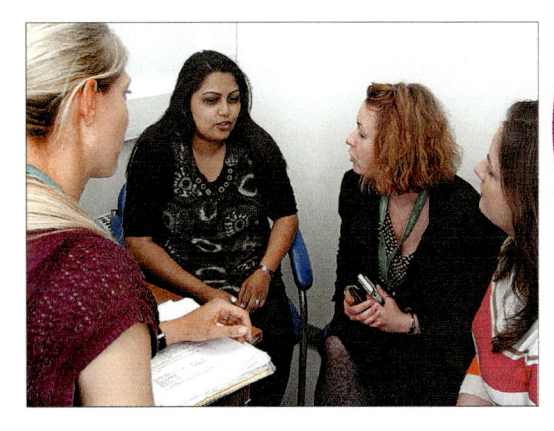

Figure 5.8 Patient care. Management involves a team: a physician, dietitian, nurse specialist, and patient discuss a problem.

The amount of time spent with an educator correlates with outcomes.

Patient education and community care

◆ The care of diabetes is based on self-management by the patient, who is advised by those with specialized knowledge.
◆ Education should begin when the patient is diagnosed.
◆ The diabetes team members include the patient, doctors, nurses, diabetes educators, dietitians, and chiropodists (Figure 5.8). Lack of motivation, expertise, or education of any one of these individuals can disrupt the quality of care.
◆ A particular challenge is the diverse socioeconomic and ethnic background of diabetic patients presenting to the educators. Culturally appropriate educational materials and illustrations, such as examples of carbohydrate servings and food groups, can be made more understandable and effective when adapted to the patient's local setting.
◆ Diabetes self-management education (DSME) is helpful, at least in the short term, in improving glycemic control and psychosocial outcomes in diabetic patients. The amount of time spent with the educator correlates with outcome.
◆ In the US, it is recommended that DSME programs fulfil the following:
  ◇ Describe the diabetes disease process and treatment options.
  ◇ Incorporate appropriate nutritional management into lifestyle.
  ◇ Incorporate physical activity into lifestyle.
  ◇ Use medications safely for maximum therapeutic effectiveness.
  ◇ Monitor blood glucose and other parameters and use the results for self-management decision making.
  ◇ Prevent, detect, and treat acute complications.
  ◇ Prevent, detect, and treat chronic complications.
  ◇ Develop personal strategies to address psychosocial issues and concerns.

- ◇ Develop personal strategies to promote health and behavior change.
- ◆ In patients with type 1 diabetes, specific education to manage carbohydrate counting (such as Dose Adjustment for Normal Eating [DAFNE]) has been shown to improve glycemic control and quality of life.

Living with diabetes

- ◆ There may be aspects of the lives of diabetes patients that have an influence on the choice of treatment (Table 5.5).

Employment

- ◆ All jobs are open to people with diabetes except a few in which the risk of hypoglycemia, due to insulin therapy, might put others at risk (Table 5.6).

Finance

- ◆ It is important that life and car insurance companies are informed of the diagnosis of diabetes or the start of insulin therapy.
  - ◇ Some brokers and companies are more accommodating than others toward insuring patients with diabetes and will offer better deals, though the premium will be dependent on the type of insurance, the nature of the therapy, the risk of hypoglycemia, and the presence of complications. Visual acuity and fields must be assessed to determine suitability for driving.
- ◆ In the UK, patients with diabetes are exempt from prescription charges.

Table 5.5 Living with diabetes. The choice of treatment may need to take into account a patient's lifestyle.

Lifestyle problems	
AREA	EXAMPLES
Employment	Shift workers
	Long working day (resulting in early breakfast, late evening meal, or erratic mealtimes)
	Skipping midday meal or having frequent business lunches
	International travel
Eating	National and cultural variations (e.g. time of main meal, varying dietary compositions)
	Individual variations (e.g. availability, preferences, affordability, dining out)
Exercise	Sportsmen and women
	Sedentary office workers
	Manual laborers
Travel	Long-haul air travel
	Means of traveling to work (e.g. cycling, long walks)
Leisure	Strenuous hobbies (e.g. sports, gardening)

Table 5.6 Employment restrictions. Some occupations are exempt from disability discrimination legislation, usually where the risk of hypoglycemia would be dangerous.

Employment exclusions, UK and USA	
EMPLOYMENT	EXAMPLES
Vocational driving	Large goods vehicle (LGV), passenger-carrying vehicles (PCV), locomotives or underground trains, professional drivers (chauffeurs), taxi drivers (variable, depending on local authority)
Civil aviation	Commercial pilots, flight engineers, aircrew, air-traffic controllers
National and emergency services	Armed forces (army, navy, air force), police force, fire brigade or rescue services, merchant navy, prison and security services
Dangerous work areas	Offshore oil-rig work, moving machinery, incinerator loading, hot-metal areas, railway tracks
Work at heights	Overhead linesmen, crane driving, scaffolding/high ladders or platforms

Sport
- Having diabetes should rarely be a bar to participation in sport. People with diabetes can play, and many excel at, most sports. CSII therapy can enable people with type 1 diabetes to perform at elite level in many sports.
- Some sports are wary of allowing patients on insulin to participate in competition such as scuba diving, motor rally driving, and boxing.
- Patients exercising intensively are at risk of hypoglycemia and should:
  - Measure blood glucose before exercise (perhaps with a general rule of not starting exercise if blood glucose is less than 5.6 mmol/L [100 mg/dL] or greater than 14 mmol/L [250 mg/dL]).
  - Take 20 g carbohydrate every 45 minutes during exercise.
  - Keep fast-acting glucose preparations in their pocket in case they feel hypoglycemic.
  - Avoid dangerous situations, such as swimming alone.

Holidays and travel
- Patients with insulin-treated diabetes who are traveling will need:
  - Insulin and insulin syringes, or pen devices or insulin pump supplies, and glucose-monitoring equipment. Bring spare insulin and syringes when possible in case one is mislaid. Insulin in various forms is widely available in most international destinations nowadays. Nevertheless it still makes sense to bring extra supplies for emergency, and people using pumps and pens should consider bringing spare 'traditional' vials of rapid-acting and basal insulin, and syringes.
  - Identification to confirm that they have diabetes (e.g. Medic Alert bracelet) and letter to confirm they need to carry syringes/devices in airplanes. The US Transportation Security Administration allows the following through the checkpoint after screening: insulin if clearly identified, syringes when accompanied by insulin or other injectables, insulin pumps, and other supplies (Figure 5.9).
  - Glucose tablets to manage or avoid hypoglycemia.
  - Medical insurance.
- Vaccinations should be done as required; there are no special needs when someone has diabetes.
- On the day of travel aim particularly to avoid hypoglycemia, as this can be very disruptive to travel arrangements, so plan to check glucose levels frequently:
  - When traveling eastwards, the day is shorter, so the insulin dose may need to be reduced, and extra snacks may be required. Plan to resume the usual insulin schedule, fitting in with the times in the particular time zone, once at the destination.
  - When traveling westwards, the day is longer and an additional insulin injection may be required; use soluble (regular insulin in the US) or rapid-acting insulin for the extra injection, take an additional meal, and monitor blood glucose carefully. Again, resume the usual schedule in the new time zone.
  - If the trip is very long, perhaps with stopovers, a change in regime may be necessary so that it is possible to use soluble (regular) or rapid-acting insulin before each meal.

Driving
- Patients with diabetes who drive a car or want to drive a car must:
  - Inform their car insurers as soon as they have been diagnosed; not to do so could invalidate any insurance. Check with other insurance brokers if the insurance premiums are increased following the diagnosis of diabetes; be prepared to 'shop around'.

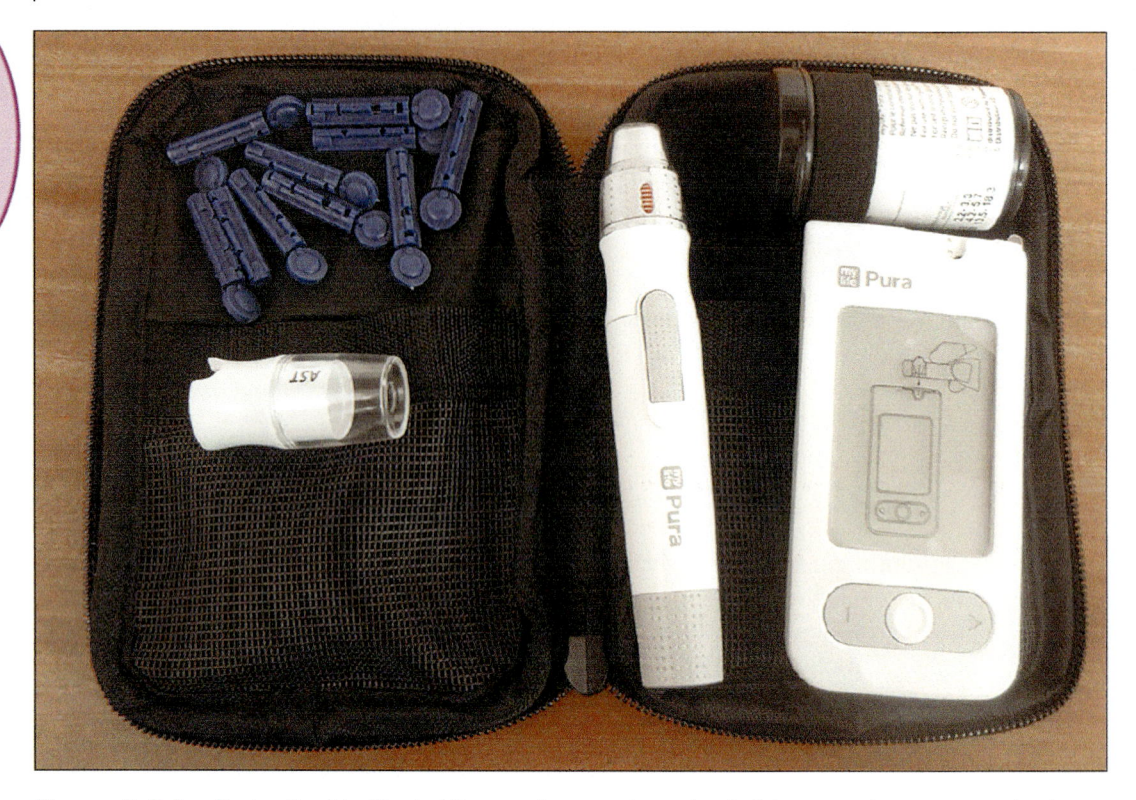

Figure 5.9 Insulin testing kit. Check airline security procedures ahead of time: some items may need to be labeled.

- ◇ Inform the licensing authority (in the UK, the DVLA; in the US, relevant state agency) if you are treated with tablets or insulin.
- ◇ The DVLA will ask the patient to sign a declaration allowing their doctor to disclose medical information about them if they are treated with insulin. In particular they will want information about hypoglycemia awareness. This point applies to motorcyclists and car drivers. Licenses restricted to 1, 2, or 3 years only are provided if diabetes is treated with insulin.
- ◆ Most people with diabetes obtain a license. Erratic control, hypoglycemia, and poor eyesight are the usual reasons for being refused a license.
- ◆ To avoid hypoglycemia patients should be educated as to the nature and treatment of hypoglycemia. They should:
  - ◇ Check their blood glucose before driving.
  - ◇ Not drive for more than 2 hours.
  - ◇ Have glucose available in the car if needed.
  - ◇ Not delay a meal or snack.
  - ◇ Stop driving if there are any suggestions that they are developing hypoglycemic symptoms.
- ◆ Patients with diabetes should not drive if they have just started insulin, have erratic control, have difficulty with hypoglycemia, or have impaired vision not corrected with glasses.
  - ◇ The American Diabetes Association has a useful set of tips aimed mainly at younger and recently qualified drivers, accessible at https://www.diabetes.org/tools-support/know-your-rights/drivers-license-information Pass the test. Check your blood glucose before getting into the car. Every time. No exceptions.
  - ◇ Stop for a diabetes red light. Treat low blood glucose and then recheck

- in 15 minutes. Do not get behind the wheel until blood glucose is in the target range.
- Slow down. Treat blood glucose even if it means being late. It's never okay to drive with a low blood glucose. Call whoever is waiting for you and explain why you'll be a little late. They'll understand.
- Always have enough fuel. Stock the car with healthy, nonperishable snacks and fast-acting sugars. And keep your diabetic supplies within easy reach.
- Pull over. Pull over immediately if you are feeling sick or low while driving. Check your blood glucose, treat yourself, wait 15 minutes, and then recheck.
- ID, please. Don't leave home without a driver's license and medical ID bracelet or necklace. Always wear medical ID.

Patients who have just started insulin, have erratic control, have difficulty with hypoglycemia, or have impaired vision not corrected with glasses should not drive.

CHAPTER 6

Diabetes and vascular disease

Macrovascular disease

- In high-income countries, macrovascular disease is a leading cause of mortality.
- The mortality rates for patients with type 2 diabetes, which varies between populations, are up to four times those of the nondiabetic population, and this excess mortality has been attributed mainly to accelerated macrovascular disease, in particular cardiovascular disease (Figure 6.1).
- Diabetes remains the commonest single cause of limb amputations, as well as the commonest cause of blindness and renal failure in middle-aged adults in high-income countries.
- Risk factors associated with a predisposition to macrovascular disease include diabetes and impaired glucose tolerance, hypertension, obesity, and dyslipidemia.
  ◇ These risk factors typically cluster in any one person, i.e. the prevalence of each factor is increased in those individuals with the other factors, leading to a self-perpetuating vicious cycle, which is further exaggerated in type 2 diabetes patients.
  ◇ These metabolic, hemodynamic, and constitutional changes are considered to be a syndrome associated with hyperinsulinemia – metabolic or insulin-resistance syndrome (see p. 43).
  ◇ Such an insulin-resistant state may be present in 25% of the nondiabetic population, and about 2–12% per year of these individuals in adult life progress to diabetes.
- Since the metabolic or insulin-resistance syndrome represents a continuum into a state associated with major clinical consequences, there are three implications for the practicing physician in identifying this syndrome in any single patient:
  ◇ Identification of any one of the changes associated with the syndrome should lead to a search for other features of the syndrome.
  ◇ The approach to the management of a person with diabetes should not be viewed simply as the management of blood glucose.
  ◇ The management of each patient with type 2 diabetes must be tailored to the particular risk factor profile identified in that individual.

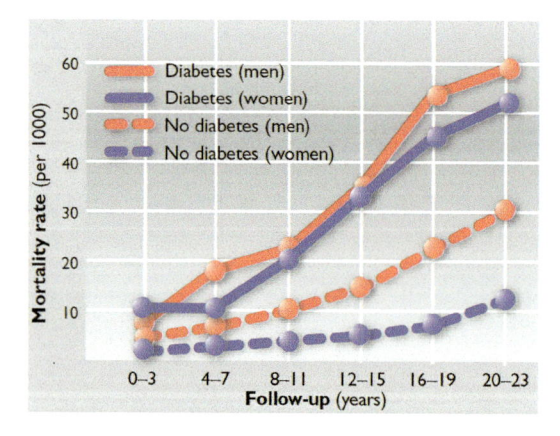

Figure 6.1 Cardiovascular risk. There is increasing risk with disease duration. Note also the relatively high risk in diabetic women, compared with nondiabetic women.

Mortality in adults with type 2 diabetes is far higher than in the nondiabetic population, largely because of cardiovascular disease.

Pathogenesis of macrovascular complications

- Normal vascular homeostasis is regulated by an intricately interrelated network of endothelial and smooth muscle cells.
  - Endothelial cells act as a semipermeable gateway; they maintain the blood in a liquid state and produce mediators that promote vascular homeostasis (notably nitric oxide and lipid factors, such as prostacyclin).
  - Contraction of smooth muscle cells regulates the vascular tone of arteriolar walls, thereby determining both systolic blood pressure and peripheral blood flow.
- In diabetes, this intricate network is disturbed, resulting in atherogenesis. Endothelial cell dysfunction occurs early in the pathology of atherosclerosis and is common in patients with traditional risk factors – even in the absence of manifest atherosclerotic lesions. Such endothelial dysfunction predicts both progression to atherosclerosis and major cardiovascular events, such as myocardial infarction.
- The pathogenesis of atherosclerosis, from the initial phase of leukocyte recruitment to late events such as rupture of vulnerable plaques, predominantly involves inflammatory processes, including the release of inflammatory mediators (Figure 6.2). This leads to an elevation of several inflammatory markers in the peripheral blood of patients with atherosclerosis, as well as patients with type 2 diabetes.
  - An example is C-reactive protein (CRP), which is an acute-phase reactant thought to be a marker

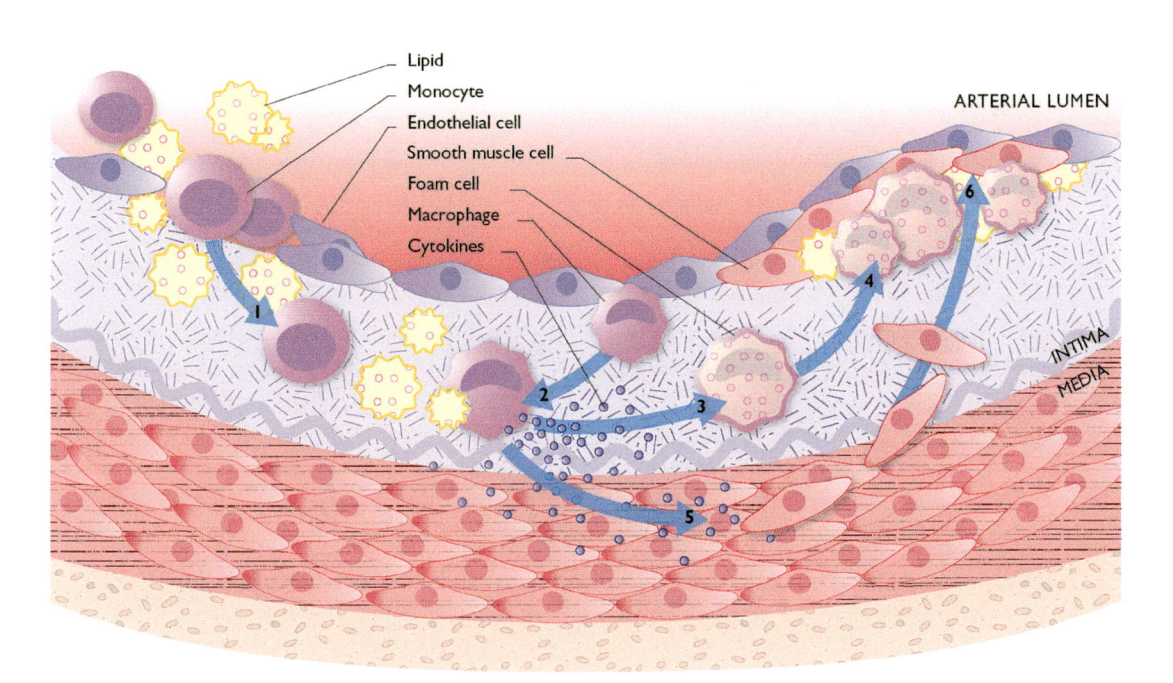

Figure 6.2 Atherosclerosis. Damage to arterial endothelium allows entry of monocytes and lipids (1) and activation of macrophages (2). The macrophages engulf the lipids, subsequently breaking down into foam cells and causing lipid accumulation on the vessel wall (3, 4). The release of cytokines stimulates migration of smooth muscle cells to form a fibrous cap (5, 6).

of vascular inflammation. CRP is localized within the atheromatous plaque and its expression precedes the recruitment of leukocytes at the surface of the vessel wall. Since levels of CRP and other pro-inflammatory mediators, such as fibrinogen, are increased in the plasma of patients with diabetes they may serve as clinical biomarkers of vascular risk.
- The pathogenesis of atherosclerosis in diabetes is as in nondiabetic subjects, but with the added burden of hyperglycemia and its impact on cell function, allied to the clustering of other risk factors found in metabolic syndrome.

Treatment and management principles for macrovascular disease

General principles
- In the diabetic patient with macrovascular disease, management is directed at alleviating symptoms, reducing mortality risk, and treating the anatomical lesion.
- To correct symptoms, consider drugs to reduce angina, including nitrates, beta-adrenoreceptor blockers, long-acting calcium channel blockers, potassium channel openers, and ranolazine.
- To reduce mortality risk, consider drugs to limit cardiovascular disease progression, including aspirin, statins, and angiotensin-converting enzyme inhibitors (ACEIs).
  - Use statins and aspirin in all diabetic patients with macrovascular disease, and consider fibrates to correct hypertriglyceridemia and increase HDL as necessary.
  - Fibrates must be used cautiously in patients taking statins because of the risk of rhabdomyolysis.
  - If statins and fibrates have to be used concurrently, fenofibrate is recommended over gemfibrozil, as gemfibrozil interferes with statin glucuronidation, thereby conferring a higher risk of myopathy and rhabdomyolysis than does fenofibrate.
- Improved glycemic control may reduce mortality risk, but care must be taken to avoid hypoglycemia.
- To correct the anatomical lesions, consider surgical intervention to improve revascularization, in order to control symptoms and improve prognosis. There are two techniques for successful cardiac revascularization:
  - Percutaneous intervention.
  - Coronary bypass surgery.
- The role of cerebrovascular revascularization should be considered in acute stroke, as for nondiabetic patients.

Glycemic targets should be individualized in people with diabetes and myocardial infarction, with particular care to avoid hypoglycemia.

Glucose control
- Patients with hyperglycemia on admission for a myocardial infarction have a poorer prognosis than patients with normoglycemia.
- In patients presenting with an acute myocardial infarction, the Diabetes Mellitus Insulin Glucose Infusion in Acute Myocardial Infarction (DIGAMI) study showed that strict glycemic control in people with diabetes improved cardiovascular outcomes (Figure 6.3).
  - Subsequent studies, however, suggested that tight glycemic control in the context of acute coronary syndromes or intensive care do not offer a survival benefit, and indeed may be deleterious, particularly if they induce hypoglycemia. Therefore many protocols now suggest intervention with insulin to lower glucose below 200

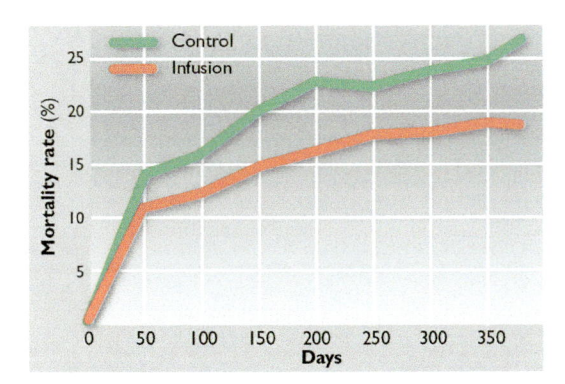

Figure 6.3 Glycemic control and cardiovascular outcomes. The DIGAMI study demonstrated decreased mortality in patients receiving insulin–glucose infusion against control patients over the course of one year.

mg/dL (11.0 mmol/L) in the UK, or 180 mg/dL (10.0 mmol/L) in the US. A glucose target of 140–180 mg/dL (7.8–10.0 mmol/L) is recommended for the majority of patients.

Glucose-lowering drugs and cardiovascular disease

- The UKPDS study suggests that in obese patients with type 2 diabetes, metformin reduces all-cause mortality and hospitalization for heart failure (hHF).
- Previous studies suggested that sulfonylureas may increase cardiovascular risk in people with diabetes, but subsequent data suggests they are cardiovascularly neutral. They can induce hypoglycemia, which can be severe in certain groups such as the elderly or renally impaired, and should be used with caution in people with known cardiovascular disease.
- Thiazolidinediones (glitazones) act via perioxisome proliferator activated receptorΓ (PPAR gamma receptors in muscle, adipose tissue, and liver to increase insulin sensitivity. They have similar glycemic effectiveness to metformin, but their use is limited due to adverse effects, including weight gain and fluid retention, which can exacerbate heart failure (and hence are contraindicated), and increased postmenopausal fractures in women. Rosiglitazone was associated with a 43% increase in MI in a meta-analysis. Pioglitazone, however, has been shown to offer modest cardiovascular protection in one RCT.
- The advent of cardiovascular outcomes trials (CVOTs) in people with diabetes treated with newer agents has highlighted the benefit of newer agents in reducing cardiovascular and renal outcomes in high-risk patients with type 2 diabetes (Table 6.1).
  - ◇ Dipeptidylpeptidase-4 inhibitors (DPP-4s, or gliptins) have shown cardiovascular safety, but no cardiovascular benefit in all CVOTs. Saxagliptin and alogliptin may exacerbate heart failure.
  - ◇ Glucagon-like peptide-1 receptor analogues (GLP-1 RA) stimulate glucose-dependent insulin secretion. They are resistant to DPP-4 degradation and are administered subcutaneously. They achieve significant reductions in HbA1c without the risk of hypoglycemia. GLP1-RAs favor weight loss and improvements in lipids and blood pressure. They can be initiated in patients with eGFR as low as 15 mL/min/1.73 m^2.
  - ◇ A meta-analysis of the seven largest trials studying 56,004 patients showed a 12% reduction in the three-point major adverse cardiovascular outcomes (3p-MACE) associated with GLP1-RAs. This observation was due to reduced rates of cardiovascular death (12%), fatal or nonfatal stroke (16%), and fatal or nonfatal MI (9%). There was also a reduction in all-cause mortality (12%) and hHF (9%).
  - ◇ Sodium glucose transporter-2 inhibitors (SGLT-2i) appear to enhance natriuresis and glycosuria-driven osmotic diuresis, with subsequent inhibition of the renin-angiotensin system contributing to blood pressure reduction. Other improvements also

Table 6.1 A summary of cardiovascular outcomes trials with antidiabetes medications in Type 2 diabetes.

Class	Drug	CVOT & total patients (n)	Median follow up (years)	Patient characteristics (all T2DM)	Outcomes
SGLT-2i	Empagliflozin	EMPA-REG Outcome (2015) n = 7020	3.1	Established CVD (99%) eGFR >30 History of: MI >50% Multivessel CVD 5% HF 10%	Lower 3p-MACE HR 0.86 (0.79–0.9) Lower CV related deaths HR 0.62 (0.49–0.77) Lower death from any cause HR 0.68 (0.57–0.82) Lower hHF HR 0.65 (0.50–0.85) No significant difference in: MI, stroke
	Canagliflozin	CANVAS Program (2017) n = 10,142	2.4	Either: 1) >30 years old + established CVD (65.6%) 2) >50 years + 2 or more CV risk factors eGFR >30	Lower 3p-MACE HR 0.86 (0.75–0.97) Lower albuminuria progression HR 0.73 (0.67–0.79) Lower composite outcome of 40% eGFR reduction, RR need, death from renal causes HR 0.60 (0.47–0.77) No significant difference in CV death, death from any cause
		CREDENCE (2019) n = 4401	2.62	Albuminuric CKD	Lower renal-specific composite of ESRD, doubling of creatinine, death from renal causes HR 0.66 (0.53–0.81) Lower ESRD HR 0.68 (0.54–0.86) Lower CV death, MI, stroke HR 0.80 (0.67–0.95) Lower hHF HR 0.61 (0.47–0.80)
	Dapagliflozin	DECLARE-TIMI 58 (2019) n = 17,160	4.2	Either: 1) Established CVD (40.6%) 2) Multiple CV risk factors (59.4%)	No significant difference in 3p-MACE HR 0.93 (0.84–1.03) Lower hHF HR 0.83 0.73 (0.61–0.88) Reduced renal events HR 0.76 (0.67–0.87) No significant difference in CV death, death from any cause

(Continued)

Table 6.1 (Continued)

Class	Drug	CVOT & total patients (n)	Median follow up (years)	Patient characteristics (all T2DM)	Outcomes
DPP-4i	Saxagliptin	SAVOR-TIMI 53 (2013) n = 16,492	2.1	History or multiple risk factors for CVD	No significant difference in 3p-MACE HR 1.0 (0.89–1.12) No significant difference in all-cause mortality, CV death, MI, stroke, hospitalisation for angina Significant increase in hHF HR 1.27 (1.07–1.51)
	Alogliptin	EXAMINE (2013) n = 5380	1.5	ACS (AMI or UA requiring hospitalization) within 15–90 days before randomization	No significant difference in 3p-MACE HR 0.96 (≤1.16) No significant difference in all-cause mortality, CV death Contributed to a nonsignificant 19% increase in hHF
	Sitagliptin	TECOS (2015) n = 14,671	3.0	Established CVD	No significant difference in 3p-MACE 4p-MACE HR 0.98 (0.88–1.09) No significant difference in hHF HR 1.0 (0.83–1.20)
	Linagliptin	CARMELINA (2018) n = 6979	2.2	High CV risk (history of vascular disease and UACR >200mg/g), and High renal risk (reduced eGFR and micro- or macroalbuminuria). ESRD patients excluded	No significant difference in 3p-MACE HR 1.04 (0.89–1.22) HR 1.02 (0.89–1.17) No significant difference for hHF HR 0.90 (0.74–1.08)
		CAROLINA (2019) n = 6042	6.3	High CV risk	Non inferior to Glimepiride in 3p-MACE HR 0.98 [0.84–1.14]; $P < .001$ for noninferiority

GLP-1 RA				
Exenatide	EXSCEL (2017) n = 14752	3.2	73.1% with established CVD	No significant difference in 3p-MACE HR 0.91 (0.83–1.00) No significant difference in CV death, fatal or nonfatal MI, fatal or nonfatal stroke, hHF, ACS hospitalization
Lixisenatide	ELIXA (2015) n = 6068	2.1	History of ACS	No significant difference in 4P-MACE HR 1.02 (95% CI 0.89–1.17) No significant difference in CV death, hHF
Liraglutide	LEADER (2016) n = 9340	3.8	Either: 1) ≥ 50 years with established CVD 2) ≥ 60 years with at least one CV risk factor	Lower 3p-MACE HR 0.87 (0.78–0.97) Lower CV related deaths HR 0.78 (0.66–0.93) Lower all-cause mortality HR 0.85 (0.74–0.97) No significant difference in hHF, nonfatal MI, nonfatal stroke
Semaglutide	SUSTAIN-6 (2016) n = 3297	2.1	83% with established CVD, CKD, or both 17% with CV risk factors	Lower 3p-MACE HR 0.74 (0.58–0.95) Lower rate of nonfatal MI HR 0.74 (0.51–1.08) Lower rate of nonfatal stroke HR 0.61 (0.38–0.99) No significant difference in CV deaths, hHF
Dulaglutide	REWIND (2019) n = 9622	5.4	≥ 50 years old 31% with established CVD 69% with CV risk factors	Lower 3p-MACE HR 0.88 (0.79–0.99) Lower rate of nonfatal stroke HR 0.76 (0.6–0.95) No significant difference in nonfatal MI, all-cause mortality
Albiglutide	HARMONY (2018) n = 9400	1.6	≥ 40 years old Established CVD	Lower 3p-MACE HR 0.78 (0.65–0.90) Lower rate of fatal or nonfatal MI HR 0.75 (0.61–0.90)

noted are reduced arterial stiffness, intravascular volume contraction, and intrarenal hemodynamic alterations. CVOT studies of empagliflozin, canagliflozin, and dapagliflozin show significant reductions in cardiovascular outcomes – meta-analysis has shown a 11% reduction in the 3p-MACE, 15% reduction in MI, 20% reduction in cardiovascular death and 23% reduction in the risk of CV death and hHf.

◆ Most recent guidance from the ADA and EASD suggest that SGLT-2i and GLP-1RAs should be used second line to metformin in people with known cardiovascular disease (Figure 6.4 and Table 6.1; see also Chapter 14).

Lipid-lowering drugs

◆ The Long-Term Intervention with Pravastatin in Ischemic Disease (LIPID) trial showed that in patients with diabetes or impaired fasting glucose, with a previous myocardial infarction or unstable angina and total plasma cholesterol level of 4.0–7.0 mmol/L (154–270 mg/dL), pravastatin reduced the incidence of cardiovascular events, including stroke.

◆ In the Cholesterol and Recurrent Events (CARE) trial, pravastatin was given to adults with myocardial infarction, total cholesterol levels less than 6.2 mmol/L (240 mg/dL) and LDL-cholesterol levels of 3.0–4.5 mmol/L (115–174 mg/dL). The primary endpoint – a fatal coronary event

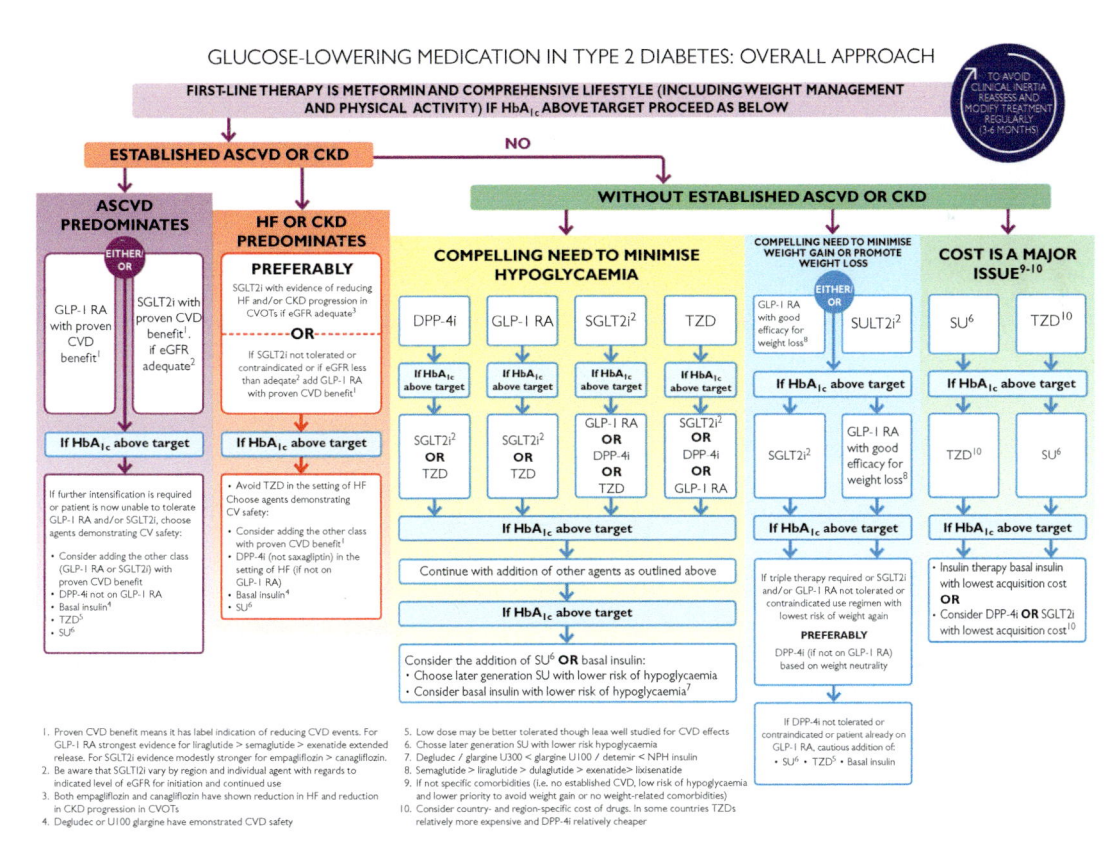

Figure 6.4 The ADA/EASD guidelines for management of Type 2 diabetes. *From Buse, JB, Wexler, DJ, Tsapas, A, et al. 2019 update to: Management of hyperglycaemia in type 2 diabetes, 2018. A consensus report by the American Diabetes Association (ADA) and the European Association for the Study of Diabetes (EASD). Diabetologia 63, 221–228 (2020). https://doi.org/10.1007/s00125-019-05039-w.*

or a nonfatal myocardial infarction – was significantly reduced with pravastatin compared to placebo. This reduction was seen in both diabetic and nondiabetic patients.
- A number of primary prevention studies of statins in people with diabetes, including the Collaborative Atorvastatin Diabetes Study (CARDS), showed that statins offered a 25–36% risk reduction in the risk of cardiovascular disease.
- With regard to fibrates, the Veterans Affairs HDL Intervention Trial (VA-HIT) showed that gemfibrozil reduced the incidence of myocardial infarction and stroke in patients, including diabetes patients, with coronary artery disease plus low HDL- and high LDL-cholesterol levels.

Revascularization procedures
- Coronary revascularization relieves symptoms and, in certain subgroups – particularly patients with advanced three-vessel or left main stem disease – improves prognosis.
- Thresholds for CT angiography or formal coronary angiography should be low in diabetes.
  ◇ This is not only because of diabetes patients' heightened risk and poorer outlook, but also because symptoms are often atypical, perhaps because of abnormalities in the perception of angina caused by autonomic neuropathy (Figure 6.5).
- Revascularization procedures in diabetes may be technically demanding and potentially hazardous because the diffuse and severe arterial disease makes clear targets for stenting or graft insertion hard to identify.
- The Bypass Angioplasty Revascularization Investigation (BARI) trial showed that coronary artery bypass grafting (CABG) resulted in a lower cardiac mortality than percutaneous transluminal coronary angioplasty (PTCA) in diabetic patients.
- However, the introduction of stenting, plus the more potent antithrombotic agents, particularly glycoprotein IIb/IIIa receptor blockers, have improved prognosis.
  ◇ In the Evaluation of PTCA to Improve Longterm Outcome by c7E3 GP IIb/IIIa Receptor Blockade (EPILOG) trial, abciximab (a platelet aggregation

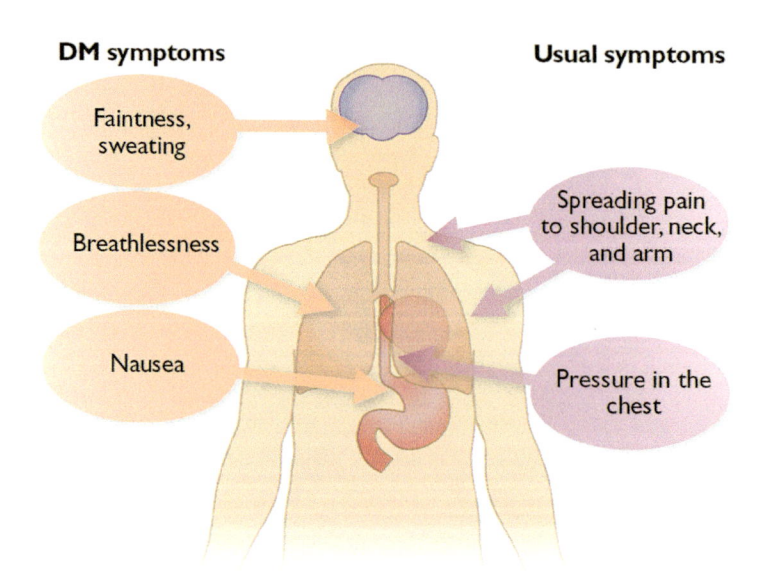

Figure 6.5 Symptoms of angina. Diabetic patients may exhibit atypical symptoms, such as weakness, faintness, sweating, nausea, and breathing difficulty, as well as reduced pain sensitivity.

inhibitor) given during PTCA was associated with a significant reduction in death or myocardial infarction in both diabetic and nondiabetic patients.
- ◇ A predefined subgroup analysis from the Evaluation of Platelet IIb/IIIa Inhibitor for Stenting (EPISTENT) trial showed that stenting combined with infusion of abciximab improved the long-term outcome in diabetic patients substantially. In a combined analysis the 1-year incidence of ischemic endpoints was comparable to that achieved in nondiabetic patients.
- ◇ The results of the EPILOG, EPISTENT, and one other study on abciximab, the Evaluation of Platelet IIb/IIIa Inhibition for Prevention of Ischemic Complications (EPIC) trial, were pooled. The combined analysis showed that abciximab reduced the mortality of diabetic patients to the level of nondiabetic patients receiving placebo (Figure 6.6).

Microvascular disease

- ◆ Whereas macrovascular disease affects both diabetic and nondiabetic people, microvascular disease is only seen in people with diabetes and a few other conditions, such as hypertension.
- ◆ Small blood vessels throughout the body are affected but the disease process has a particular clinical impact at three sites:
  - ◇ Retina (retinopathy).
  - ◇ Renal glomerulus (nephropathy).
  - ◇ Nerve sheaths (neuropathy).

Pathogenesis of microvascular complications

- ◆ The cause of diabetic microvascular disease is not known, but several factors are understood to play a role (Table 6.2).
- ◆ In some ways the factors causing this form of vascular disease are similar to those involved in macrovascular disease, for example:
  - ◇ Hypertension is a risk factor in renal and eye disease.
  - ◇ Smoking is a risk factor in renal disease.

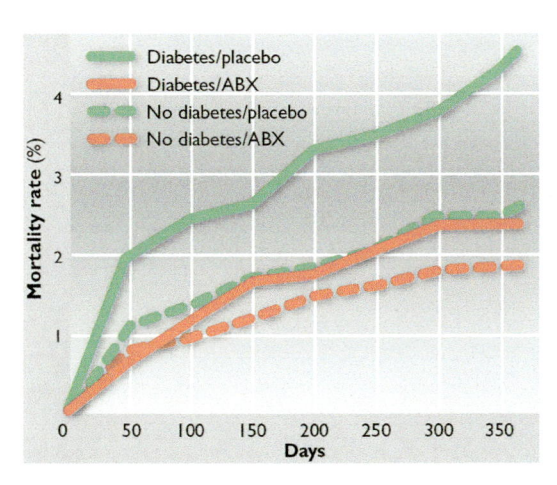

Figure 6.6 Abciximab therapy and PTCA. Combined data from the three placebo-controlled trials, EPISTENT, EPILOG, and EPIC, showed that abciximab (ABX) substantially decreased the mortality of diabetic patients. *From Bhatt DL, et al. 2000.*

Table 6.2 Causes of microvascular disease. There is a direct causal link between hyperglycemia and microangiopathy, although there are several other contributing factors.

Factors associated with the pathogenesis of microvascular complications
Hyperglycemia
Protein glycation
Advanced glycation end products (AGE)
Reactive oxygen species (ROS)
Activation of cell NFκB
Sorbitol accumulation in cells
Activation of cell protein kinase C
Hemodynamic changes

Hyperglycemia appears not to be a major factor in macrovascular disease, but is critical in the development of microvascular disease. Hypertension is just as important in predisposing to microvascular disease as hyperglycemia, and all the five modifiable factors targeted by therapy are relevant:
- ◇ Hyperglycemia.
- ◇ Hypertension.
- ◇ Hyperlipidemia.
- ◇ Lack of exercise.
- ◇ Smoking.

◆ While hyperglycemia is the primary metabolic dysfunction in microvascular complications, the main target is the endothelial cell (Figure 6.7).

Hyperglycemia is critical in the development of microvascular disease.

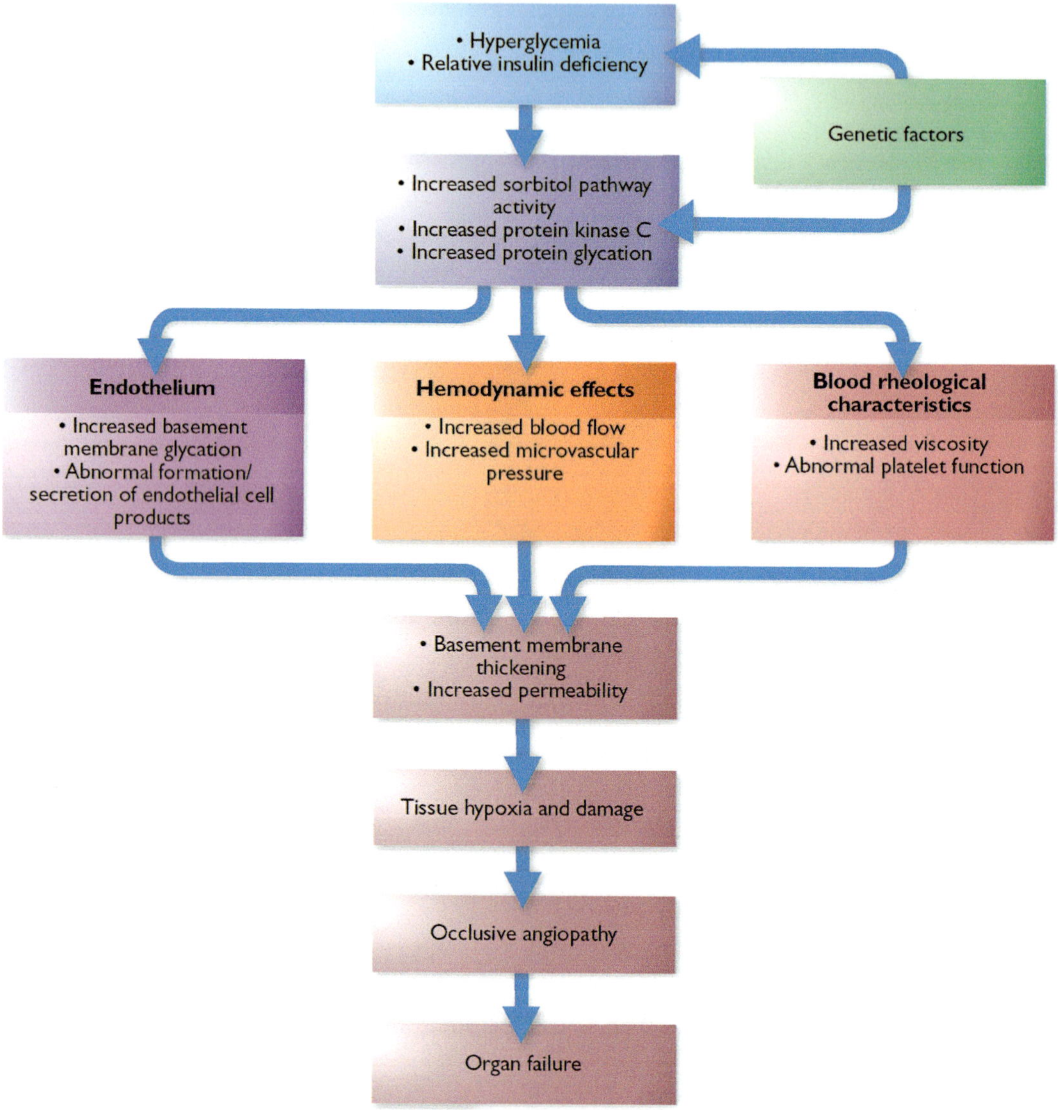

Figure 6.7 Pathogenesis of diabetic microangiopathy. Excess glucose causes an array of abnormalities, eventually leading to basement membrane thickening, endothelial cell changes, and pericyte cell death.

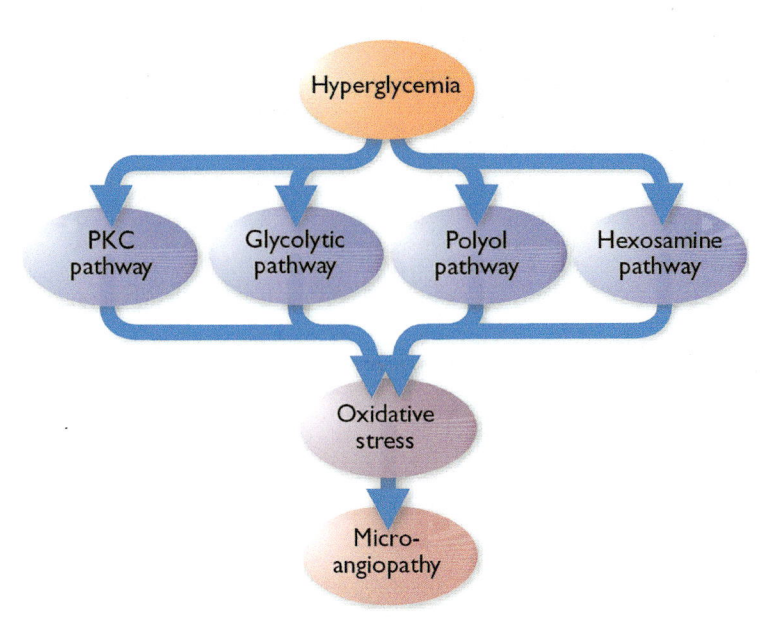

Figure 6.8 Oxidative stress pathways. Hyperglycemia leads to oxidative stress and diabetic complications via several seemingly independent mechanisms: polyol pathway activation, advanced glycation end product (AGE) formation, protein kinase C (PKC) activation, and hexosamine pathway activation.

Hyperglycemia

- Hyperglycemia predisposes to diabetic microvascular disease; reducing hyperglycemia can limit that progression and prevent disease development, as illustrated by DCCT for type 1 diabetes and UKPDS for type 2 diabetes:
  - In terms of reducing risk for microvascular complications, the DCCT showed that intensive glycemic control in type 1 diabetes reduced the risk of developing retinopathy in the primary prevention cohort (no retinopathy at baseline) by 76%, microalbuminuria by 34%, and neuropathy by 71% compared to conventional treatment.
  - In the UKPDS study of newly diagnosed type 2 diabetic patients, intensive glycemic control was associated with a reduced risk of microvascular endpoints, including microalbuminuria retinopathy.
  - In the Kumamoto study on slim type 2 diabetic Japanese patients, those in the intensive glycemic treatment group had a 76% risk reduction for retinopathy and 57% for microalbuminuria in the primary prevention cohort.
- There are several possible mechanisms linking hyperglycemia and diabetic microvascular disease (Figure 6.8).

High intracellular glucose

- When glucose is high inside a cell, most of it is metabolized by glycolysis, first to glucose-6-phosphate, then to fructose-6-phosphate, and on through the glycolytic pathway. Some fructose-6-phosphate is diverted into the hexosamine pathway in which it is converted to N-acetyl glucosamine, which can modify gene expression.
- At the same time, high intracellular glucose causes increased mitochondrial production of reactive oxygen species (ROS). ROS can cause strand breaks in nuclear DNA, which can reduce the activity of key enzymes and activate less beneficial pathways.
- Broadly, the consequence of high intracellular glucose is that the cell is stressed and mounts an antistress response to try to restore homeostasis.

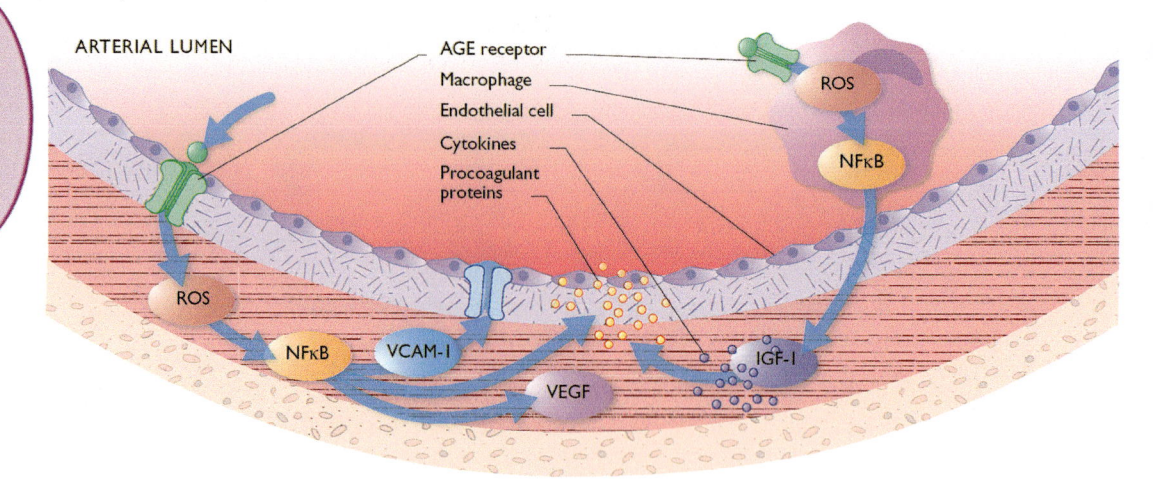

Figure 6.9 AGE reactions. The interaction of advanced glycation end products (AGE) with arterial wall components increases vascular permeability and wall thickness, the expression of procoagulant activity, the generation of reactive oxygen species (ROS), and the endothelial expression of adhesion molecules. NFκB, a transcription factor; IGF-1, insulin-like growth factor 1; VEGF, vascular endothelial growth factor; VCAM-1, vascular cell adhesion molecule-1.

Advanced glycation end products

- Long-term modification of proteins by protein glycation and oxidation leads to the formation of advanced glycation end products (AGEs) (Figure 6.9). AGE precursors damage cells via:
  ◊ Modification of intracellular proteins, including proteins involved in regulation of gene transcription.
  ◊ Modification of extracellular matrix molecules on diffusion out of cells, which alters matrix-cell signaling and causes cellular dysfunction.
  ◊ Modification of circulating blood proteins which bind to AGE receptors and activate them, causing inflammation and vascular pathology.
- Tissue levels of AGE increase with age, and can be derived from exogenous sources such as food and tobacco smoke.

Reactive oxygen species

- Increased production of ROS causes reduced availability of nitric oxide, with loss of its anti-inflammatory, antiproliferative, and antiadhesive properties.
- Activation of NFκB: this critical complex involved in cellular immune responses can be activated by oxidative stress and binding of AGEs to cell receptors on inflammatory cells including macrophages. AGE engagement with these AGE receptors (RAGE) promotes expression of pro-inflammatory cytokines, procoagulants and vasoconstriction.

Sorbitol accumulation

- Aldose reductase normally reduces toxic aldehydes in the cell to inactive alcohols, but when the glucose concentration in the cell is high, aldose reductase also reduces that glucose to sorbitol, which is later oxidized to fructose (Figure 6.10).
- In the process of reducing high intracellular glucose to sorbitol, the aldose reductase consumes the cofactor NADPH. NADPH is also the essential cofactor for regenerating a critical intracellular antioxidant, reduced glutathione.
- By decreasing reduced glutathione, the polyol pathway increases susceptibility to intracellular oxidative stress.
- As a result, there is a cellular 'pseudohypoxia' as well as accumulation of the osmotically active sorbitol. Sorbitol can damage these cells.

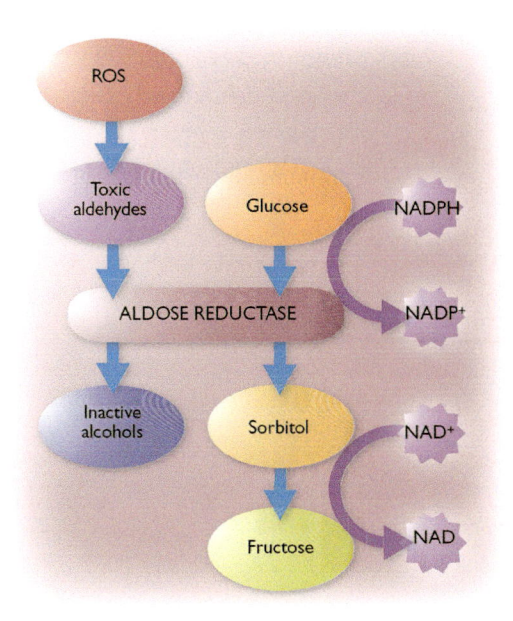

Figure 6.10 Sorbitol conversion. Aldose reductase reduces toxic aldehydes generated by ROS to inactive alcohols, and excess glucose to sorbitol, subsequently oxidizing the sorbitol to fructose, and using NADPH and NAD⁺ as co-factors. However, this consumption of NADPH can lead to decreased glutathione reductase and further oxidative stress.

◆ Aldose reductase inhibitors limit sorbitol formation.

Activation of protein kinase C-beta
◆ High glucose inside a cell increases the synthesis of diacylglycerol, which is a critical activating cofactor for protein kinase C-beta (PKC-β), an enzyme which regulates vascular permeability, contractility, and proliferation.
◆ PKC-β activation by high intracellular glucose influences gene expression pathologically. For example, the vasodilator producing endothelial nitric oxide synthase (eNOS) is decreased, while the vasoconstrictor endothelin-1, implicated in diabetic eye disease, is increased.

Glucose + NADPH + H⁺ leads to (aldose reductase) Sorbitol + NADP⁺.

Hemodynamic changes
◆ In diabetes there is increased blood viscosity and shear stress, with plugging of capillaries by activated leukocytes, as well as chronic hypoxia due to closure and nonperfusion of capillaries with proliferation of new vessels.
◆ Activation of pro-adhesive mechanisms in retinopathy can cause white cells to plug capillaries with consequent problems with perfusion. New vessels grow to bring blood back to the periphery, but these new vessels are inadequate at revascularizing ischemic areas, grow from the venous side of the retinal circulation, bleed easily, and cause the growth of fibrous tissue.

Treatment and management principles for microvascular disease

◆ Microvascular disease is influenced by several modifiable factors, including hyperglycemia, hypertension, dyslipidemia, and smoking.
◆ Microvascular disease is also influenced by several unmodifiable factors, including:
  ◇ Duration of diabetes. Complications tend to manifest themselves 10–20 years after diagnosis in young patients. A patient who does not develop renal disease by 30 years postdiagnosis is unlikely to develop that complication. Retinopathy can be present at diagnosis of type 2 diabetes, probably because the patient had unrecognized diabetes for several years prior to diagnosis.
  ◇ Genetic factors. Diabetic siblings of diabetic patients with renal and eye disease have a 3–5-fold increased risk of the same complication compared to siblings of patients without renal or eye disease. Patients with diabetes due to a glucokinase polymorphism associated with raised fasting glucose

but minimal postprandial hyperglycemia rarely develop microvascular complications.

◇ Racial factors. Some races are at higher risk of microvascular complications than others. For example, in the US, the rank order of risk is Pima American Indians > Hispanic/Mexican origin > US African origin > US European origin patients.

Reducing the risk of vascular disease

◆ In the diabetic patient without vascular disease, management is directed at reducing risk for these complications, primarily by addressing a set of modifiable risk factors (Figure 6.11).

◆ Prevention of microvascular complications reduces morbidity in diabetic patients, while reduction of cardiovascular risk is of prime importance, since this is the major contributor to both mortality and morbidity.

◇ The Multiple Risk Factor Intervention Trial (MRFIT) showed increasing likelihood of death from cardiovascular disease, according to the number of risk factors present (Figure 6.12).

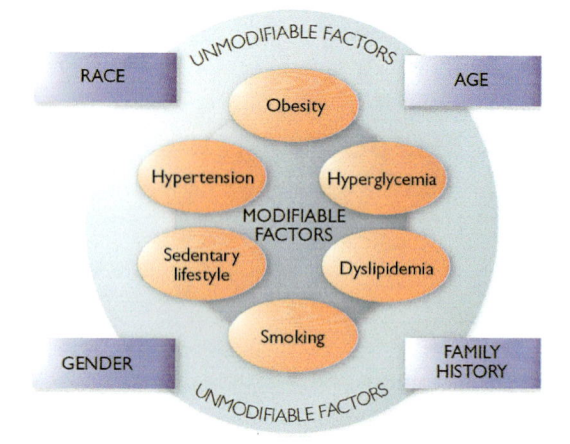

Figure 6.11 Risk factors in vascular disease. Risk factors can be either modifiable by therapy or life-style changes, or – as with age or gender – not modifiable.

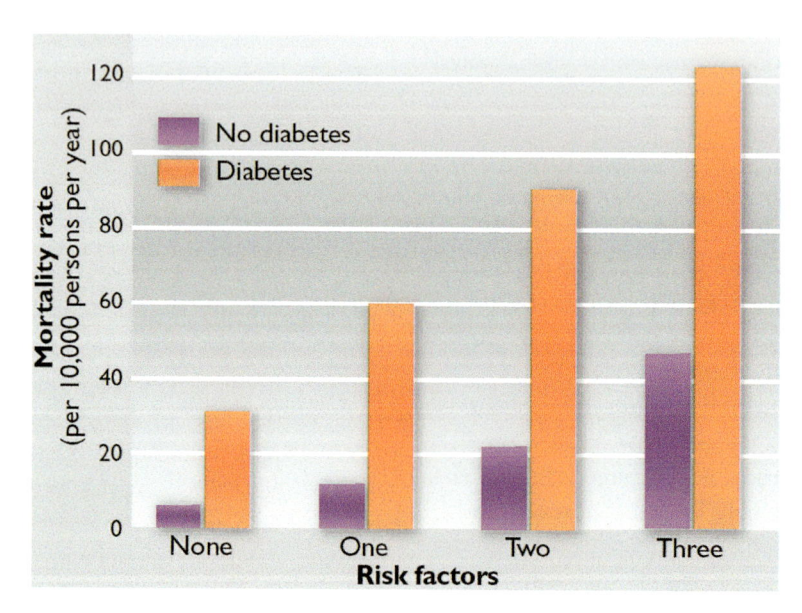

Figure 6.12 Cardiovascular risk. Among the 347,978 men aged 35–57 years screened for inclusion in the MRFIT trial were 5163 who reported taking medication for diabetes. In both diabetic and nondiabetic men, the number of risk factors (dyslipidemia, hypertension, or smoking) independently predicted cardiovascular disease (CVD) mortality, with the diabetic patients having a higher CVD death rate than nondiabetics with one or even two other cardiovascular risk factors.

Obesity and sedentary lifestyle

- Central to the prevention of cardiovascular disease is behavior modification (Figure 6.13).
- Diet and exercise are always advocated, though their importance has been cast aside by many patients because of the difficulty in achieving the goals – as compared with the relative ease of taking pills, or doing nothing – to address hypertension and dyslipidemia.
- Dietary recommendations include limiting saturated fat to <7% of total caloric intake, having two or more servings of fish per week to provide polyunsaturated fatty acids, and incorporating fruits, vegetables, legumes, low-fat dairy products, and whole grains into meals.
- Aim for 150 minutes per week of moderate intensity aerobic physical activity (50–70% maximum heart rate); in the absence of contraindications, people with type 2 diabetes should be encouraged to perform resistance training three times per week. (American Diabetes Association [ADA] guidelines).

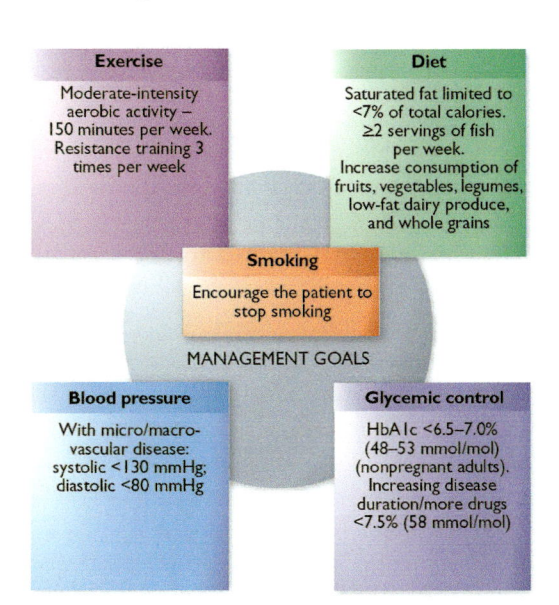

Figure 6.13 Prevention and management. A combination of behavior modification and tight glycemic and blood pressure control can significantly reduce cardiovascular risk.

Management Goals

Exercise: Moderate-intensity aerobic activity – 150 minutes per week. Resistance training 3 times per week.

Diet: Saturated fat limited to <7% of total calories. ≥2 servings of fish per week. Increase consumption of fruits, vegetables, legumes, low-fat dairy produce, and whole grains.

Smoking: Encourage the patient to stop smoking

Blood pressure: With micro/macro-vascular disease: systolic <130 mmHg; diastolic <80 mmHg

Glycemic control: HbA1c <6.5–7.0% (48–53 mmol/mol) (nonpregnant adults). Increasing disease duration/more drugs <7.5% (58 mmol/mol)

Hypertension

- The UKPDS trial concluded that tight blood pressure (BP) control in patients with hypertension and type 2 diabetes achieves a clinically important reduction in the risk of diabetes-related deaths and complications.
- The initial therapy for borderline hypertension in diabetes patients (within 10 mmHg of the target pressure) is exercise (30 minutes brisk walking per day) and sodium restriction (<100 mmol or <2.3 g per day). Weight loss also improves BP, partly by reducing insulin resistance.
- If the BP target – which varies with a number of factors, including age and recommending agency – has not been reached with these non-pharmacological measures, thiazide diuretics, angiotensin-converting-enzyme inhibitors (ACEIs), angiotensin-receptor blockers (ARBs), beta-blockers, and/or calcium-channel blockers should be employed.
- Particular care should be taken when initiating therapy in patients aged above 70 years, or if there is postural hypotension, hypovolemia, or renal impairment.
- UK NICE guidelines recommend ACEIs in general, but for Afro-Caribbean patients recommend ACEIs plus either a diuretic or calcium-channel blocker. These three agents are first- and second-line therapy and can then be used in any combination to achieve the target.
- Multiple studies, such as the Hypertension Optimal Treatment (HOT) trial, UKPDS, and the Anti-Hypertensive and Lipid-Lowering Treatment to Prevent Heart Attacks Trials (ALLHAT), have shown that two or more antihypertensive agents are usually needed.
- For most patients, ACEIs are the initial treatment of choice, assuming the patient can tolerate them. The second drug of choice is either a calcium-channel blocker (based on the ASCOT study) for a patient without nephropathy, or a thiazide diuretic (based on the ALLHAT).

- Women who are pregnant or might become pregnant should avoid ACEI and ARB drugs and start with calcium-channel blockers.
- In the ALLHAT, there was no significant difference in the risk of fatal coronary heart disease and nonfatal myocardial infarction between a thiazide, ACEI, and calcium-channel blocker.
- An ACEI reduced the risk of microalbuminuria in type 2 diabetes patients with hypertension and normoalbuminuria in the Bergamo Nephrologic Diabetes Complications Trial (BENEDICT), so it can be argued that the renoprotective effect makes ACEIs the first choice.
- ACEIs are also debatably the initial drug of choice, based on a cardioprotective effect, in patients aged over 55 years with type 2 diabetes and a cardiovascular risk of at least 20% in the next 10 years.
- The Micro-HOPE study demonstrated decreasing risk of major vascular events with ramipril in diabetes patients with a previous cardiovascular event.
  - 577 people with diabetes aged 55 years or older, with a previous cardiovascular event or at least one other cardiovascular risk factor, were randomly assigned ramipril (10 mg/day) or placebo. The study was stopped after 4.5 years.
  - Ramipril lowered the risk of the combined primary outcome by 25%, myocardial infarction by 22%, stroke by 33%, total mortality by 24%, and overt nephropathy by 24%. The cardiovascular benefit of ramipril was greater than that attributable to the decrease in blood pressure.
- The IDNT and RENAAL studies suggested that ARBs offer a reduction in development and progression of renal disease in patients with diabetic nephropathy, and hence ARBs can also be considered first line in patients with diabetic nephropathy. The commonest reason for withdrawing an ACEI is a chronic dry cough, which reflects angioedema of the bronchus.
- With either ACEIs or ARBs, it is recommended that serum potassium and creatinine be checked 1–2 weeks after starting, since hyperkalemia and further renal dysfunction can ensue if concomitant renal artery stenosis is present.
- Alpha-adrenergic blockers are useful as add-on medications to control BP. Beta adrenergic blockers may be used, although their adverse metabolic risk with hyperglycemia and dyslipidemia is a caution. Further options include calcium-channel blocking agents and thiazides (Table 6.3). Potassium-sparing diuretics can also be used at this stage.
- Short-acting calcium-channel blockers should be avoided.

Dyslipidemia
- Different therapies are available depending on the nature of the dyslipidemia (Table 6.4).
- The Collaborative Atorvastatin Diabetes Study (CARDS) showed that statins can reduce the risk of a first cardiovascular event (Figure 6.14).
- In type 2 diabetic patients who had no previous history of cardiovascular disease but with either hypertension, albuminuria, retinopathy, or were currently smoking, atorvastatin 10 mg daily resulted in primary prevention of acute coronary events and stroke. Mean LDL-cholesterol at entry was 3.04 mmol/L (117.4 mg/dL) for the atorvastatin group and 3–02 mmol/L (116.6 mg/dL) for the placebo group; and at the end of the study these were 2.11 mmol/L (81.5 mg/dL) and 3.12 mmol/L (120.5 mg/dL) respectively.
- Statins and aspirin are currently recommended:
  - Either simplistically for all diabetes patients aged 40 years or more, or
  - For patients with LDL-C >2.5 mmol/L or 100 mg/dL, or,
  - Using a personalized approach, for those diabetes patients with a 20% 10–year risk of progression to macrovascular disease.

Table 6.3 Drug therapy for hypertension. Of the six main classes of antihypertension drugs used in diabetes ACEIs are the drug of choice, partly because they tend to give the greatest BP reduction and improved cardiovascular outcomes. However, there is substantial variation among individuals.

Antihypertensive agents for type 2 diabetes

DRUG CLASS	ADVANTAGES	DISADVANTAGES
ACEIs	Reduce microalbuminuria Improve cardiovascular outcomes Beneficial in heart failure	Can cause hyperkalemia Can worsen renal function if with renal artery stenosis
Thiazide diuretics	Inexpensive	Can cause hypokalemia Usually not effective when serum creatinine reaches 159.1 µmol/L (1.8 mg/dL)
ARBs	Decrease risk of progression of micro-albuminuria and later stages of nephropathy	Can cause hyperkalemia Can worsen renal function if with renal artery stenosis
Beta-blockers	Reduce cardiovascular outcomes especially postmyocardial infarction	Hyperglycemia and dyslipidemia Can reduce adrenergic symptoms accompanying hypoglycemia
Calcium-channel blockers	Effective	Can cause peripheral edema
Alpha-blockers	Effective	Can cause postural hypotension

Table 6.4 Dyslipidemia therapies. Different drugs are used for different lipid abnormalities.

Pharmacological management of adverse lipid profile

LIPID ABNORMALITY	DRUG
Elevated LDL-cholesterol	Statins Ezetimibe Niacin Bile acid sequestrants
Elevated triglycerides	Fibrates Fish oils Ezetimibe Niacin
Low HDL-cholesterol	Niacin Fibrates

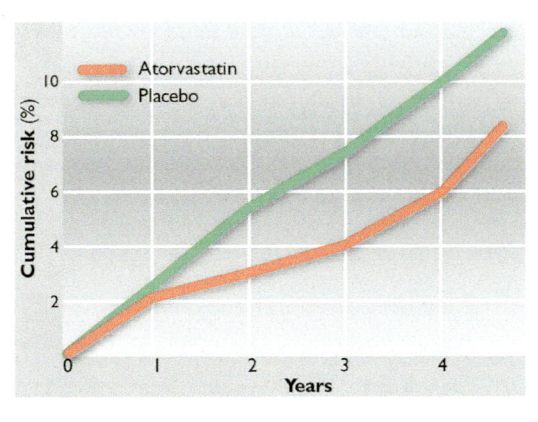

Figure 6.14 Effect of statins. Diabetes patients taking atorvastatin demonstrated reduced cardiovascular and mortality risk. *From the CARDS study: Colhoun H, et al. 2004.*

◆ High doses of statins have a greater benefit than low doses in the absence of side-effects so treatment with simvastatin 40 mg or atorvastatin 20 mg is often recommended, even when the lipid target has been achieved with a lower dose.

◆ Fibrates to correct hypertriglyceridemia and increase HDL are also suggested.
◇ The Fenofibrate Intervention and Event Lowering in Diabetes (FIELD) study found that fenofibrate therapy reduced lower-limb amputation events in patients with type 2 diabetes (Figure 6.15).

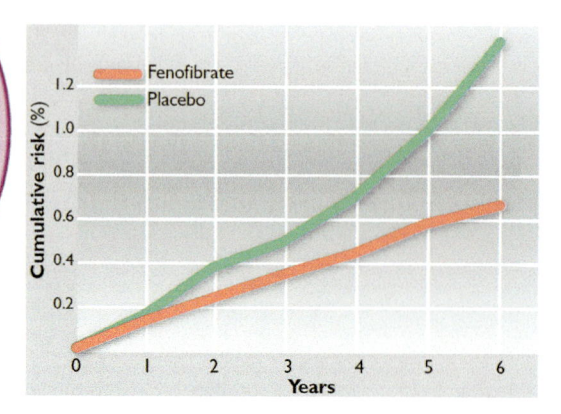

Figure 6.15 Effect of fibrates. Fenofibrate lowered the long-term risk of minor amputations for diabetes patients. *From the FIELD study: Rajamani K, et al.*

- Fibrates must be used cautiously in patients taking statins because of the risk of rhabdomyolysis.
- If statins and fibrates have to be used concurrently, fenofibrate is recommended over gemfibrozil because of a lower risk of myopathy and rhabdomyolysis. This greater risk is because gemfibrozil interferes with statin glucuronidation.
- Other medications such as ezetimibe and bile acid sequestrants play a role when desired lipid levels are not achieved with statins and fibrates.
- More recently, proprotein convertase subtilisin/kexin type 9 (PCSK9) inhibitors have been used to treat people who are poorly responsive or intolerant to statins. They are given as a monthly injection and offer significant LDL-cholesterol lowering effects. There role in diabetes dyslipidaemia is being explored.
- The mode of action of statins, fibrates, and other lipid-lowering drugs is shown in Figure 6.16.

Smoking

- Stopping smoking reduces the risk of cardiovascular disease by up to 70% in nondiabetic subjects and the same is probably true in patients with diabetes.
- All patients of any age should be advised against smoking. This is especially true in children who are at greatest risk of starting to smoke.
- At the annual review smoking habits should be documented and patients encouraged to stop or reduce the numbers of cigarettes.
- Counseling in combination with nicotine supplements is more effective at reducing smoking than nicotine supplements alone.
- Nicotine replacement therapy, bupropion or varenicline are therapies to aid smoking cessation, but should be prescribed

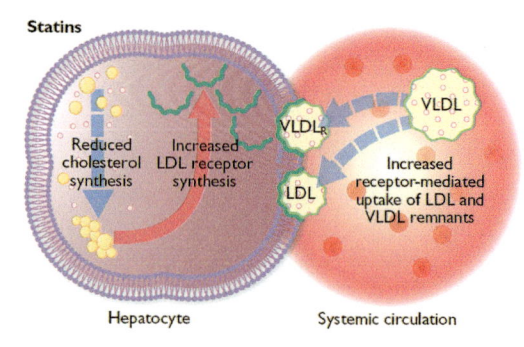

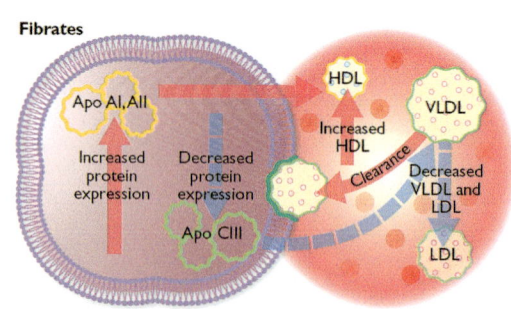

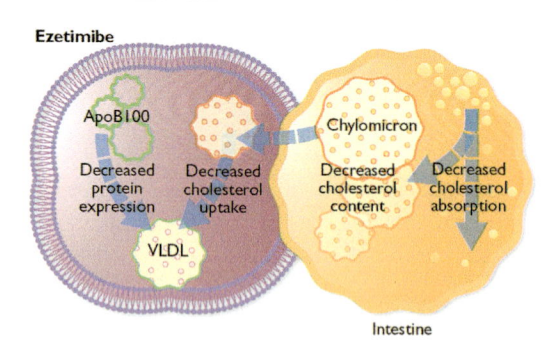

Figure 6.16 Lipid-lowering drugs. Very-low-density lipoproteins (VLDL) are precursors of cholesterol-rich, atherogenic LDL. Some drugs target the metabolism of VLDL by affecting apolipoprotein expression, some improve the clearance of LDL from the circulation, and others increase HDL production.

for short periods, in combination with counseling and with strict adherence to guidelines, such as avoiding their use in depression.

Hyperglycemia
- Glycemic control can be assessed by measuring the average blood glucose levels with glycated hemoglobin (HbA1c).
  - Glycation of hemoglobin occurs as a nonenzymatic two-step reaction, resulting in the formation of a covalent bond between the glucose molecule and the terminal valine of the beta chain of the hemoglobin molecule.
  - The percentage of hemoglobin glycated is related to the prevailing glucose concentration, intracellular glucose metabolism, and the lifespan of the red cell.
  - Glycated hemoglobin is expressed as a percentage of the normal hemoglobin (normal range approximately 4–6% [DCCT] or 20–42 mmol/mol [IFCC] depending on the technique of measurement).
  - HbA1c provides an index of the average blood glucose concentration over the life of the hemoglobin molecule (over a 6–12-week period). The level of HbA1c provides an index of hyperglycemia, and thus diabetes control, over that period.
  - The figure will be misleading if the lifespan of the red cell changes, either due to altered red cell survival, as in renal failure, or an abnormal hemoglobin, as in thalassemia.
- HbA1c estimations have been standardized and the improved accuracy, allied to the poor reproducibility of oral glucose tolerance tests, has led to suggestions that HbA1c could be used as a screening test to alert physicians to the possibility of diabetes.
  - In broad terms, HbA1c levels >6.5% (48 mmol/mol) are associated with a risk of diabetic microvascular disease (retinopathy), while lower levels, even into the normal range, are associated with an increased risk of macrovascular disease.
  - ADA guidelines aim for HbA1c <7.0% (53 mmol/mol) (nonpregnant adults). UK NICE guidelines aim for HbA1c <6.5% (48 mmol/mol) initially; later with increasing disease duration and more drugs aim less low, i.e. <7.5% (58 mmol/mol). Glycemic targets, however, should be individualized according to the patients preferences and comorbidities.
- Glycated plasma proteins (fructosamine) can also be measured as an index of control and relate to a shorter period of diabetes control (2–3 weeks).
  - This can be of value in patients with a hemoglobinopathy or in pregnancy (when hemoglobin turnover is changeable) and other situations that require rapid changes of treatment.
- Strict glycemic control did not reduce macrovascular complications in the UKPDS by a statistically significant degree in the first 15 years, but did so thereafter.
  - Type 1 diabetic patients followed from the original DCCT showed that tight glycemic control resulted in less cardiovascular disease (i.e. nonfatal myocardial infarction, stroke, death from cardiovascular disease, confirmed angina, or the need for coronary artery revascularization), compared to conventional treatment.
- By contrast, tight glycemic control has a marked effect on the onset of microvascular complications in both type 1 and type 2 diabetes patients. However, only 11% of the variation in microvascular complication risk is attributable to HbA1c change.
- Choice of agent after metformin is guided by patient preferences, and comorbidity (Figure 6.4).

Antithrombotic agents
- Statins are currently recommended for all diabetes patients aged >40 years; some

- physicians prefer to individualize cardiovascular disease risk, starting statins when this is in excess of 10% over 10 years.
- Following recent studies, the case for aspirin in those under 65 years of age without cardiovascular disease is much less clear. The UK NICE guidelines point out that aspirin is not licensed for primary prevention treatment.
- The balance of benefit must be set against the risk of hemorrhage when on aspirin, and both will vary for different individuals with diabetes.

CHAPTER 7

Diabetic neuropathy

Prevalence and classification

- Diabetic neuropathy is the most common complication of diabetes, conferring high morbidity.
- It is thought to be the result of several interrelated factors. Vascular abnormalities have been implicated in acute neuropathies, but without categorical evidence.
- It is difficult to estimate the prevalence of diabetic neuropathy, as it has a variety of manifestations and there are multiple diagnostic criteria; it varies from 20% of people with diabetes using simple clinical tests, such as perception of vibration, to >80% with more formal testing.
- Because of the variety in its presentation, several classification schemes are used to describe neuropathy (Table 7.1), such as the following:
  ◇ Chronic sensory nerve disorders, which are usually distal symmetrical polyneuropathies and are the most common presentations of diabetic neuropathy.
  ◇ Acute sensory nerve disorders, which are usually asymmetrical, transient mononeuropathies.
  ◇ Acute motor neuropathies, which are uncommon.
  ◇ Autonomic neuropathy; the most common clinical manifestation of which is erectile dysfunction.
- An alternative classification scheme is to describe the neuropathy as diffuse (distal symmetric sensorimotor polyneuropathy, autonomic neuropathy) or focal (mononeuropathy, mononeuropathy multiplex, plexopathy, radiculopathy, cranial neuropathy).

Table 7.1 Classification of neuropathy.
This scheme classifies sensory neuropathies as distal symmetric polyneuropathy, focal neuropathy, and diabetic amyotrophy. Autonomic neuropathies may be classified by the affected system, with motor neuropathies classified by the muscles that are involved.

Summary of diabetic neuropathy
SENSORIMOTOR NEUROPATHY
Distal symmetric polyneuropathy
Focal neuropathy
Diabetic mononeuropathy (cranial, truncal, peripheral nerves)
Mononeuropathy multiplex
Diabetic amyotrophy
AUTONOMIC NEUROPATHY
Hypoglycemic unawareness
Abnormal pupillary function
Cardiovascular autonomic neuropathy
Vasomotor neuropathy
Sudomotor neuropathy (sweat glands)
Gastrointestinal autonomic neuropathy
Gastric atony
Diabetic diarrhea or constipation
Fecal incontinence
Genitourinary autonomic neuropathy
Bladder dysfunction
Sexual dysfunction

Diagnosis

- The earliest functional change in diabetic nerves is delayed nerve conduction velocity.
- The earliest histological change is segmental demyelination caused by damage to Schwann cells. In the early stages, axons are preserved, implying prospects of recovery, but at a later stage irreversible axonal degeneration develops.
- The diagnosis of neuropathy can be made with such modalities as nerve conduction velocity and electromyography.
- In the outpatient setting, simpler tools are needed to diagnose diabetic neuropathy. Several neuropathy screening instruments, which involve scorecards grading physical exam findings (such as the presence or absence of ankle reflexes or vibration perception) have been developed, and vary in ease of use (Table 7.2).
- The Semmes-Weinstein 5.07 (10 gram) monofilament has been widely accepted as a screening tool for diabetic neuropathy (Figure 7.1).
    ◇ The monofilament is applied perpendicularly to nine sites on the plantar

Table 7.2 Screening instruments. An example scorecard for staging diabetic foot disorders in order to assess the level of severity and the risk of problems.

Diabetic foot risk assessment chart		
FEET (appearance)	RIGHT	LEFT
	Normal ☐	Normal ☐
	Abnormal (**1**) ☐	Abnormal (**1**) ☐
	Deformed (**1**) ☐	Deformed (**1**) ☐
	Dry skin, callus (**1**) ☐	Dry skin, callus (**1**) ☐
	Infection, fissure (**1**) ☐	Infection, fissure (**1**) ☐
ULCER		
	Absent ☐	Absent ☐
	Present (**1**) ☐	Present (**1**) ☐
ANKLE REFLEXES		
	Present ☐	Present ☐
	Present/reinforcement (**0.5**) ☐	Present (**0.5**) ☐
	Absent (**1**) ☐	Absent (**1**) ☐
VIBRATION (detected at first toe)		
	Present ☐	Present ☐
	Reduced (**0.5**) ☐	Reduced (**0.5**) ☐
	Absent (**1**) ☐	Absent (**1**) ☐
Total	☐ /8	☐ /8

Source: Adapted from Feldman EL. Diabetes Care, 1994.

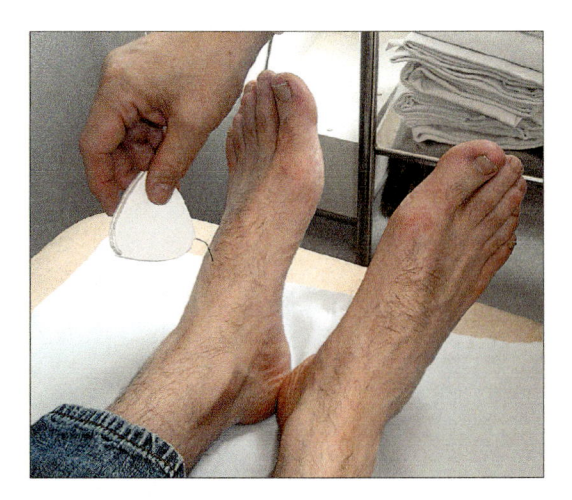

Figure 7.1 Neuropathy screening. Foot examination for sensation in a diabetic patient using a microfilament. A thorough annual foot examination by a health care professional is recommended for all diabetes patients.

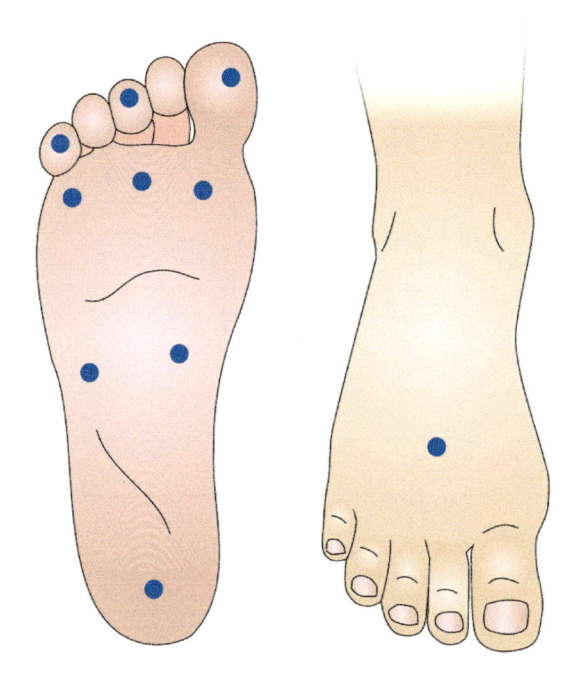

Figure 7.2 Monofilament testing. The Semmes–Weinstein monofilament test is performed at 10 sites on the foot. The filament exerts 10 grams of force when bowed against the skin for one second. Patients who cannot reliably detect this are considered to have lost protective sensation.

surface and one on the dorsal surface of the foot, with enough force to cause it to buckle; a variation is to apply it at only two sites – the plantar aspect of the first and fifth metatarsal heads (Figure 7.2).
  ◇ If the patient is unable to feel the monofilament at these locations, this has 80% sensitivity and 86% specificity for diagnosing diabetic neuropathy.

Chronic sensory polyneuropathy

- Diabetic neuropathies are usually sensory and most commonly bilateral, symmetrical, peripheral, and chronic (see Figure 7.3).
  ◇ Chronic symmetrical sensory polyneuropathy is the most common form.
- Sensory deficits first appear in the distal lower extremities. A slowing in nerve conduction is the first physiological change, and occurs even before symptoms appear.
- Early clinical signs are impaired vibration sense (using a 128-Hz tuning fork), pain sensation (deep before superficial), paresthesias, and temperature sensation in the feet.
  ◇ At later stages patients may complain of a feeling of 'walking on cotton wool' and can lose their balance when walking in the dark, owing to impaired proprioception.
- Involvement of the hands is less common and results in a 'stocking and glove' sensory loss.
- Complications include unrecognized trauma at pressure points, beginning as blistering due to an ill-fitting shoe or a hot water bottle, and leading to ulceration.
- Unbalanced traction by the long flexor muscles leads to a characteristic foot, with a high arch and clawed toes.

Clinical patterns of diabetic peripheral neuropathy

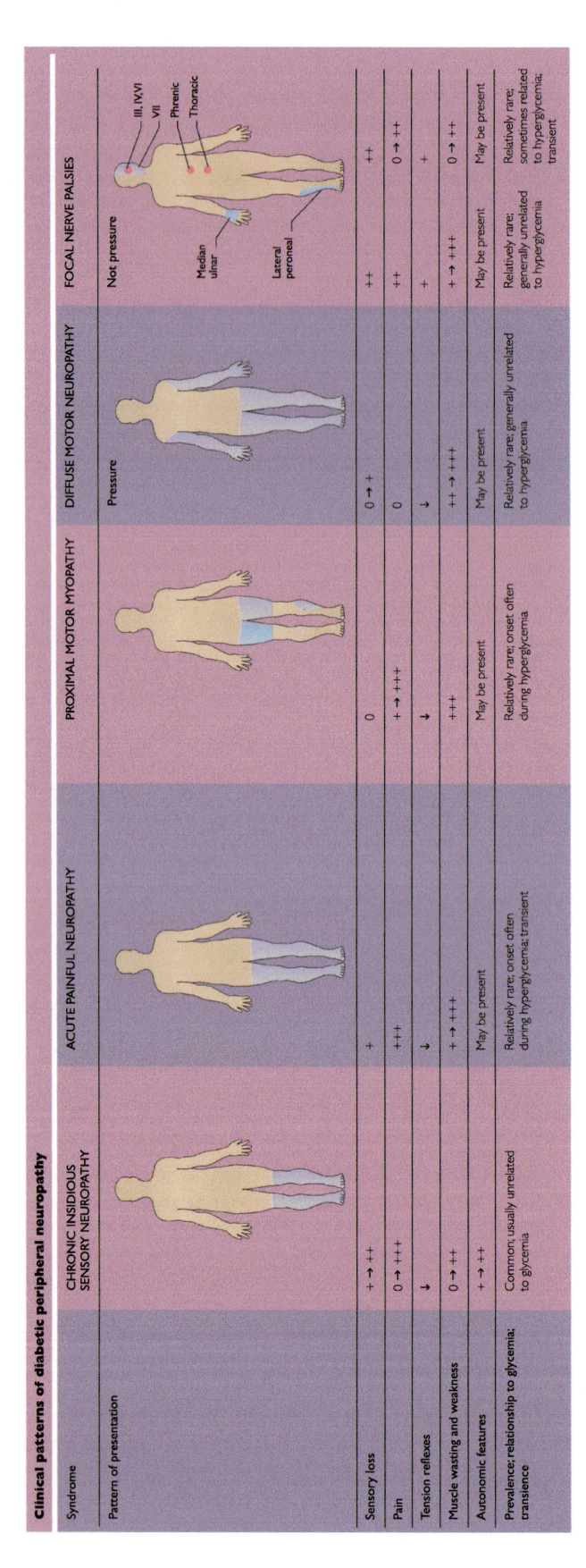

Syndrome	CHRONIC INSIDIOUS SENSORY NEUROPATHY	ACUTE PAINFUL NEUROPATHY	PROXIMAL MOTOR MYOPATHY	DIFFUSE MOTOR NEUROPATHY	FOCAL NERVE PALSIES
Pattern of presentation				Pressure	Not pressure
Sensory loss	+ → ++	+	0	0 → +	++
Pain	0 → +++	+++	+ → +++	0	++
Tension reflexes	↓	↓	↓	↓	+
Muscle wasting and weakness	0 → ++	+ → +++	+++	++ → +++	+ → ++
Autonomic features	+ → +++	May be present	May be present	May be present	May be present
Prevalence; relationship to glycemia; transience	Common; usually unrelated to glycemia	Relatively rare; onset often during hyperglycemia; transient	Relatively rare; onset often during hyperglycemia	Relatively rare; generally unrelated to hyperglycemia	Relatively rare; generally unrelated to hyperglycemia	Relatively rare; sometimes related to hyperglycemia; transient

Focal nerve palsies labels: III, IV/VI; VII; Phrenic; Thoracic; Median ulnar; Lateral peroneal.

Figure 7.3 Clinical patterns. Note that different forms of diabetic neuropathy can coexist in the same patient.

- ◇ This change in turn leads to abnormal pressure distribution, resulting in callus formation under the first metatarsal head or on the tips of the toes and perforating neuropathic ulceration (see Chapter 10).
- ◆ Neuropathic arthropathy (Charcot's joints) may sometimes develop in any joint, but most often affects the ankle or mid-tarsal joints (see Chapter 10).

Early clinical signs of chronic sensory polyneuropathy are an impaired sense of vibration, pain, and temperature in the feet.

Acute sensory neuropathy

- ◆ Although some of the symptoms of acute and chronic sensory neuropathy are similar, there are differences in the mode of onset, signs, and prognosis (Figure 7.3). Acute neuropathies may be either:
  - ◇ Diffuse and painful.
  - ◇ Focal.
- ◆ In either event they are usually transient.
- ◆ A diffuse, painful neuropathy is uncommon (5%). The patient describes burning or crawling pains in the feet, shins, and anterior thighs and muscular leg cramps, all typically worse at night, and pressure from bedclothes may be intolerable (allodynia). Painful neuropathy may present at diagnosis or develop after sudden improvement in glycemic control. It usually resolves spontaneously after 3 months and resolves in 90% of cases at 2 years.
  - ◇ A more chronic form, developing later in the course of the disease, is sometimes resistant to almost all forms of therapy. There is no diagnostic test so alternative diagnoses such as vitamin B12 deficiency, alcohol, HIV-related, drug-related (isoniazid, nitrofurantoin), porphyria, and cancer-related neuropathy should be considered.
  - ◇ Muscle wasting is not a feature and objective signs can be minimal.
- ◆ Focal mononeuritis and mononeuritis multiplex (multiple mononeuropathy) can affect any nerve in the body. Typically the onset is abrupt and sometimes painful.
- ◆ Isolated cranial nerve palsies are more commonly seen in the elderly and are rare in children.
  - ◇ Involvement of the third cranial nerve is the most common, with characteristic pupillary sparing, i.e. pupillary reflexes are often retained owing to sparing of pupillomotor fibers. It usually presents with unilateral ophthalmoplegia that spares lateral eye movement, and pain above or behind the eye. However, pain may be absent or mild in half of the cases.
  - ◇ The sixth cranial nerve is also commonly involved.
  - ◇ The fourth and seventh cranial nerves are affected less often and not more frequently than in nondiabetic patients.
  - ◇ Full spontaneous recovery is the rule for most episodes of focal cranial nerve involvement, even in the elderly.
- ◆ Isolated peripheral nerve palsies are more commonly seen in diabetic than nondiabetic individuals. Lesions are more likely to occur at sites for external pressure palsies or nerve entrapment (e.g. the median nerve in the carpal tunnel). Carpal tunnel syndrome is a common cause for sensory symptoms in the hands in diabetes, and is twice as common in people with diabetes than in those without.
- ◆ Radiculopathy (i.e. involvement of a spinal root) may occur. Thoracic radiculopathy presents as dermatomal pain and loss of sensation. Hyperesthesia can occur. Spontaneous resolution usually occurs in 6–24 months.

Diabetic peripheral neuropathy can be acute or chronic.

Acute motor neuropathy

- Diabetic amyotrophy is a rare motor neuropathy that is more prevalent in older men.
- It presents as weight loss, depression, and painful wasting of the quadriceps muscles.
  - Depression may be severe and resolves as the weight increases.
  - The wasting may be marked, causing severe proximal weakness, and knee reflexes may be diminished or absent. The affected area is often extremely tender.
  - Extensor plantar responses sometimes develop and cerebrospinal fluid (CSF) protein content is elevated.
  - The presentation may be unilateral; the contralateral thigh can be involved immediately following or months after the initial insult.
- Diabetic amyotrophy is usually associated with periods of poor glycemic control and may be present at diagnosis. It resolves like an acute sensory neuropathy with the same management regimen.
- There is some suggestion that diabetic amyotrophy may be the result of ischemic damage to the nerves from an immune mediated microvasculitis. The use of immunosuppression, however, has not consistently shown benefit in improving severity or duration of symptoms.
- Nondiabetic causes for the amyotrophy must be excluded, including spinal lesions.

Autonomic neuropathy

- Diabetic autonomic neuropathy (DAN) can affect almost every organ system (Table 7.3). It affects both the sympathetic and parasympathetic nervous systems and can be disabling.

Table 7.3 Symptoms of autonomic neuropathy. Symptoms vary according to the nerves and organ systems affected.

Clinical manifestations of diabetic autonomic neuropathy	
ORGAN SYSTEM	MANIFESTATION
Cardiovascular	Postural hypotension, tachycardia, sudden cardiac death
Gastrointestinal	Esophageal dysmotility, gastroparesis, diarrhea, constipation, incontinence
Genitourinary	Erectile dysfunction, retrograde ejaculation, bladder dysfunction
Neuroendocrine	Hypoglycemia unawareness
Sudomotor	Dry skin, impaired skin blood flow, gustatory sweating
Pupillary	Abnormal reflexes

- Asymptomatic autonomic changes can be demonstrated on laboratory testing in many patients, but because of its variable manifestation, it can escape clinical recognition.
- Patients with severe autonomic neuropathy have an increased mortality, possibly due to cardiac arrhythmia, especially in those with marked prolongation of the QTc interval on ECG.

Cardiovascular system
- Autonomic neuropathy results in tachycardia at rest and loss of sinus arrhythmia. Cardiovascular reflexes including the Valsalva maneuver are impaired.
- A fixed heart rate that does not respond to exercise should alert one to cardiovascular autonomic neuropathy.
- Silent ischemia is more common in patients with DAN.
- Myocardial infarction should be considered in people with diabetes who present with unexplained nausea, vomiting, breathlessness or diaphoresis even if there is no chest pain.

- DAN is associated with impaired dilation of coronary arteries and can predispose to arrhythmias.
- Impaired blood pressure regulation is another manifestation of DAN.
  ◇ The normal diurnal blood pressure variation is lost, so that patients have supine hypertension at night.
  ◇ Postural hypotension, where there is an orthostatic fall in systolic blood pressure by more than 20 mmHg, results from loss of sympathetic tone to peripheral and splanchnic arterioles. Patients complain of dizziness, feeling faint, blurring of vision, or loss of consciousness.
- Early cardiovascular DAN may not be clinically apparent, and may require diagnostic tests for evaluation. Most of these techniques rely on the impaired heart-rate variability and blood pressure responses.
  ◇ The heart rate response to standing can be ascertained by continuous ECG monitoring. The R-R interval is then measured after standing at beats 15 and 30. The ratio of the R-R interval at beat 30:15 is normally >1.03 since a tachycardia is followed by reflex bradycardia.

Diabetic autonomic neuropathy can escape clinical recognition because of its variable manifestation.

Gastrointestinal tract
- Gastroparesis results in delayed gastric emptying. Solid-phase emptying occurs in the antrum, and if affected in diabetic patients, results in gastric retention.
  ◇ Vagal neuropathy can cause gastroparesis, often asymptomatic, but sometimes resulting in intractable vomiting. Other milder symptoms are early satiety, nausea, bloating, and abdominal pain.
  ◇ Scintigraphic gastric emptying studies are used to diagnose gastroparesis, although acute hyperglycemia may give false positive results.
- Diarrhea often occurs at night with urgency and incontinence. Small intestinal bacterial overgrowth (SIBO) in the stagnant bowel, pancreatic exocrine insufficiency, malabsorption, and incontinence can lead to diarrhea and steatorrhea.

Bladder involvement
- DAN can lead to decreased bladder sensation and reduced voiding frequency.
  ◇ This can result in bladder enlargement, bladder stasis, loss of tone, and incomplete emptying (predisposing to infection) with eventual urinary retention.
  ◇ Patients experience dribbling and urinary incontinence.
  ◇ A postvoiding residual of more than 150 ml indicates bladder dysfunction and can be ascertained by postvoiding catheterization or postvoiding ultrasonography.

Erectile dysfunction
- Erectile dysfunction is a common complication of diabetes resulting from autonomic neuropathy, vascular disease, or more often a combination of both. Acute illness, for whatever reason, can lead to transient ED.
- A careful history should determine the nature of erectile dysfunction to establish the ability to obtain erections, penetration, and ejaculation, or combinations of these problems.
- Common presentations in diabetes are:
  ◇ Incomplete erections.
  ◇ Absent emissions due to retrograde ejaculation in patients with autonomic neuropathy.
- Erectile dysfunction in diabetes has many causes including anxiety, depression, alcohol excess, drugs, primary or

secondary gonadal failure, and hypothyroidism, and is more common with age.
- ◇ History and examination should focus on these possible causes.
- ◇ Blood should be taken for luteinizing hormone (LH), follicle-stimulating hormone (FSH), testosterone, prolactin, and thyroid function.
- ◆ Sexual dysfunction is may also be a feature in women though the management has not yet been determined.

Neuroendocrine disturbances
- ◆ In patients with longstanding diabetes, there is loss of the adrenergic symptoms of hypoglycemia that usually precede neuroglycopenia. The counter-regulatory responses of glucagon and catecholamines are impaired.
- ◆ Patients have hypoglycemia unawareness, which increases the risk of hypoglycemic coma.

Sudomotor dysfunction
- ◆ Upper body hyperhidrosis and lower body anhidrosis are seen in DAN.
- ◆ Gustatory sweating (especially after cheese or wine) is an often unrecognized manifestation.
- ◆ The dry and cracked skin commonly seen in diabetes contributes to the development of skin infection.

Pupillary effects
- ◆ In DAN, there is decreased pupillary diameter in dark adaptation that might result in difficulty during night driving.

Treatment and management

- ◆ The management of diabetic neuropathies depends on the nature of the neuropathy.

Acute sensory neuropathies
- ◆ The first step is to explore other nondiabetic causes, in particular alcohol excess, and vitamin B12 deficiency, which is sometimes seen in long term metformin use.
- ◆ Once other conditions have been reasonably excluded, four factors are important:
  - ◇ Reassurance about the high likelihood of remission within months.
  - ◇ Management of blood glucose control, often with insulin even when glucose control is not bad.
  - ◇ Medications: the treatment of choice for acute painful neuropathy is pregabalin (recommended in the USA) or duloxetine (recommended in the UK), or, when such therapy is unsuccessful, both in combination. Other treatments include tricyclic antidepressants, gabapentin, and carbamazepine, which all reduce the perception of neuropathic pain. Topical capsaicin-containing creams help some patients, but can discolor clothes. Epidurals may be required for chronic unremitting pain.
  - ◇ Many vitamins, including vitamin B, are used without clear evidence of their benefit.

Focal sensory mononeuropathies
- ◆ It is important first to explore nondiabetic causes.
- ◆ Once diabetes is identified as the likely cause, four factors are important:
  - ◇ Reassurance about the high likelihood of remission within months.
  - ◇ Management of blood glucose control, with the introduction of insulin should optimum control of either glucose or the pain be difficult.
  - ◇ Symptomatic relief such as eye patches for diplopia, or wrist splints for carpal tunnel syndrome.
  - ◇ Consider surgery for carpal tunnel syndrome and radiculopathy to decompress the lesions should pain not resolve.

Acute motor neuropathies
- ◆ Management is similar to that for acute mononeuropathies and includes
  - ◇ Reassurance regarding likelihood of remission.

- Blood glucose control using insulin therapy.
- General care including bed rest when muscle wasting is severe.
- Antidepressant therapy when the depression is severe.

Autonomic neuropathy

Cardiovascular system
- Patients with orthostatic hypotension should be instructed not to get up suddenly from a reclining position.
- The use of compression stockings in waking hours helps to increase venous return from the periphery and may alleviate orthostatic hypotension.
- Debilitating hypotension can be helped by the sympathomimetic, midodrine, or the mineralocorticoid, fludrocortisone. Treatment has to be adjusted to minimize symptoms and at the same time avoid the development of supine hypertension or congestive heart failure.

Gastrointestinal tract
- Optimization of blood glucose levels can improve gastric motility.
- Frequent small meals with reduced fat content helps in gastroparesis.
- Metoclopramide and domperidone (not available in the US) have antiemetic effects and are helpful in gastroparesis. Erythromycin stimulates motilin receptors and improves gastric emptying.
- Broad-spectrum antibiotics such as doxycycline or metronidazole are useful for bacterial overgrowth and can improve diarrhea. The antidiarrheal drug loperamide and diphenoxylate offer symptomatic relief.
- A laparoscopically implanted gastric pacemaker can improve gastric emptying.

Erectile dysfunction is a common complication of diabetes. Patients require counseling as well as treatment.

Bladder involvement
- Urinary retention can be improved by cholinergic agents such as oxybutynin.
- Incomplete bladder emptying leading to distention will benefit from intermittent catheterization.
- Urinary tract infections should be treated with antibiotics.

Erectile dysfunction
- All patients require counseling irrespective of the cause of the erectile dysfunction. Therapy for erectile dysfunction includes:
  - Phosphodiesterase type-5 (PDE5) inhibitors. A therapeutic trial of these agents, including sildenafil citrate, should be considered in most impotent diabetic patients who do not suffer from angina or previous myocardial infarction (concurrent use of nitrates is a contraindication). These drugs enhance the effects of nitric oxide on smooth muscle and increase penile blood flow. About 60% of patients benefit (Figure 7.4).

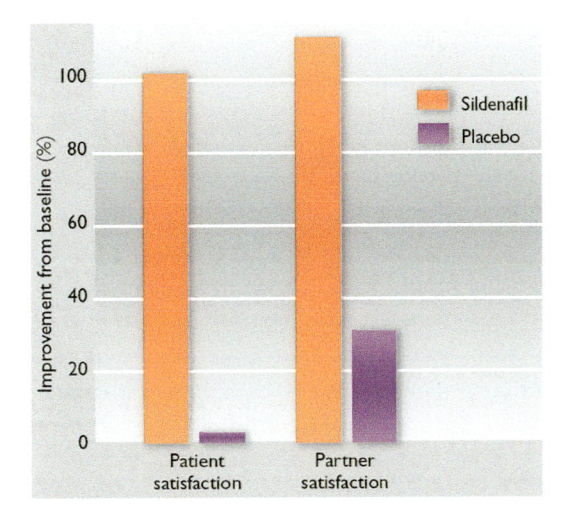

Figure 7.4 Oral therapy for erectile dysfunction. Sildenafil (Viagra) is usually regarded as a first-line drug for the treatment of erectile dysfunction. Response rates against placebo are high, with over 60% success in trials.

Side-effects, including headaches and altered vision, are not uncommon. If a PDE5 inhibitor succeeds it is worth trying without it after a few months, since sometimes potency will continue unaided after confidence is restored. Psychological factors are important and long-acting agents such as tadalafil can be helpful, as they reduce the need to plan precise treatment periods.

◇ Prostaglandin E-1 preparations. These agents promote penile blood flow when applied topically to the urethra or as an intracavernosal injection. Alprostadil given after suitable training via a small pellet inserted into the urethra has a lower success rate than intracavernosal injection of the same drug, but is less invasive. If the partner is pregnant, barrier contraception must be used to keep prostaglandin away from the fetus.

◇ Intracavernous injection. Patients can be trained to inject either alprostadil or papaverine (a smooth muscle relaxant), sometimes given with phentolamine and thymoxamine (alpha-adrenoreceptor blockers). The dose should be increased incrementally until a satisfactory response is obtained. Side effects include local reactions (e.g. discomfort, hematoma, fibrosis) and priapism. Patients should be given contact details for urgent treatment should erection last for more than 3 hours. To treat priapism, insert a large butterfly needle into the cavernous tissue and aspirate blood with a large syringe until detumescence has occurred.

◇ Vacuum devices. These provide a non-pharmacological aid. A perspex tube with a seal in the base is placed over the penis and a vacuum pump draws blood into the penis to achieve tumescence, which is then maintained by slipping a rubber band over the base of the penis (then removing the tube) until intercourse is complete.

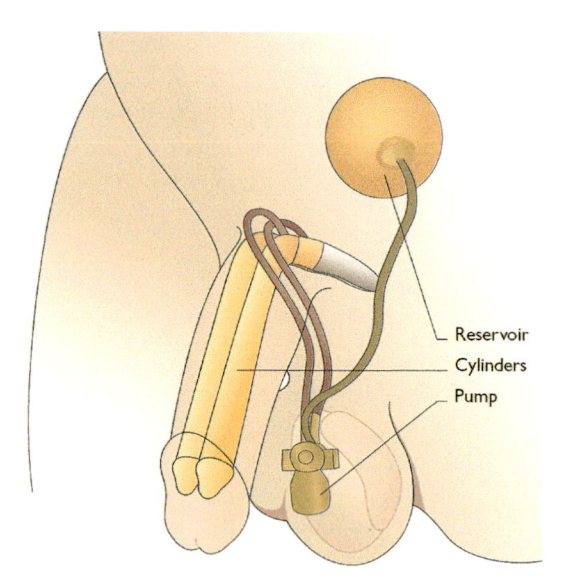

Figure 7.5 Penile implant surgery. There are a number of prosthetic options available: this shows a three-piece inflatable implant consisting of a pair of cylinders implanted in the penis, a pump bulb implanted in the scrotum, and a reservoir placed within the abdomen.

◇ Surgery. A proportion of patients find none of these solutions of value, especially if they have vascular disease. Patients with erectile dysfunction unresponsive to drug therapy can achieve penetration by means of a semirigid plastic rod inserted surgically into the penis. Other more sophisticated devices can generate an erect penis when required, using a hydraulic system (Figure 7.5).

◇ Constriction of venous outflow. Constriction of venous outflow from the penis by application of an elastic band around the base of the penis can enhance the firmness of an erection, but on its own will lead to an engorged penis without unidirectional rigidity (the so-called 'wand' effect). Whether application of a constricting band in association with a PDE5 inhibitor will enhance the success of the latter remains to be proven, but it may be worthwhile as a trial.

CHAPTER 8

Diabetic eye disease

Overview

- Patients with diabetes are at risk of eye disease including:
  - *Retinopathy*. About 5% of patients in the past became blind after 30 years of diabetes, and diabetes is the commonest cause of blindness in the population up to 65 years of age.
  - *Maculopathy*. Increased permeability of the capillaries and microaneurysms in the retina can result in accumulation of fluid and thickening in the macular area.
  - *Cataracts*. The lens may be affected by reversible osmotic changes in patients with acute hyperglycemia, causing blurred vision. Senile cataracts develop 10 years earlier in diabetic patients, compared to non-diabetic subjects.
  - *Glaucoma*. Glaucoma is more prevalent in diabetes due to new vessel formation in the iris (rubeosis iridis). Open-angle glaucoma is not more prevalent in diabetes.
  - *Ocular nerve palsies*. Ocular palsies of the third and sixth cranial nerves can occur. Like other causes of mononeuritis, these palsies are acute and transient, always resolving within 2 years and usually within 4 months.

Natural history

- Duration of diabetes is one of the best predictors of retinopathy:
  - Patients who have had type 1 diabetes for 5 years or less rarely have evidence of retinopathy.
  - After 5–10 years of diabetes, close to 30% of type 1 diabetes patients have retinopathy.
  - After 20–30 years, about 95% of patients have retinopathy, and 30–60% of these progress to sight-threatening proliferative retinopathy (Figure 8.1).

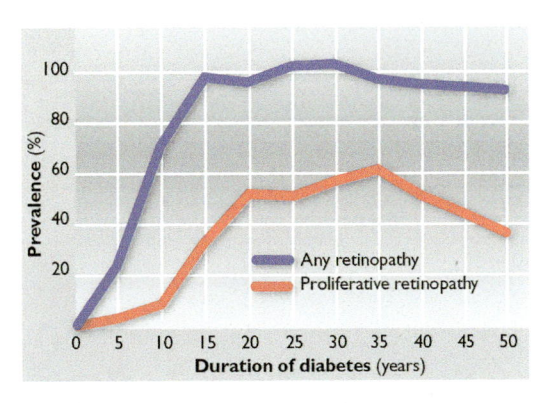

Figure 8.1 Prevalence of diabetic retinopathy in type 1 diabetes. Data from the Wisconsin Epidemiologic Study of Diabetic Retinopathy (WESDR) reported by Klein et al. showed that by 25 years following the onset of the disease, almost all patients had developed some sort of retinopathy with over 50 percent having vision-threatening proliferative retinopathy. *From Klein, et al. (2008)*.

- In type 2 diabetes, 20% of newly diagnosed patients already have diabetic retinopathy, and most will subsequently develop the condition.
- Without treatment, 50% of patients with proliferative retinopathy become blind within 5 years.
- At least annual dilated eye examinations with digital retinal photography by trained professionals are recommended (Table 8.1).
- Diabetic retinopathy can be classified into nonproliferative (NPDR) and proliferative (PDR).
  - NPDR comprises: microaneurysms, 'dot and blot' hemorrhages, hard exudates, 'cottonwool spots', and intraretinal microvascular abnormalities (IRMAs), while venous beading, neovascularization, vitreous/preretinal hemorrhages, and traction-induced retinal detachment are found in PDR (107).
  - A suggested grading of diabetic retinopathy used in the UK is shown in Table 8.2.

Retinopathy is more likely with increasing duration of diabetes.

Nonproliferative diabetic retinopathy

- Diabetic retinopathy is caused by progressive damage to the blood vessels that supply the retinal tissues (Figures 8.2 and 8.3). Early changes are detectable by fluorescein angiography (Figure 8.4).
  - Hyperglycemia leads to tissue hypoxia and reduced retinal function.
  - Leucocyte adhesion to the capillary wall results in occlusion and reduced blood flow, and ultimately greater hypoxia and ischemia.
  - Capillary nonperfusion can also cause compensatory dilation and microaneurysms in other vessels.
  - Basement membrane thickening, endothelial cell damage, and degeneration of the pericytes supporting the blood vessel wall cause

Table 8.1 Eye examinations. Regular screening is important in order to detect early changes indicative of retinopathy.

Recommended ophthalmologic examination
TYPE 1 DIABETES
First examination within 3–5 years after diagnosis of diabetes once patient is age 10 years or older (since some evidence suggests that prepubertal duration of diabetes may be important in the development of microvascular complications, use clinical judgment)
Yearly routine follow-up at the minimum (more frequent if abnormal findings)
TYPE 2 DIABETES
First examination at the time of diagnosis of diabetes
Yearly routine follow-up at the minimum (more frequent if abnormal findings)
PREGNANCY IN PRE-EXISTING DIABETES
First examination prior to conception, then during first trimester
Follow-up is at physician discretion pending results of first-trimester examination
RETINOPATHY AND MACULAR EDEMA
Ophthalmology referral in patients with macular edema, severe NPDR, or any form of PDR

Table 8.2 Grading of retinopathy.

R GRADE	RETINOPATHY LEVEL	CLINICAL FEATURES
R0	No retinopathy	Normal fundus
R1	Background retinopathy	Microaneurysms Retinal hemorrhages Exudates Cotton wool spots Venous loop
R2	Preproliferative retinopathy	Multiple blot hemorrhages Intraretinal microvascular anomalies Venous beading Venous reduplication
R3A	Active proliferative retinopathy	New vessels on the disc New vessels elsewhere New preretinal or vitreous hemorrhage New tractional retinal detachment
R3S	Stable treated proliferative retinopathy	Stable features previously noted from above
P1	Laser photocoagulation	Laser photocoagulation scars
U	Ungradeable	May be due to cataract or poor concordance with instructions
	MACULOPATHY LEVEL	
M0	No maculopathy	Normal macular area
M1	Maculopathy	Exudate within 1 disc diameter of macula Group of exudates within the macula Microaneurysms or hemorrhages within 1 dis diameter of macula, with visual acuity 6/12 or worse

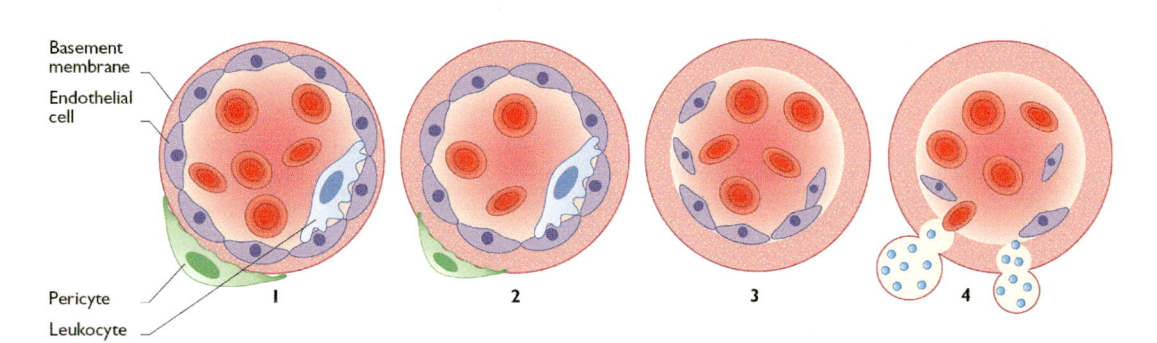

Figure 8.2 Capillary changes. (1) Leukocyte adhesion; (2) basement membrane thickening and reduced blood flow; (3) pericyte and endothelial cell death; and (4) increased permeability.

breakdown of the blood-retina barrier and increased permeability of the retinal capillaries.
◇ Leakage of plasma, proteins, and growth factors such as VEGF gives rise to cell edema and new vessel growth, respectively.

◆ In NPDR, hemorrhages and microaneurysms can be seen:
  ◇ Clinically, microaneurysms are visible through the ophthalmoscope as round dots.
  ◇ By 20 years of diabetes, virtually all fundi show at least the occasional microaneurysm on ophthalmoscopy.

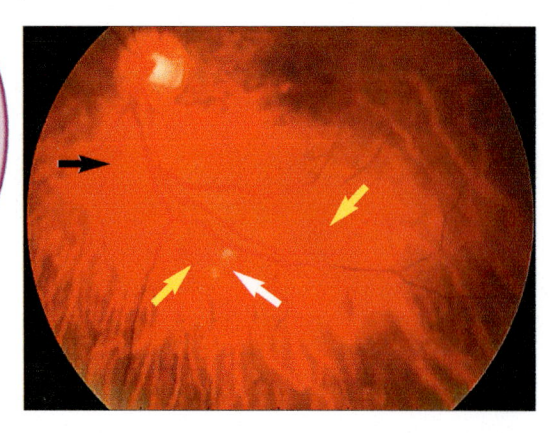

Figure 8.3 Moderate nonproliferative diabetic retinopathy. Retinal fundus photograph showing IRMA (black arrow), hemorrhages (yellow arrows), and cotton-wool spots (white arrow).

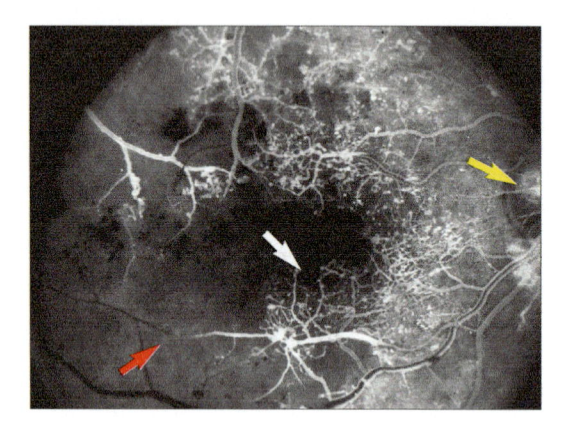

Figure 8.4 Fluorescein angiography. This photograph shows retinal ischemia and capillary nonperfusion (red arrow), microaneurysms, and vascular pruning (white arrow). There is an area of neovascularization on the optic nerve (yellow arrow), which is often associated with extensive retinal ischemia. *Courtesy Michael J. Tolentino, Palm Beach Eye Center, Lakeland, Florida, USA.*

- ◇ When a microaneurysm ruptures, it may give rise to flame-shaped hemorrhages if in the superficial layers of the retina, or to 'dot and blot' hemorrhages in the deeper layers. The 'dot and blot' hemorrhages might be difficult to distinguish from microaneurysms just by using the ophthalmoscope.
- ◆ Exudation of fluid rich in lipids and protein causes hard exudates to form. These have a bright yellow-white color with an irregular outline and a sharply defined margin.
- ◆ In more advanced stages of NPDR, cotton-wool spots, venous beading and loops, and IRMAs can be seen. These features are associated with a high risk of progression to PDR and are sometimes termed preproliferative retinopathy.
  - ◇ Cotton-wool spots (also called soft exudates) appear as gray or white fluffy-looking lesions in the nerve fiber layer of the retina that result from nerve fiber infarction, and are also a feature of hypertensive retinopathy.
  - ◇ Venous beading denotes sluggish circulation in the retina.
  - ◇ IRMAs are dilated capillaries shunting blood through nonperfused areas.

Proliferative diabetic retinopathy

- ◆ In PDR, new blood vessels grow on the retinal surface in response to growth factors released from ischemic areas. These new vessels are fragile and bleed easily, so PDR is characterized by neovascularization, vitreous hemorrhage (Figure 8.5), or retinal detachment.
  - ◇ The neovascularization often arises from retinal veins, and may be seen on or near the optic disc (NVD) or elsewhere (NVE). New vessels either are superficial on the retina or grow forward into the vitreous.
  - ◇ Hemorrhages can be preretinal or vitreous. A vitreous hemorrhage can cause loss of vision. Ophthalmoscopy shows a featureless, gray haze. Partial recovery of vision is the rule as the blood is reabsorbed, but repeat bleeding may occur.
  - ◇ Fibrous proliferation associated with new vessel formation can distort the retina and the vision. Such changes may give rise to traction bands that contract, producing retinal detachment.

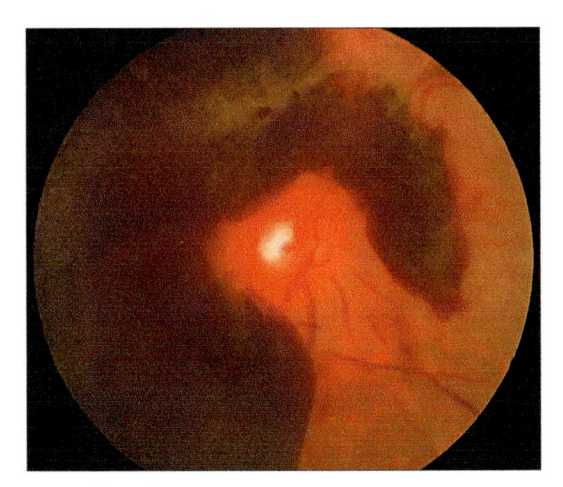

Figure 8.5 Vitreous hemorrhage. If vitreous hemorrhage is associated with visible neovascularization, this is considered high-risk PDR and would require panretinal photocoagulation. *Courtesy Rishi P. Singh, Cole Eye Institute, Cleveland Clinic.*

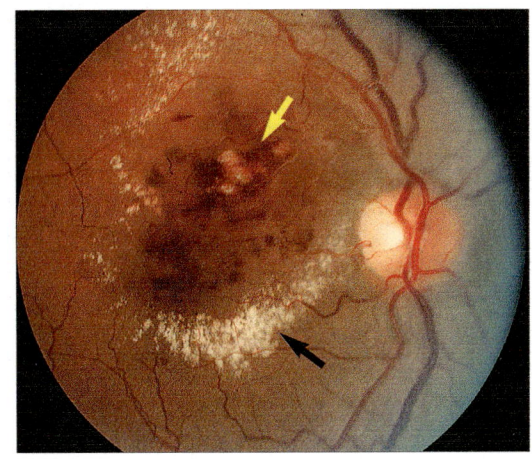

Figure 8.6 Maculopathy. Retinal fundus photograph showing exudates (black arrow), hemorrhage (yellow arrow), and edema in the area of the macula. *Courtesy Rishi P. Singh, Cole Eye Institute, Cleveland Clinic.*

Diabetic maculopathy

- Maculopathy is retinal damage concentrated at the macula, which can threaten central vision. It is a particular characteristic of type 2 diabetes.
- There are three types of maculopathy:
  ◇ Exudative.
  ◇ Edematous.
  ◇ Ischemic.
- Of these types, edematous may be difficult to visualize with direct ophthalmoscopy and ischemic is the least responsive to laser therapy.
- Macular edema (Figure 8.6) is the first feature of maculopathy and may in itself cause permanent macular damage, if not treated early. It can result in deterioration of visual acuity – especially if the fovea centralis is involved – even in the absence of significant findings by ophthalmoscopy, since retinal thickening is not easily detected by this method.
  ◇ Diabetic macular edema can be seen in any level of diabetic retinopathy.
- It is essential to screen diabetes patients regularly for changes in visual acuity.

Cataracts

- Cataract is characterized by a gradual clouding of the lens; senile cataracts are the most common form. Cataracts are 60% more common in diabetic than in nondiabetic patients.
- Cataracts result in reduced visual acuity that cannot be improved by viewing through a pinhole. In the early stages they are usually asymptomatic, but if left untreated can cause blindness.
- Myotonic dystrophy and steroid therapy, which are associated with increased risk of diabetes, are in turn associated with cataracts.
- Juvenile or 'snowflake' cataracts are rare (about 1%), diffuse, rapidly progressive cataracts associated with very poorly controlled diabetes and amenable to surgery.
- Posterior subcapsular cataracts are more common in diabetic than nondiabetic patients.
- It is thought that with hyperglycemia, glucose in the aqueous humor enters the lens cells, is converted to sorbitol, and leads to osmotic swelling.

Glaucoma

- Neovascularization of the iris that can lead to neovascular glaucoma is a potentially serious ophthalmological complication in diabetes. New iris vessels form at the pupillary border, then progress into the angle of the anterior chamber.
- Neovascular glaucoma occurs when there is closure of the angle by the fibrovascular structures.
- Diabetes is the second leading cause of neovascular glaucoma.

Ocular nerve palsies

- Third nerve palsies are the most common cranial neuropathy in diabetes. Pupillary sparing is characteristic in diabetes, with preservation of the pupillary reflexes.
- External ocular palsies of the sixth nerve can also occur.
- Like other causes of mononeuritis, these palsies are acute and transient, almost always resolving within 2 years and usually within 4 months.
  - Some 10% are bilateral or multiple and they can recur.

Treatment and management

- Medical treatment to limit diabetic eye disease development or progression involves aggressive treatment of blood glucose and blood pressure levels.
- In the DCCT, type 1 diabetic patients who were in the intensive glycemic control group had a 76% reduction in the rate of development of any retinopathy in those who did not have retinopathy at baseline (primary prevention cohort) and a 54% reduction in progression in those with established retinopathy (secondary intervention cohort) compared with the conventional treatment group.
- The benefit of tight glycemic control has been demonstrated for type 2 diabetes as well.
  - In the UKPDS, there was a 21% reduction in the 1-year rate of progression of retinopathy.
- There is currently no specific medical treatment for diabetic retinopathy.
  - Based on the Early Treatment Diabetic Retinopathy Study (ETDRS), aspirin treatment does not alter the progression of retinopathy.
  - Smoking worsens the rate of retinopathy progression.
  - Some evidence suggests that ACEIs are of particular value in hypertension and the threshold for introduction of these agents should be low.
  - Intravitreal anti-vascular endothelial growth factor (anti-VEGF) injections have proved valuable in clinically significant macular edema.
- Development or progression of retinopathy may be accelerated by a sudden, rapid improvement in glycemic control, pregnancy, and in those with nephropathy; these groups need frequent monitoring. The glucagon-like receptor-1 analogue, Semaglutide, has been associated with a progression of retinopathy, possibly due to rapid improvement in glucose control.
- All patients with retinopathy should be examined regularly by an ophthalmologist. The ophthalmologist may perform fluorescein angiography to define the extent of the problem.
- Early referral is essential in the following circumstances:
  - Deteriorating visual acuity.
  - Hard exudates encroaching on the macula.
  - Preproliferative changes (cotton-wool spots or venous beading).
  - New vessel formation.
  - Acute vitreous hemorrhage.
- Maculopathy and proliferative retinopathy are often treatable by retinal laser

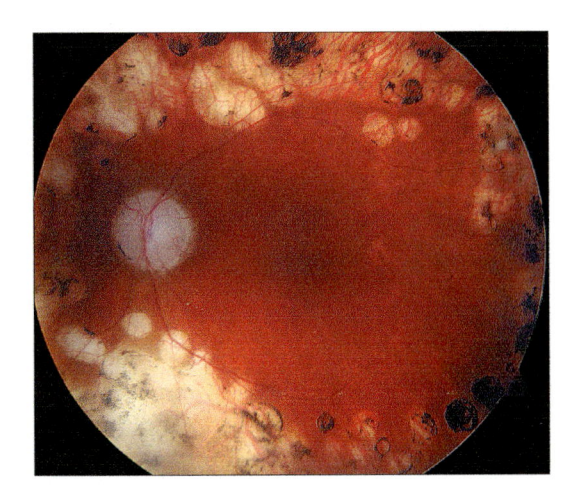

Figure 8.7 Laser treatment. Retinal fundus photograph of laser photocoagulation for proliferative diabetic retinopathy. *Courtesy Rishi P. Singh, Cole Eye Institute, Cleveland Clinic.*

photocoagulation (Figure 8.7); in the latter condition, early effective therapy reduces the risk of visual loss by about 50%. Treatment of NVD is particularly successful using panretinal photocoagulation.
- Vitrectomy surgery can be performed to try to salvage vision after vitreous hemorrhage and to treat traction-induced retinal detachment.
- Vascular endothelial growth factor (VEGF) is a potent driver of vascular proliferation. Anti-VEGF drugs (aflibercept, bevacizumab) cause regression of proliferative retinopathy, and studies show that anti-VEGF is as good as laser photocoagulation for PDR. In vitreous hemorrhage where laser photocoagulation cannot be undertaken, anti-VEGF treatment may delay or reduce the need for vitrectomy.
- Visual aids should be considered for all patients with reduced vision. These include insulin injection pens, talking glucose meters, powerful illumination, magnifying glasses, audiobooks, and guide dogs. Support systems for the visually impaired can be contacted, including charitable organizations and occupational therapy centers.

Sudden improvement in glucose levels can accelerate retinopathy.

Diabetic maculopathy
- Patients should be referred to a specialist if there is an unexplained change in visual acuity or hard exudates within two disc diameters of visual fixation.
- Patients with clinically significant macular edema may benefit from focal laser photocoagulation.
- The efficacy and safety of intravitreal anti-VEGF as therapy for diabetic macular edema has been shown in a number of clinical trials to be sight saving. Indeed for diabetic macular edema, anti-VEGF therapy offers the best chance of improving visual acuity.

Cataracts
- In the UKPDS, intensive glycemic control was associated with a 34% reduction in cataract extraction compared to conventional treatment.
- The patient should be referred to a specialist for cataract removal when loss of vision interferes with their daily life.
- Cataract surgery with intraocular lens implantation is successful 90–95% of the time in restoring vision.
- Patients should be carefully selected since there are potential complications in diabetic patients.
  ◇ After cataract surgery in diabetic patients, there is an increased incidence of neovascularization of the iris and of neovascular glaucoma.
  ◇ In the presence of active proliferative retinopathy, care must be exercised given the risk of deterioration of the retinopathy. In this instance, laser therapy may have to be given concurrently.

Glaucoma

◆ The treatment of neovascularization of the iris and neovascular glaucoma may include a combination of the following: photocoagulation, topical and systemic antiglaucoma drugs, topical steroids, topical atropine, filtration surgery.

All patients with retinopathy should have a regular ophthalmic examination.

CHAPTER 9

Diabetic kidney disease

Overview

- The kidney can be damaged by diabetes in three main ways:
  - Glomerular damage.
  - Ischemia resulting from hypertrophy of afferent and efferent arterioles.
  - Ascending infection.
- Clinically significant nephropathy usually appears between 15 and 25 years after diagnosis and rarely develops >30 years from diagnosis.
- Nephropathy affects 25–35% of patients diagnosed under the age of 30, but recent data suggests this percentage is falling. It is the main cause of end stage renal disease (ESRD) in Europe, accounting for more than 30% (40% in the US) of new renal replacement therapy.
  - Some ethnic groups, such as Native Americans, African Americans, and South Asians are at particular risk.
- Patients with type 2 diabetes develop nephropathy less frequently than those with type 1 diabetes, however more than 80% of patients with diabetes who do need renal replacement in the US have type 2 diabetes, since this is much more prevalent than type 1.
- Both proteinuria and diabetic nephropathy are associated with an increased risk of developing macrovascular disease.
- There is a strong genetic effect predisposing to nephropathy.

Albuminuria is a marker of cardiovascular risk.

Natural history

- The progression of diabetic nephropathy toward end-stage renal failure proceeds through five stages.
  - Stage 1: Functional changes.
  - Stage 2: Structural changes.
  - Stage 3: Microalbuminuria.
  - Stage 4: Overt clinical nephropathy (macroalbuminuria).
  - Stage 5: End-stage renal disease.
- After initial microalbuminuria, intraglomerular pressure is raised and subsequently, frank proteinuria develops with renal dysfunction (Figure 9.1).
- Diabetic nephropathy does not become symptomatic until renal dysfunction is severe.

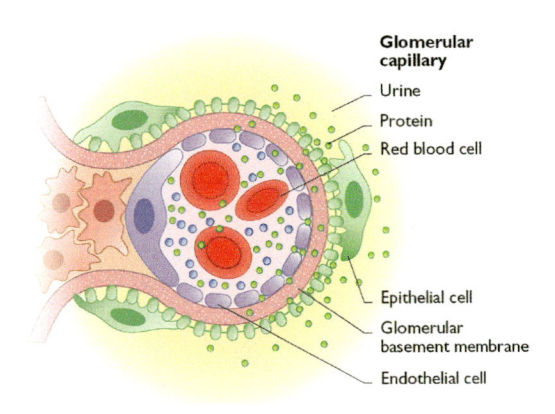

Figure 9.1 Albuminuria. Thickening of the basement membrane is the earliest detectable glomerular change. Damage to this membrane and adjacent capillary wall cells permits leakage of proteins into the urine.

DOI: 10.1201/9781003240341-9

Stage 1: Functional changes

- Glomerular filtration rate (GFR) is increased (hyperfiltration), due to an increase in intraglomerular pressure and in glomerular capillary surface area.
- The increase in GFR is related to the degree of hyperglycemia, and GFR usually falls as blood glucose levels improve, though it remains elevated in a proportion of patients.
- Serum creatinine is usually normal or decreased in this stage of hyperfiltration.

Stage 2: Structural changes

- Initially, the glomerular basement membrane is thickened. Afferent arteriolar vasodilatation leads to intraglomerular hypertension.
- Intraglomerular hypertension damages the glomerular capillaries. Increased intraglomerular pressure causes shearing forces, which results in increased secretion of extracellular mesangial matrix material (Figure 9.2). This process leads to glomerular hypertrophy, then glomerulosclerosis.

Stage 3: Microalbuminuria

- This is the earliest clinically detectable stage of diabetic nephropathy, and is sometimes called the stage of incipient nephropathy.
- Disruption of protein cross-linkages alters the glomerular filter, with progressive leakage of large molecules into the urine (Figure 9.3).
  - Small quantities of albumin can be detected in the urine and can be estimated on a 24-h sample or more practically as an albumin/creatinine ratio from the first-voided urine sample (Table 9.1).

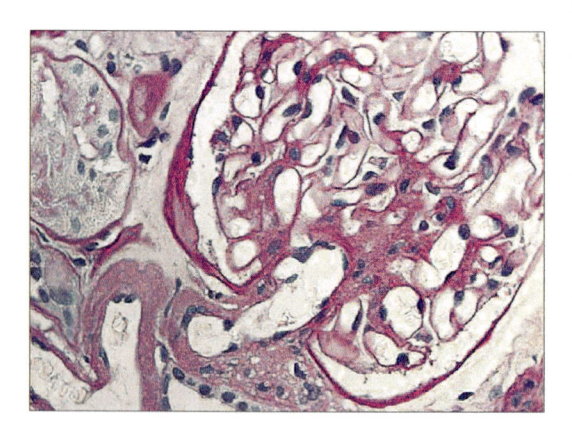

Figure 9.2 Early changes of diabetic nephropathy. There is mesangial expansion (pink-stained region), accompanied by basement membrane thickening. *Courtesy Barts Health NHS Trust.*

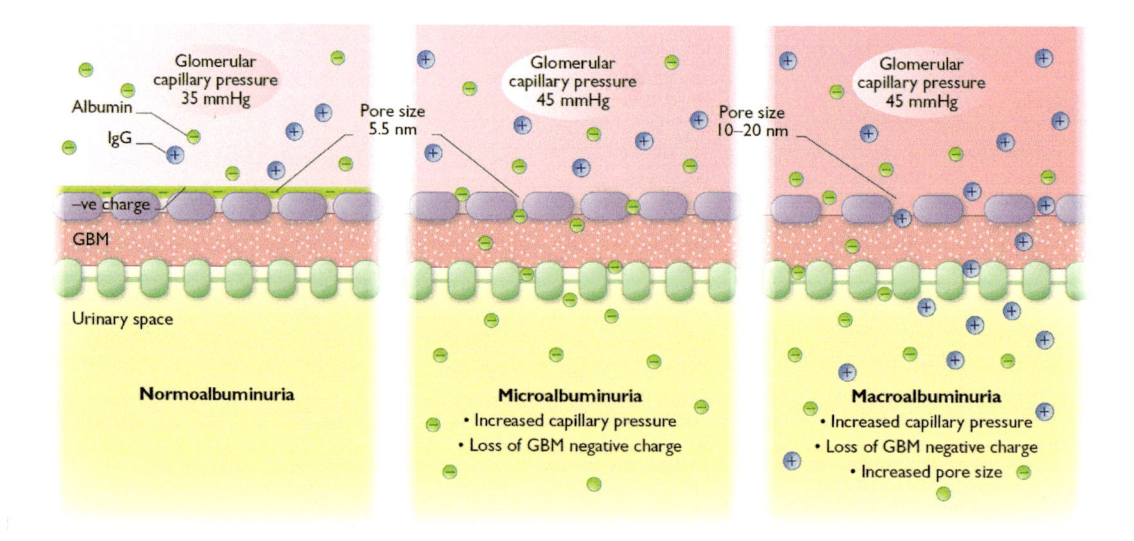

Figure 9.3 Glomerular particle filtration. Rising glomerular pressure leads to loss of the negative charge on the glomerular basement membrane (GBM) and increases pore sizes. This consequently enables passage of plasma proteins, such as albumin and IgG, which is normally restricted.

Table 9.1 Definition of microalbuminuria. Microalbuminuria is defined as the excretion of between 30 and 300 mg of albumin a day in the urine.

Values for albuminuria				
	URINE ALBUMIN CREATININE RATIO (ACR) (MG/MMOL)	URINE ALBUMIN CREATININE RATIO (ACR) (MG/G)	24 HOUR URINE (MG/24HRS)	TIMED URINE COLLECTION (MCG/MIN)
Normal	<3	<30	<30	20
Microalbuminuria	3–30	30–300	30–300	20–200
Macroalbuminuria	>30	>300	>300	>200

- Microalbuminuria may be tested for by radioimmunoassay or by using sensitive dipsticks.
- It is a predictive marker of progression of nephropathy in type 1 diabetes (conferring a 20-fold increased risk of developing overt proteinuria or reduced GFR over 10 years), and less strongly in type 2 diabetes (5-fold increased risk over 10 years).
- It is a marker of macrovascular complications in both type 1 and type 2 diabetes.
- Left untreated, about 80% of type 1 diabetics with sustained microalbuminuria will progress to overt nephropathy in 10–15 years.
- Microalbuminuria worsens with uncontrolled glucose levels, elevated blood pressure, infections of the urinary tract, high protein intake, and exercise. It is therefore recommended to repeat testing for microalbuminuria if the initial test is positive.

Albuminuria is the hallmark of diabetic nephropathy.

Stage 4: Overt clinical nephropathy
- As glomerular filtration falls, blood pressure and serum creatinine rise, and proteinuria increases above 300 mg/day, but not usually to levels associated with nephrotic syndrome.

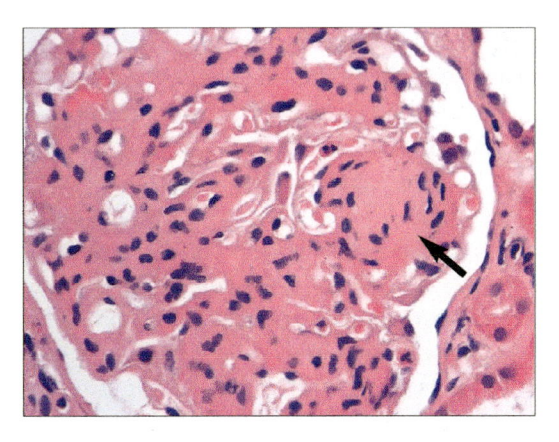

Figure 9.4 Late changes of diabetic glomerulosclerosis. More severe changes are apparent, with nodular lesions (arrow) within the mesangium, characterized by accumulation of homogeneous eosinophilic material (rounded acellular masses known as Kimmelstiel-Wilson nodes). *Courtesy Barts Health NHS Trust.*

- When overt nephropathy is left unattended in type 1 diabetes, GFR falls and end-stage renal disease (ESRD) develops in 50% of patients in 10 years, and about 75% in 20 years.
- Light-microscopic changes of glomerulosclerosis become manifest, both diffuse and nodular; the latter is known as the Kimmelstiel-Wilson lesion (Figure 9.4).

Stage 5: End-stage renal disease
- Patients with ESRD typically show:
  ◇ Raised BUN.
  ◇ Raised creatinine.

- Decreased creatinine clearance.
- Anemia (normochromic normocytic).
- Altered calcium metabolism (low calcium, high phosphate).
- Dyslipidemia.
- Hypertension.
- Symptoms of uremia – anorexia, fatigue, edema, pruritus, breathlessness, pericarditis.

Diagnosis of nephropathy

◆ Albuminuria is the hallmark of diabetic nephropathy.
◆ The urine in all people with diabetes should be checked for the presence of albumin (Figure 9.5).
   ◇ Screening for microalbuminuria is recommended annually for type 1 diabetic patients with diabetes duration of >5 years, and in type 2 patients at the time of diagnosis, since good glycemic control, early antihypertensive treatment, and the use of an ACEI at this stage may delay progression of nephropathy.
◆ Serum creatinine determination for eGFR is also recommended annually.
◆ There is no definitive test to verify that the nephropathy is due to diabetes, so other possible causes should be considered, including myeloma, autoimmune nephritis, and chronic pyelonephritis (Table 9.2).
◆ Patients with diabetes can have renovascular disease leading to renal dysfunction, in which case they may not have proteinuria and are at risk of adverse responses to ACEIs. Renal biopsy might be considered to exclude a nondiabetic cause of nephropathy, but in practice it is rarely necessary.

Table 9.2 Differential diagnosis. There is a range of differentiating tests to exclude nondiabetic kidney disease.

Tests for nondiabetic causes of nephropathy
Urine microscopy for casts (vasculitis), red cells (nephritis), and culture (infection)
Serum protein electrophoresis (monoclonal bands = myeloma), calcium, phosphate, alkaline phosphatase, urate, ESR (raised ESR = myeloma or vasculitis), CRP
Serum for autoantibodies (vasculitis), excluding antinuclear autoantibodies and complement 4 levels
Renal ultrasound (large kidneys = polycystic; small kidneys = chronic pyelonephritis)

Urinary tract infections

◆ Urinary tract infections are more common in diabetes. However, in well-controlled diabetes, some studies have not found a higher risk of infection compared to that in nondiabetic patients.
◆ Infections may develop because of urinary stasis from autonomic neuropathy affecting bladder function or from impaired host defenses.
◆ Once a urinary tract infection develops, the complication rate is higher in diabetic than in nondiabetic patients, including the risk of pyelonephritis.
◆ Untreated infections in diabetic patients can lead to renal papillary necrosis, a rare condition in which renal papillae are shed in the urine. It should be suspected in patients who have fever, flank pain, poor response to antibiotics, and rapidly deteriorating renal function.

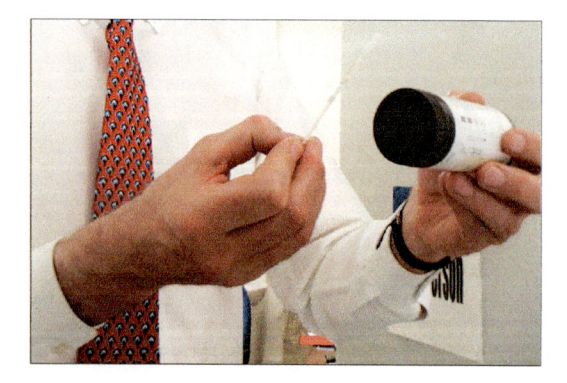

Figure 9.5 Urine strip testing for proteinuria. Persistent proteinuria is the hallmark of diabetic nephropathy; detection of hematuria suggests a different cause, such as menstruation, urinary tract infection, or vasculitis.

Treatment and management

- Management of diabetic nephropathy extends from the management of microalbuminuria to prevent disease progression through to the management of ESRD.

- The management of diabetic nephropathy is similar to that of other causes of chronic kidney disease, with a particular focus on treatment of hypertension (Figure 9.6).

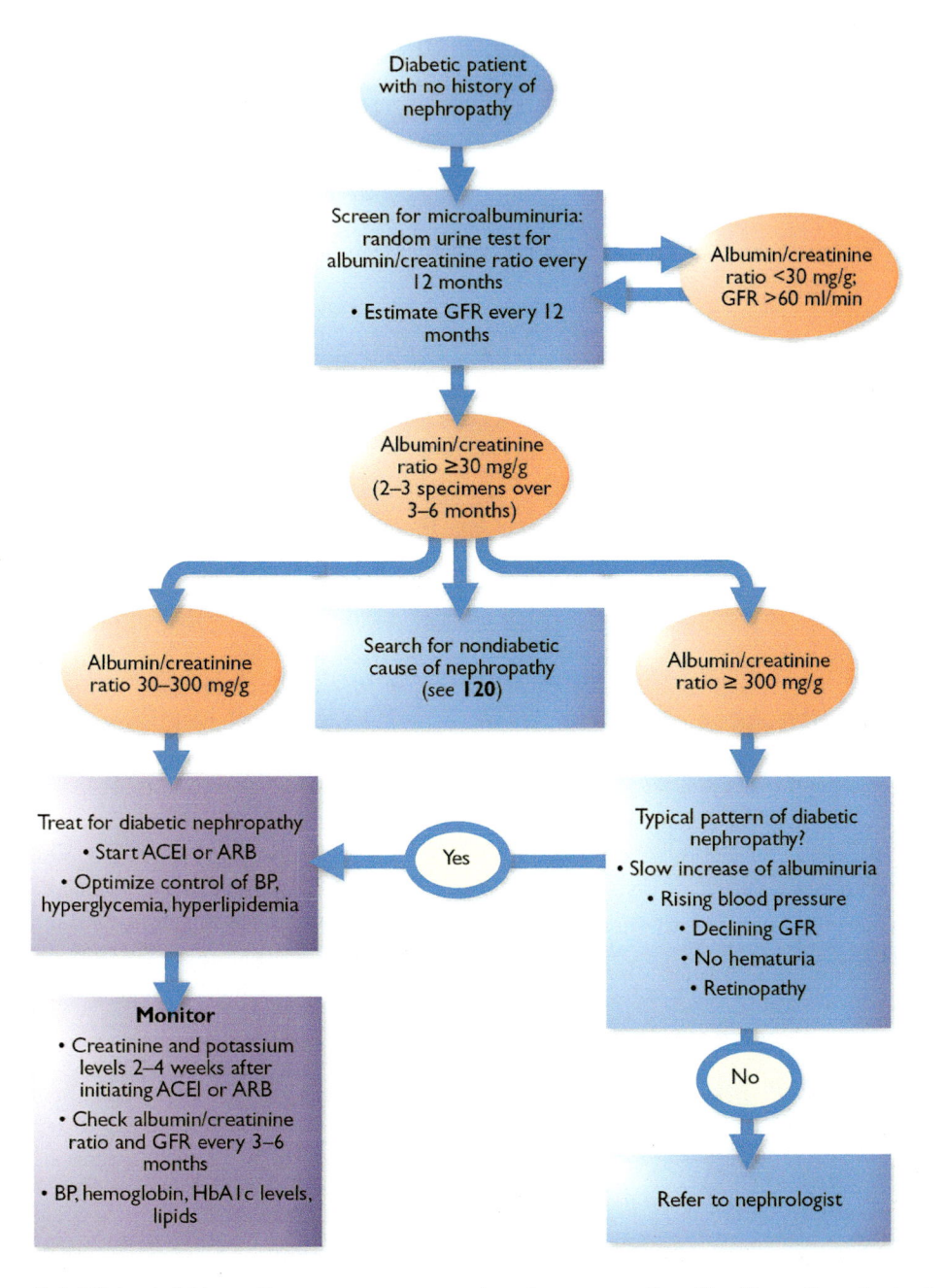

Figure 9.6 Diabetic kidney disease management in primary practice. Algorithm with routes to diagnosis, monitoring, and control. Control of hypertension and hyperglycemia is essential in patients with nephropathy. Angiotensin-converting enzyme inhibitors (ACEIs) and angiotensin-receptor blockers (ARBs) delay the progression of renal disease and have antiproteinuric and renoprotective effects.

◇ Particular attention must be paid to macrovascular risk factors and complications as well as the increased risk of neuropathy and retinopathy in patients with diabetic kidney disease.

Look out for macrovascular risk factors in patients with diabetic renal disease.

General therapy
- Once renal dysfunction has been established therapy should include:
  ◇ Phosphate binders such as calcium carbonate.
  ◇ Vitamin D analogs once serum parathyroid hormone increases.
  ◇ Erythropoietin once hemoglobin falls significantly.
  ◇ Multivitamins.

Blood glucose
- Intensive glucose control is helpful in the earlier stages of renal involvement (Figure 9.7):
  ◇ In the DCCT, intensive glycemic control in type 1 diabetes patients reduced the occurrence of microalbuminuria by 39% and of overt proteinuria by 54% (Figure 9.8).
  ◇ In the UKPDS intensive glycemic control led to a 30% reduction in microalbuminuria risk.

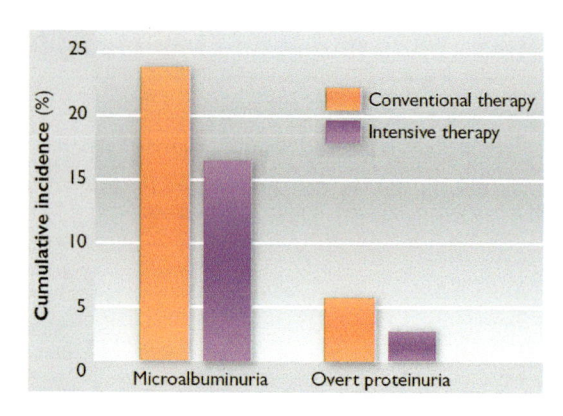

Figure 9.8 Nephropathy event rates. The DCCT showed that stringent glycemic control dramatically reduced the risk of developing diabetic nephropathy.

  ◇ In the Steno-2 study there was a 61% reduction in progression to clinical nephropathy with intervention directed at glucose, lipids, and blood pressure.
- Therapy should aim to achieve an HbA1c of <7.0% (53 mmol/mol) or <6.5% (48 mmol/mol) (in the US) (individualized to the patient), without causing severe hypoglycemia.
- However, the initiation of intensive glucose control after the onset of overt proteinuria or renal insufficiency is often ineffective in preventing progression to ESRD.
- Once eGFR has fallen below 30 mls/min/1.73m2, metformin should not be used, while the dose of other agents should be monitored carefully.

Newer glucose-lowering drugs in diabetic kidney disease

- Cardiovascular outcomes trials (CVOTs) of newer agents in T2D have led to a wealth of cardiovascular and renal outcome data which have informed clinical practice.
- Several studies of SGLT-2i in diabetic kidney disease suggest significant benefit independent of glucose control (Table 9.3).

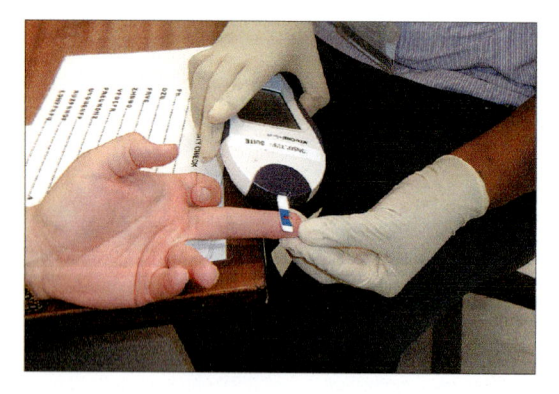

Figure 9.7 Capillary blood glucose measurement. Optimal glycemic control is helpful in the early stages of kidney disease.

Table 9.3 CV and renal outcome studies with SGLT-2i.

Trial Intervention (N) Median Follow Up	Study Population Characteristics — General	Study Population Characteristics — Renal	Cardiovascular Outcomes	Renal Outcomes
Dapagliflozin				
DECLARE TIMI 58 Dapagliflozin 10mg vs placebo N = 17160 4.2 years	T2D (100%) Established CVD (40.6%) CV risk factors (59.4%) ACE-I/ARB (86.7%)	eGFR (ml/min/1.73²) mean 85 ≥90 (47.6%) 60–90 (45.1%) <60 (7.4%) Albuminuria (mg/g) <30 (69.1%) ≥30 - ≤30 (23.9%) >300 (6.9%)	**17% reduction CV death or hHF** (HR 0.83; [0.73–0.95]; p = 0.005) **No effect on MACE** (HR 0.93, [0.84–1.03], p = 0.17) No significant difference in CV death, death from any cause	**47% RRR in the renal composite ∑** (HR 0.53; [0.43–0.66]; P < 0.0001) **59% RRR in risk of ESKD or renal death** (HR 0.41; [0.20–0.82]; p = 0.012) **Reduced eGFR decline at 3.4 years**
DAPA-CKD Dapagliflozin 10mg vs placebo N = 4304 2.4 years	T2D (67.5%) Established CVD (37%) Nearly all patients on an ACE-I/ARB	eGFR (ml/min/1.73²) mean eGFR 43.1 ≥60 (10%) 45 - <60 (31%) 30 - <45 (44.1%) <30 (14.5%) Albuminuria (mg/g) Range 200–5000 >1000 (48.3%) Mean/median 949	**29% reduction in the composite of death from CV causes or hHF** (HR 0.71; [0.55–0.92]; p = 0.009) **31% reduction in death from any cause** (HR 0.69; 0.53–0.88 p = 0.004)	**44% reduction in the renal composite ±** (HR 0.56; [0.45–0.68]; p <0.001)
DAPA-HF N = 4644 18.2 months	T2D (45%) NYHA 2,3,4, EF ≤40% Majority of patients on ACE-I/ARB	eGFR (ml/min/1.73²) eGFR >30 Mean 66 <60 (40.6%)	25% reduction in CV death or hHF HR 0.75, [0.65–0.85] p <0.001) 17% reduction in all-cause mortality (HR 0.83; [0.71–0.97])	**39% nonsignificant reduction in worsening renal function ±** (HR = 0.71; [0.44–1.16]; p = 0.17) **Smaller eGFR decline per year** (dapagliflozin -1.09 (−1.41, −0.78) vs. placebo -2.87 (−3.19, −2.55) (p <0.001)

(Continued)

Table 9.3 (Continued)

Trial Intervention (N) Median Follow Up	Study Population Characteristics General	Renal	Cardiovascular Outcomes	Renal Outcomes
Empagliflozin				
EMPA-REG OUTCOME Empagliflozin 10mg/15mg vs placebo 3.1 years N = 7020	T2D (100%) Established CVD (99%) ACE-I/ARB (80.7%)	eGFR (ml/min/1.73²) eGFR>30 Mean 74.1 45–59 (17.8%) 30–44 (7.7%) Albuminuria (mg/g) 30–300 (28.7%) >300 (11%)	14% reduction in 3p-MACE¥ (HR 0.86; [0.74–0.99]) 38% RRR in CV death (HR 0.62; [0.49–0.77]; p <0.001) 35% reduction in hHF (HR 0.65; [0.50–85]; p = 0.002) 32% reduction in death from any cause (HR 0.68; [0.57–0.82]; p <0.001). No effect on MI/stroke	46% reduction in composite renal outcome ≠ (HR 0.54; [0.40–0.75]; p <0.001) 39% reduction in incident or worsening of nephropathy μ (HR 0.61; [0.53–0.70]; p <0.001)
EMPEROR REDUCED Empagliflozin 10mg vs placebo N = 3730 16 months	T2D (50%) EF ≤ 40% EF <30% (73%) >30% (27%) hHF in last 12 months or NT-proBNP of at least 1000 pg per milliliter (79%) Majority on ACEi/ARB	eGFR (ml/min/1.73²) mean 62 eGFR <60 (48%)	25% reduction in hHf or CV death (HR 0.75; [0.65–0.86]; p <0.001)	50% reduction in renal composite § (HR 0.50; [0.32 to 0.77]; significance level not specified)
Canagliflozin				
CANVAS Program (CANVAS and CANVAS-R trials) Canagliflozin 100mg/300mg vs placebo N = 10 142 2.4 years	T2D (100%) Established CVD (65.6%) CV risk factors (34.4%)	eGFR (ml/min/1.73²) Egfr >30 Mean eGFR 76.5 Albuminuria (mg/g) Median 12.3 30–300 (22.6%) >300 (7.6%)	14% reduction in 3p-MACE¥ (HR 0.86; [0.75–0.97]; p = 0.02) No significant difference in CV death, death from any cause	40% reduction in the composite renal outcome∞ (HR 0.60; [0.47–0.77]; p <0.01) 27% reduction in albuminuria progression (HR 0.73; [0.67–0.79]; p <0.001)

Diabetic kidney disease

110

CREDENCE Canagliflozin 100mg Vs placebo N = 4401 2.62 years	T2D (100%) ACE-i/ARB (100%)	**eGFR (ml/min/1.73⁻)** eGFR >30 mean 56.2 **Albuminuria (mg/g)** 300–5000	31% reduction in CV composite× (HR 0.69 [0.57–0.83]; P <0.001) 20% reduction in CV death, MI, stroke (HR 0.80; [0.67–0.95]; p = 0.01)	34% reduction in renal-specific composite≠ (HR 0.66; [0.53–0.81]; p <0.001) 32% reduction in ESRDΩ (HR 0.68 [0.54–0.86]; p = 0.002) 40% reduction in doubling of serum Creatinine (HR 0.60; [0.48–0.76]; p <0.001)
Sotagliflozin				
SCORED trial Sotagliflozin vs Placebo N = 10500 95 days	T2D (100%) CKD and one additional cardiovascular risk factor RAAS inhibitor (88%)	**eGFR (ml/min/173²)** median 44.5 <30 (7%) 30–45 (44%) ≥45 (48%) **Albuminuria (mg/g)** Median 74 <30 (35%) 30 to <300 (33%) ≥300 (32%)	26% reduction in CV deaths, hHF, urgent HF visits (HR 0.74; [0.63–0.88], p = 0.0004)	29% reduction in renal composite ϴ (HR 0.71; [0.46–1.08]; significance level not specified)
Ertugliflozin				
VERTIS-CV Ertugliflozin 5mg/15mg vs placebo N = 8,246 3.5 years	T2D (100%) Established ASCVD Known coronary artery disease: 76%, prior MI: 48%, known CVD: 23%	**eGFR (ml/min/173²)** eGFR >30 Mean 76 60–89 (53%) 30–59 (22%) **Albuminuria (mg/g)** <30 (60%) >30 (40%)	3% reduction in 3p-MACE (HR 0.97 [0.85–1.11]; p <0.001)	19% reduction in renal composite ≠ (HR 0.81; [0.63–1.04]; P = 0.08)

∑ **Renal composite**: eGFR decline of more/equal 40% to less 60 ml/min/1.73 m2, ESKD (dialysis for >90 days, kidney transplantation or confirmed sustained eGFR<15 ml/min/1.73 m² or death from renal causes

± **Worsening renal function**: eGFR decline of ≥50%, ESKD, or death from renal causes

μ **Worsening/incident nephropathy**: Progression to severely increased ACR, doubling of serum creatinine and an eGFR <45 ml/min/1.73 m2, initiation of RRT or death from renal disease)

¥ **3p-MACE**: non-fatal MI, non-fatal stroke, death from CV causes

∞ **Renal composite**: sustained 40% reduction in eGFR, the need for RRT or death from renal causes

× **Cardiovascular composite**: CV death or hospitalization for heart failure

≠ **Renal specific composite**: ESRD, doubling of creatinine, death from renal causes

Ω **ESRD**: Chronic dialysis for >30 days, kidney transplantation, eGFR<15ml/min/1.73m² sustained for >30 days

§ **Renal composite**: RRT, transplant, sustained eGFR reduction of 40% or more, eGFR<15ml/min/1.73 m2 in per 1.73 m².

ϴ **Renal composite**: ≥50% decrease in eGFR, RRT, renal transplantation, sustained eGFR <15 ml/min/1.73 for ≥30 days

Diabetic kidney disease

- ◇ Specific renal outcomes with canagliflozin in patients with T2D were examined in the CREDENCE study. 4401 patients had albuminuric CKD (mean eGFR 56.2 ml/min/1.73m^2), and included patients with eGFR ≥30 ml/min/1.73m^2. Median ACR was 927 mg/g. Canagliflozin was associated with a 34% reduction in the renal specific composite (doubling of baseline creatinine, ESRD, or death from renal causes). Canagliflozin reduced 3p-MACE by 20% and hHF by 39%. The numbers needed to treat (NNT) to prevent one case of doubling of serum creatinine, ESRD, or death from renal or cardiovascular cause was 21.
- ◇ Meta-analysis confirms favorable effects of SGLT2i on the renal composite of doubling of serum creatinine (eGFR 40% decline), renal replacement therapy initiation, or renal-related death. The pooled NNT for renal outcomes was 67. SGLT2i also reduce albuminuria progression, and the benefits are present across all stages of CKD, irrespective of baseline albuminuria. The effects appear to be strongest among those patients with albuminuria, and the effect is additive to ACEI or ARB use.
- ◇ Current UK and US licensing allows canagliflozin initiation in patients with type 2 diabetes with eGFR >30 ml/min/1.73m^2, and can be continued in eGFR <30 ml/min/1.73m2 in the presence of albuminuria >300 mg/day, unless dialysis is initiated.
- ◇ ADA-EASD consensus guidelines recommend that SGLT2i can be used in any patient with T2D with HF or CKD.
- ◇ In contrast to ACEI/ARBs, renoprotective effects of SGLT-2i are thought to be mediated by tubuloglomerular feedback, natriuresis, and glucose-induced osmotic diuresis, which reduce intraglomerular pressure.

- ◆ Studies of GLP-1RAs in DKD are shown in (Table 9.4).
  - ◇ GLP-1RAs have shown promising results in CVOTs. Meta-analysis of the seven large GLP-1 trials of 56,004 patients, showed a 12% reduction in 3p-MACE. Composite renal outcome was reduced by 17% for all GLP1-RA, mainly due to a reduction in new macroalbuminuria.
  - ◇ These nephroprotective properties of GLP-1RAs have been linked to their direct actions on blood pressure, glucose, and weight, but also to improving endothelial dysfunction and inflammation. They may cause an initial eGFR reduction upon administration, with subsequent plateauing. Human GLP-1RAs are approved for use at eGFR ≥ 15mL/min/1.73m^2.

Blood pressure
- ◆ Tight control and aggressive treatment of blood pressure (target 130/80 mmHg) reduce the rate of progression to renal failure (Figure 9.9).
- ◆ In patients with nephropathy, it can be argued that ACEIs and ARBs are preferred.
- ◆ ACEIs are specifically indicated in type 1 diabetes where there is any degree of albuminuria (with or without hypertension).
- ◆ ARBs have a role when there is intolerance to ACEIs, and are the drug class recommended in patients with type 2 diabetes, hypertension, and any degree of albuminuria.
  - ◇ In type 2 diabetes with hypertension and nephropathy, ARBs prevented the progression of microalbuminuria to overt nephropathy in the Irbesartan in Patients with Type 2 Diabetes and Microalbuminuria (IRMA-2) study (Figure 9.10).
  - ◇ ARBs also reduced the incidence of doubling of serum creatinine and the risk of developing ESRD in those who had later stages of nephropathy in the Irbesartan Type 2 Diabetic

Table 9.4 Studies of GLP-1RAs in DKD.

Study	LEADER	AWARD-7	REWIND	SUSTAIN-6	PIONEER-5
Drugs studied	Liraglutide vs Placebo	Dulaglutide 0.75-1.5mg vs Insulin Glargine	Dulaglutide 1.5mg vs Placebo	Subcutaneous Semaglutide vs Placebo	Oral Semaglutide vs Placebo
Characteristics	N = 9340 64% male Mean age: 64	N = 577 52% male Mean age: 65	N = 9901	N = 3297 61% male Mean age: 65	N = 3183 Age >50
	72.4% established CVD Mean HbA1c 8.7% (72 mol/mol) Mean BP 167/77 mmHg Mean eGFR 80 20.7% eGFR 30-59 2.4% eGFR < 30 26.3% UACR>30 mg/g 10.5% UACR >300 mg/g	Mean HbA1c 7.5-10.5% Mean BP 137/75mmHg Mean eGFR 38 26% eGFR 45-60 35% eGFR 30-45 31% eGFR <30 29% UACR >30 mg/g 46% UACR >300 mg/g	CVD or risk factors mean eGFR 76.9 7.9% UACR >30 mg/g	83% established CVD, CKD, or both 17% CV risk factors Mean HbA1c 8.7% Mean BP 136/77 mmHg CKD stage 3-5 25.2% eGFR 30-59 2.9% eGFR ≤30 12.7% UACR >300 mg/g	Established CVD or CKD and >50 CV risk factors and >60 26.9% eGFR <60
ACE/ARB	82%	90-94%		83.5%	
Median Duration	3.84 years	52 weeks	5.4 years	2.1 years	15.9 months
Outcome	**22% lower composite renal outcome** (new onset macroalbuminuria, doubling serum creatinine, eGFR <45, need for RRT or renal death) (HR 0.78; [0.67-0.92]; p =0.003) **26% reduction in new macroalbuminuria** (HR 0.74; [0.60-0.91] p = 0.004) No statistically significant reduction to the composite of the doubling of the serum creatinine level, use of RRT or death from renal disease 13% lower new microalbuminuria (HR 0.87; [0.83-0.93]; p <0.001)	eGFR decline (ml/min) -3.3 insulin glargine -0.7 dulaglutide 0.75mg ✱ -0.7 dulaglutide 1.5mg ✱ eGFR decline (ml/min) in UACR >300 mg/g group -5.5 insulin glargine -0.7 dulaglutide 0.75mg -0.5 dulaglutide 1.5mg ✱ **UACR reduction** -13% insulin glargine -12.3% dulaglutide 0.75mg -29% dulaglutide 1.5mg ✱ ✱ p <0.05 (vs insulin glargine)	**15% lower composite renal outcome** (new macroalbuminuria, eGFR reduction of 30% or more from baseline, need for RRT) (HR 0.85; [0.77-0.93]; p=0.0004) **23% reduction in new macroalbuminuria** (HR 0.77; [0.68-0.87]; p = 0.0001) No statistically significant reduction to the composite of sustained eGFR reduction of 30% and RRT.	**36% lower new or worsening nephropathy** (new macroalbuminuria (urinary ACR >300 mg/g), doubling serum creatinine, eGFR <45 ml/min/1.73, need for RTT or renal death) (HR 0.64; [0.46-0.88]; p = 0.005) **46% reduction in new macroalbuminuria with semaglutide** (HR 0.54; [0.34-0.77]; p = 0.001) UACR reduction 0.75; 0.66-0.85 (semaglutide 0.5 mg) 0.66; 0.58-0.75 (semaglutide 1·0 mg) Lower 3p-MACE (HR 0.74; [0.58-0.95]) Lower rate of nonfatal MI (HR 0.74;[0.51-1.08]) Lower rate of nonfatal stroke (HR 0.61; [0.38-0.99]) No significant difference in CV deaths, hHF	Non inferior to placebo for 3p-MACE No composite renal outcome pre-specified No significant difference in eGFR reduction and renal death

Diabetic kidney disease

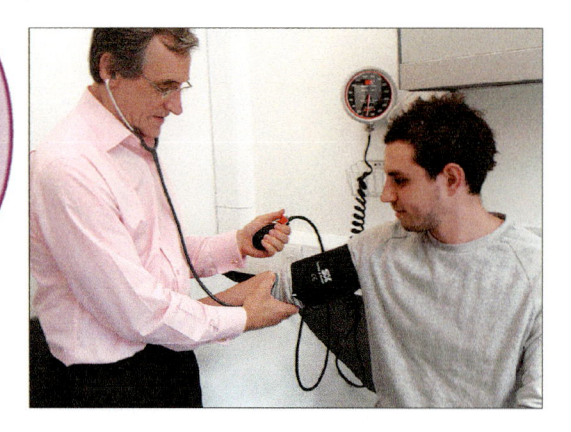

Figure 9.9 Blood pressure measurement. Control of hypertension reduces the rate of progession to renal failure.

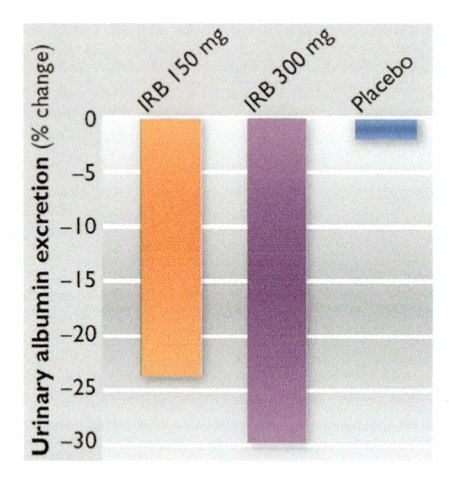

Figure 9.10 Irbesartan in patients with diabetes and microalbuminuria. The IRMA-2 study showed that patients receiving daily irbesartan were significantly less likely to develop diabetic nephropathy than those in the placebo group.

Nephropathy Trial (IDNT) and Reduction of Endpoints in NIDDM with the Angiotensin II Antagonist Losartan (RENAAL) trial.
- Combining ACEIs with calcium-channel blockers or thiazide diuretics may provide superior blood pressure control. Combining ACEI and ARBs, however, results in poorer renal outcomes and a high risk of hyperkalemia.
- Loop diuretics may be used in preference to thiazides once nephropathy is established, usually around a serum creatinine of 160 μmol/L (1.8 mg/dL).

- Combination therapy is usually required to achieve the blood pressure target.
- Beta-adrenoreceptor blockers should be considered in all patients with coronary artery disease and in patients after a myocardial infarction, since these agents improve survival.
  ◇ The beta-blocker atenolol reduced microvascular complications in diabetic patients in the UKPDS.
  ◇ However, beta-blockers are third-line treatment in the management of hypertension in diabetes – certainly for type 2 diabetes. For example, losartan reduced cardiovascular mortality more than did atenolol in patients with diabetes and hypertension in the Losartan Intervention for Endpoint Reduction (LIFE) study (adjusted risk reduction of 13% after 66 months).
  ◇ Care should be taken in patients on insulin therapy as beta-adrenergic blocking agents may mask some epinephrine-induced symptoms of hypoglycemia, though sweating may be more pronounced.
- Aldosterone receptor antagonists – a study of the aldosterone receptor antagonist, finerenone, in 5734 patients with T2D and CKD – showed some positive benefits.
  ◇ Patients included had eGFR 25–60 mls/min/1.73m2, and urine ACR 30–300 mg/g, and maximum tolerated ARB or ACEI therapy.
  ◇ The primary composite outcome was kidney failure, a sustained decrease of at least 40% in the eGFR from baseline, or death from renal causes was reduced by 18% in the finerenone group. Hyperkalemia necessitating cessation of finerenone occurred in 2.3% of patients treated.

Lipids
- Once proteinuria is established, the risk of macrovascular disease is sufficient to warrant use of statins, if the patient is

not already on them. Even if the usual picture of dyslipidemia in diabetes is that of hypertriglyceridemia, low HDL-cholesterol, and LDL-cholesterol that is within normal levels, elevated LDL-cholesterol is common in patients with marked proteinuria.
- Mortality in patients with ESRD is usually due to cardiovascular disease.
- Treatment with statins at high dose (or less commonly statins with fibrates) is often needed to achieve targets: LDL-cholesterol <2.59 mmol/L (100 mg/dL), triglycerides <1.7 mmol/L (150 mg/dL), and HDL-cholesterol to 1.17 mmol/L (45 mg/dL).
- The risk of myositis is increased in renal impairment when calcineurin inhibitors with statins or fibrates are used.

Smoking
- Smoking predisposes to diabetic nephropathy and should be particularly avoided once nephropathy is established due to the risk of macrovascular disease.

Protein restriction
- A reduction in protein intake may reduce hyperfiltration, intraglomerular pressure, and proteinuria.
- Earlier studies showed that very low-protein diets slowed the decline in GFR, however, with the advent of antihypertensive and renoprotective agents such as ACEIs, protein restriction is probably ineffective.

Renal replacement therapy

- Once the creatinine rises, in association with deteriorating creatinine clearance and GFR, referral to renal physicians is appropriate, and renal replacement should be considered, especially if symptoms develop.
- Plotting the inverse of creatinine against time gives an indication as to the rate of progression of renal dysfunction so that renal replacement can be planned in advance (Figure 9.11).
- There are three forms of renal replacement:
  ◇ Continuous ambulatory peritoneal dialysis (CAPD).
  ◇ Hemodialysis.
  ◇ Transplantation.

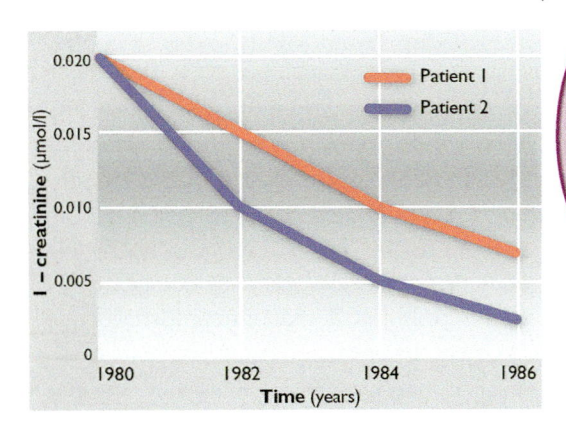

Figure 9.11 Progression of renal dysfunction. Once GFR has fallen by 50% or more, serum creatinine begins to increase. Plots of inverse creatinine against time in two type 1 diabetes patients, each 15 years from diagnosis, with persistent proteinuria, show a linear decline at a consistent rate for each patient.

In 2018, 785,883 Americans had kidney failure and needed dialysis or a kidney transplant to survive. 247,000 people are currently living with kidney failure resulting from diabetes.

Peritoneal dialysis
- Management of ESRD may be made more difficult by the fact that patients often have other complications of diabetes such as blindness, autonomic neuropathy, or peripheral vascular disease. Arteriovenous fistulas tend to calcify rapidly and hence PD may be preferable to hemodialysis. However, in some countries such as the US where many dialysis centers are available, or where there are barriers to

self-care, hemodialysis seems to be the more common modality.
- PD is relatively inexpensive compared with hemodialysis and avoids fluctuations in intravascular volume, a problem seen in patients with cardiac disease or autonomic neuropathy. Vascular access is not required.
- This form of dialysis provides greater freedom for the patient compared to hemodialysis.
- The dialysate often contains hypertonic glucose, and since the dialysis is a continuous process, hyperglycemia can be a problem.
- Peritonitis is a complication seen with PD.

Hemodialysis
- Hemodialysis is the renal replacement used in 80% of patients with diabetes with ESRD in the US.
- Hemodialysis requires vascular access, usually via an arteriovenous fistula. Because of problems with calcification and atherosclerosis, a synthetic graft is sometimes needed.
  ◇ Vascular access should be established sooner than in nondiabetic patients since retinopathy, neuropathy, hypertension, and glycemic control become more difficult to manage when diabetic patients have uremia.
  ◇ Once eGFR reaches 20 mls/min/1.73m^2, a rapid decline in kidney function may ensue such that dialysis may be needed in less than a year.
- Hemodialysis is more prone to induce hypotension than is PD.
- Peripheral necrosis of digits can be a particular problem.

Transplantation
- Renal transplant involves obtaining the kidney from a cadaver or, from a living-related or living-unrelated donor.
- Patient survival and quality of life is superior compared to dialysis. In diabetes both patient survival and graft survival are reduced compared with nondiabetic patients.
- Among transplant recipients who do not have diabetes, posttransplant diabetes mellitus (PTDM) is common due to the use of immunosuppression such as corticosteroids and calcineurin inhibitors. PTDM increases risk of graft loss and mortality, and should be actively screened for and treated.
- Assessment of the patient to exclude life-limiting comorbidity, including macrovascular disease, is vital before a transplant is performed.
- Cardiovascular disease is still the most common cause of death in patients who undergo transplantation.
- Graft and patient survival have improved with time for both living-donor and cadaveric transplants, but is still better with living-donor compared with nonexpanded criteria (deceased) donors (non-ECD) and expanded criteria (deceased) donors (ECD) (Figures 9.12 and 9.13).
  ◇ ECD refers to donors with a higher risk of kidney graft failure, such as donors who are over 60 years old, or aged more than 50 years with at least two of the following: hypertension history, serum creatinine >132.6 μmol/L (1.5 mg/dL), or cause of death from cerebrovascular accident.

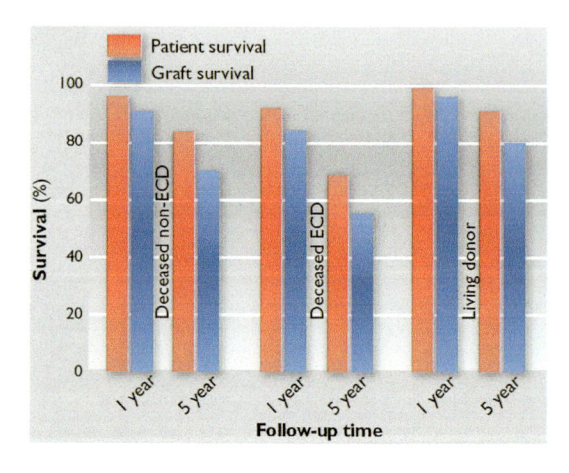

Figure 9.12 Transplant survival. Five-year survival (2002–2007) of both patient and graft was clearly better for recipients of living-donor organs than for those of deceased-donor organs. ECD = expanded criteria donor (i.e. higher failure risk); non-ECD = non-expanded criteria donor.

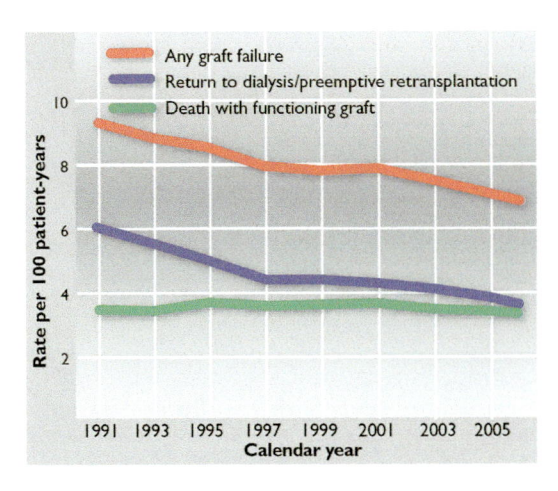

Figure 9.13 Transplant failure rates. These have gradually improved. In the USA, by 2006, there were 6.9 graft failures (including death with function) per 100 patient-years with a functioning transplant.

Pancreas transplant or islet cell implantation

◆ A segmental pancreatic graft is sometimes performed at the same time as a renal graft in patients with type 1 diabetes (simultaneous pancreas and kidney transplant [SPK]). Careful selection of patients is required, but graft survival and insulin independence at 5 years can approach 80% in good centers.

◆ Islet cell transplantation can also be performed around the time of renal transplantation in people with type 1 diabetes, especially if the person has poor hypoglycemia awareness.

These topics are also discussed in Chapter 15.

CHAPTER 10

Skin and musculoskeletal complications of diabetes

Skin manifestations of diabetes

Overview
- There are a number of cutaneous conditions which are associated with diabetes (Table 10.1).
- Some of these are related to the impact of diabetes and others are seen in the setting of medication use.
- The impact of diabetes on the skin occurs through different mechanisms but the most important is the direct and indirect (through advanced glycation end products) impacts on keratinocytes, connective tissue, and the immune system.
- The most common cutaneous manifestations seen with diabetes are noted.

Table 10.1 Most frequent skin disorders seen in type 1 and type 2 diabetes.

Most frequent skin disorders among type 1 and type 2 DM	
TYPE 1 DIABETES MELLITUS	**TYPE 2 DIABETES MELLITUS**
Necrobiosis lipoidica diabeticorum	Generalized granuloma annulare
Diabetic bullae	Scleredema diabeticorum
Vitiligo vulgaris	Diabetic dermopathy
Periungual telangiecstasia	Acathosis nigricans
–	Acrochordons
–	Psoriasis

Conditions seen with insulin resistance
Acanthosis nigricans
- This is one of the most common and well known of the skin manifestations seen with type 2 diabetes, specifically with insulin resistance. It can be seen in up to 74% of adult patients who are obese.
- It is more commonly seen in those with darker skin color.
- Acanthosis nigricans also be seen with malignancies such as gastric adenocarcinoma.
- The underlying cause is likely related to insulin activation of IGF-1 on keratinocytes and fibroblasts.
- Lesions are described as hyperpigmented and velvety, involving the skin folds of the neck, axilla, and groin (Figure 10.1).
- Often weight loss can produce improvement. Medications for diabetes such as metformin have been shown to have benefit.
- Systemic retinoid or topical keratolytics can be utilized to treat.

Diabetic dermopathy
- This is seen in more than 1/3 of patients with diabetes and is most commonly seen in men older than 50 years of age. Usually this is a later manifestation in the disease course so patients often have been affected by one or more of the microvascular complications of diabetes.
- The pathophysiology is unclear at this time.
- Appears as small (<1 cm) hyperpigmented oval atrophic macules on the pretibial

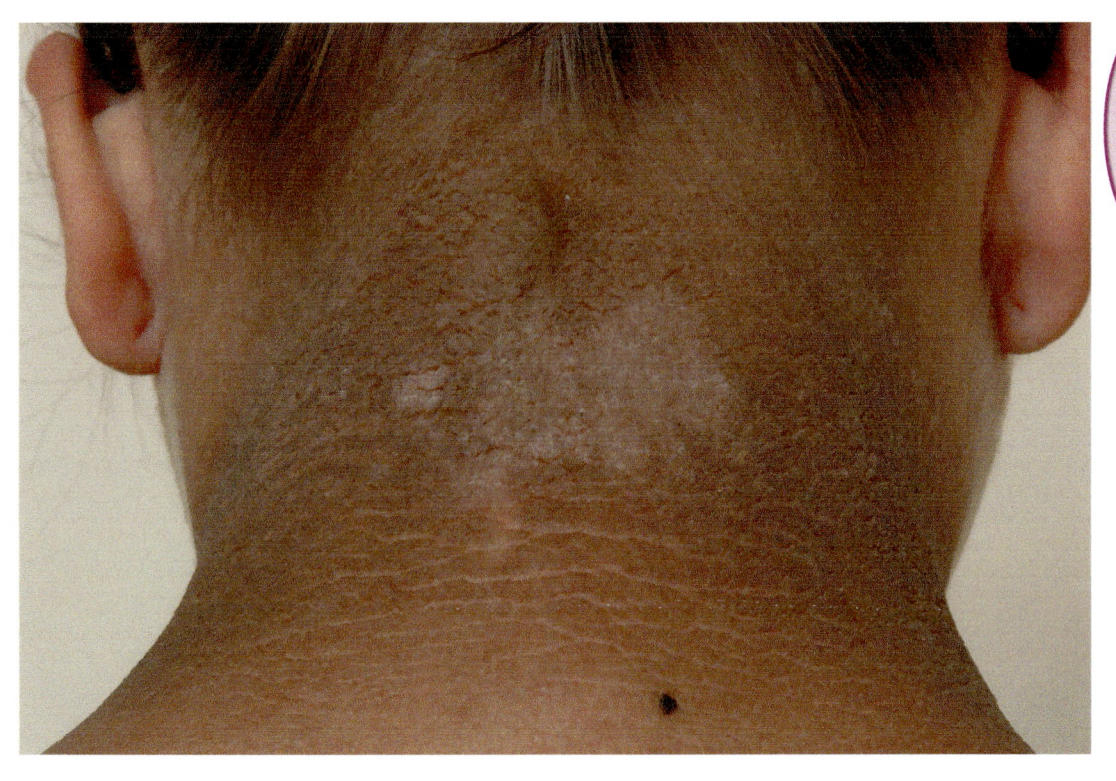

Figure 10.1 Acanthosis nigricans involving the neck. *Courtesy of Dr. Allison Vidimos, Cleveland Clinic, photographer: Janine Sot.*

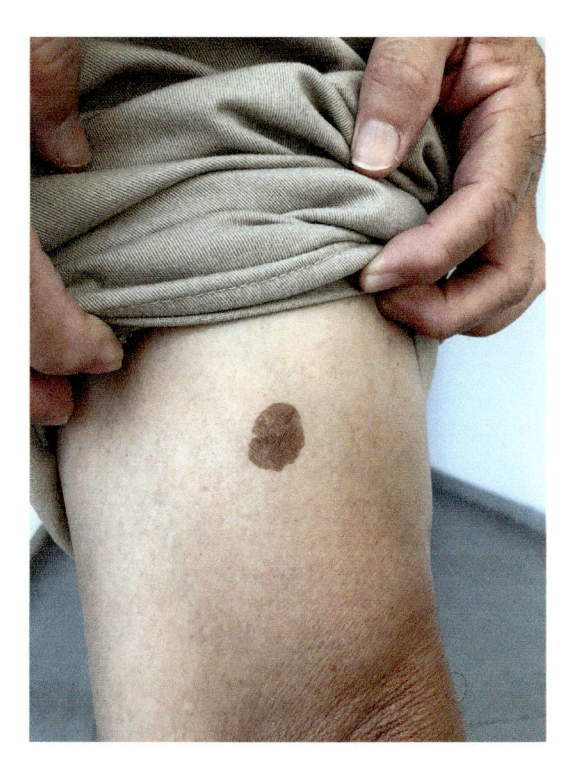

Figure 10.2 Diabetic dermopathy involving the leg.

area of the legs (Figure 10.2). Initially there is a scale on the lesions, which then dissipates after about 18–24 months.
- Typically these lesions are not treated as they will self-resolve and are asymptomatic.

Acrochordons
- These benign neoplasms involving the skin, seen in upwards of 40% of the general population, are typically associated with insulin resistance. They can result in pain or itching, particularly if there is rubbing against clothes or other materials. They tend to increase in number with age.
- The development of lesions appears to be associated with various hormonal growth factors such as tissue growth factor and epidermal growth factor.
- Lesions are small and soft, typically pedunculated, and involve areas where there are folds in the skin such as the

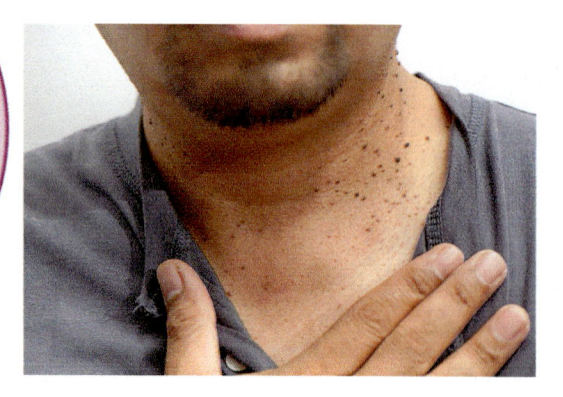

Figure 10.3 Acrochordons involving the folds of the neck.

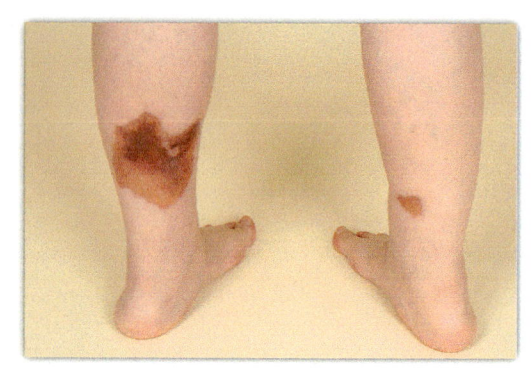

Figure 10.4 Necrobiosis lipoidica on the legs.
Courtesy of Dr. Golara Honari, Cleveland Clinic, photographer: Janine Sot.

neck, axilla, and inguinal regions. They can be flesh colored to hyperpigmented (Figure 10.3).
♦ There are a number of treatments available including excision, cryotherapy, and electrodessication. Additionally, weight loss can help with the prevention of formation of further lesions.

Conditions mainly associated with type 1 diabetes

Necrobiosis lipoidica
♦ This is a rare disorder that is typically seen in type 1 diabetes and can precede or be seen at the same time or after the diagnosis of diabetes. It impacts only about 0.3–1.2% of individuals with diabetes. There does not seem to be a correlation between the duration of the diabetes and the development of the lesion. Predominance is in females and it is typically seen in those between 30–40 years of age, although mean appear to have a worse course. Over time, these lesions can develop squamous cell cancers.
♦ The underlying cause appears to be vascular disease as significant changes in the vascularization of the skin is seen in the lesions
♦ Initially the lesions are typically small reddish-brown papules (Figure 10.4). These will enlarge and typically develop a central atrophy, and many will go on to ulcerate. Over time, the coloration becomes more yellowish with a darker rim. There is typically involvement of the pretibial surface.
♦ This will typically involve a multidisciplinary team including dermatology, infectious disease, endocrinology, and wound care as well. There is not a specific treatment, although corticosteroids have been used. Various biologics have been used with varying success. Critically, appropriate wound care if needed. Surgery typically is not helpful. Improvement in diabetic control also does not necessarily assist in resolution. The majority (over 80%) will still be present at 12 years out.

Vitiligo
♦ This is an autoimmune disorder which leads to depigmentation of the skin. It can be seen in the absence of diabetes but is much more common in those with diabetes. When present, there are often other autoimmune diseases that can be detected including thyroid and rheumatology condition.
♦ There is an aberrant response of T-cells against melanocytes leading to their destruction.
♦ The result is patches of depigmentation on the skin, typically resulting in white lesions (Figure 10.5). These can occur anywhere on the body but most frequently involves the extremities and the face as opposed to the trunk.

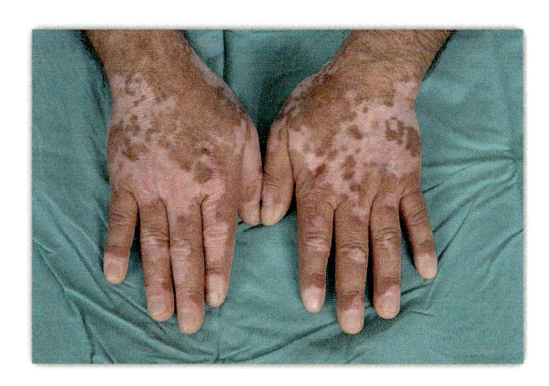

Figure 10.5 Vitiligo involving the hands. *Courtesy of Dr. Pooja Khera, Cleveland Clinic, photographer: Janine Sot.*

- The treatment is targeted against the T-cell response but only moderately effective. This includes phototherapy, topical therapies with corticosteroid and calcineurin inhibitors, and grafting of melanocytes. There is a significant psychosocial burden as well associated with the condition, which needs to be considered.

Diabetic bullae

- These are also known as bullosis diabeticorum and are typically associated with type 1 diabetes, but can be seen in all types of diabetes. They are also found more commonly in men. They are rare, typically seen in only 0.5% of individuals and are associated with a longer course of diabetes.
- There is no consensus currently on the underlying pathophysiology of the formation of these lesions.
- They appear as asymmetric transparent bullae located on the extremities, typically legs and feet with a noninflamed base. They are painless and contain a clear fluid. The size can be up to a few centimeters (Figure 10.6).
- These lesions will typically resolve over the course of a few weeks without intervention or scarring. The major concern is prevention of infection at the site of the bullae.

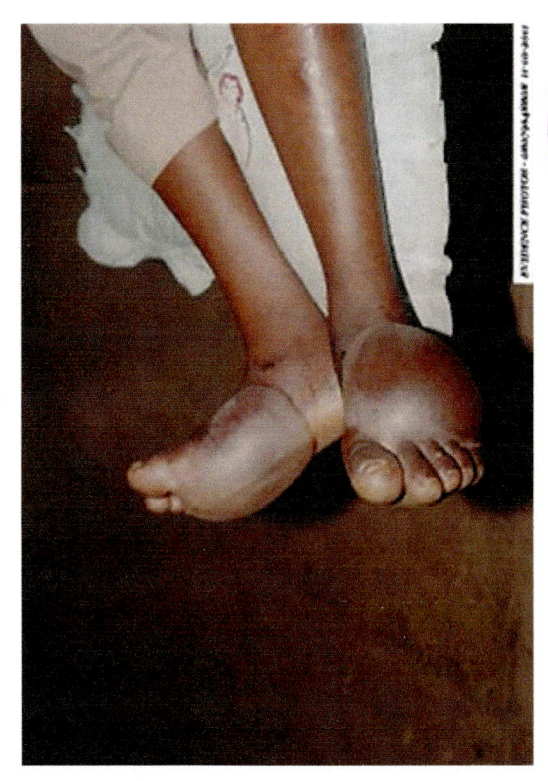

Figure 10.6 Large diabetic bullae involving the feet bilaterally. *From Bello, Fatima et al. 2 Cases of Bullosis Diabeticorum following Long-Distance Journeys by Road: A Report of 2 Cases. Case reports in endocrinology. Vol. 2012 (2012): 367218. doi: https://doi.org/10.1155/2012/367218.*

Other conditions associated with diabetes

Granuloma annulare

- This lesion is thought to have an association with diabetes as it is more commonly seen in those with diabetes, and diabetes is more commonly found in patients with it (upwards of 20%). It can have a subcutaneous, localized, or generalized form. It appears to impact younger and middle-aged women and can precede the diagnosis of diabetes.
- There is no clear etiology for the condition.
- Typically, these lesions appear as red rings with a normal center (Figure 10.7). In the localized form, it will typically involve just the hands and feet while the generalized form will involve the entirety

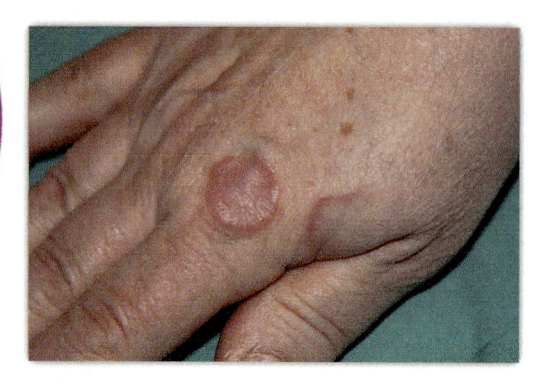

Figure 10.7 Granuloma annulare involving the hand. *Courtesy of Dr. Pooja Khera, Cleveland Clinic, photographer Janine Sot.*

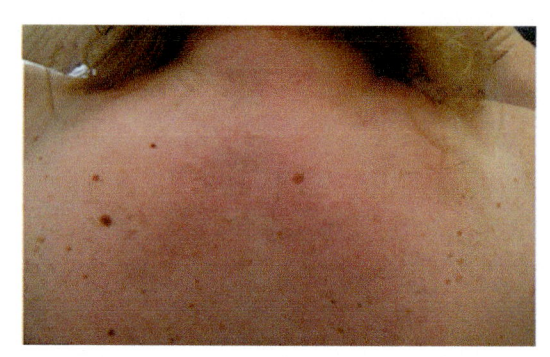

Figure 10.8 Scleroderma diabeticorum involving the upper back. *From Foti, Rosario et al. Clinical and Histopathological Features of Scleroderma-like Disorders: An Update. Medicina (Kaunas, Lithuania). Vol. 57,11 1275. 20 Nov. 2021. doi:10.3390/medicina57111275.*

of the body. The subcutaneous form is typically seen in children and presents as nodules.
- These lesions will self-resolve in a couple of years, but use of corticosteroids can be of help or phototherapy.

Scleroderma diabeticorum
- This is typically a painless thickening and hardening of skin that is often seen in those with diabetes, typically when it is poorly controlled and of longer duration. This can be seen in upwards of 14% of individuals with diabetes. It is more common in middle-aged men.
- The lesions are felt to be related to increased insulin levels and glycosylation of collagen, which leads to increased cross-linking and resistance to degradation, hence the thickening of the skin.
- These appear as thick erythematous plaques typically involving the upper back and neck (Figure 10.8), although other areas can be affected but typically not the hands and feet. There is often not a clear delineation between the affected and nonaffected skin.
- Therapies are of limited utility with the condition, although corticosteroids, phototherapy, and immune modulating treatments have been tried. Phototherapy appears to be the most efficacious.

Psoriasis
- This is a chronic inflammatory disorder of the skin that can impact up to 9% of individuals with diabetes. When diagnosed younger, there appears to be a risk factor for the future development of diabetes. It typically presents in those between 15–30 years of age.
- The persistent inflammation seen in the condition leads to uncontrolled keratinocyte proliferation with abnormal vascularization of the dermis.
- The lesions are erythematous, indurated with scales typically, and can appear on any part of the body (Figure 10.9). There are a number of different subtypes of psoriasis but the most common is psoriasis vulgaris, otherwise known as plaque-type psoriasis.
- A mild to moderate case can be treated with corticosteroids, vitamin D, and phototherapy while a more severe case will typically involve systemic therapy with biologics and small-molecule drugs.

Conditions associated with diabetes medications
- There are a number of lesions that can be seen associated with diabetes medications, traditionally insulin.

- Notably, there can also be local and systemic allergic reactions that can be seen with any of the diabetes medications.

Lipohypertrophy
- The most common adverse effect of insulin use is lipohypertrophy, which can impact up to 30% of individuals who utilize insulin.
- The lesion arises in the setting of excessive insulin injection into an area. Insulin, as a growth factor, causes localized hypertrophy of the adipocytes.
- There are therapeutic implications of the lesion as well, as injecting insulin into the area will result in erratic absorption of the medication.
- Initially these lesions can appear as small nodules underneath the skin and then grow to involve a larger area (Figure 10.10).

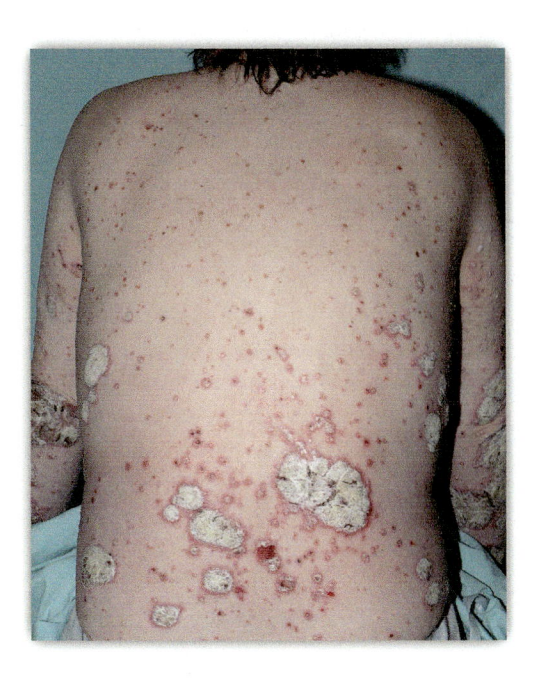

Figure 10.9 Psoriasis on the back of a patient. *Courtesy of Dr. Anthony Fernandez, Cleveland clinic, photographer: Janine Sot.*

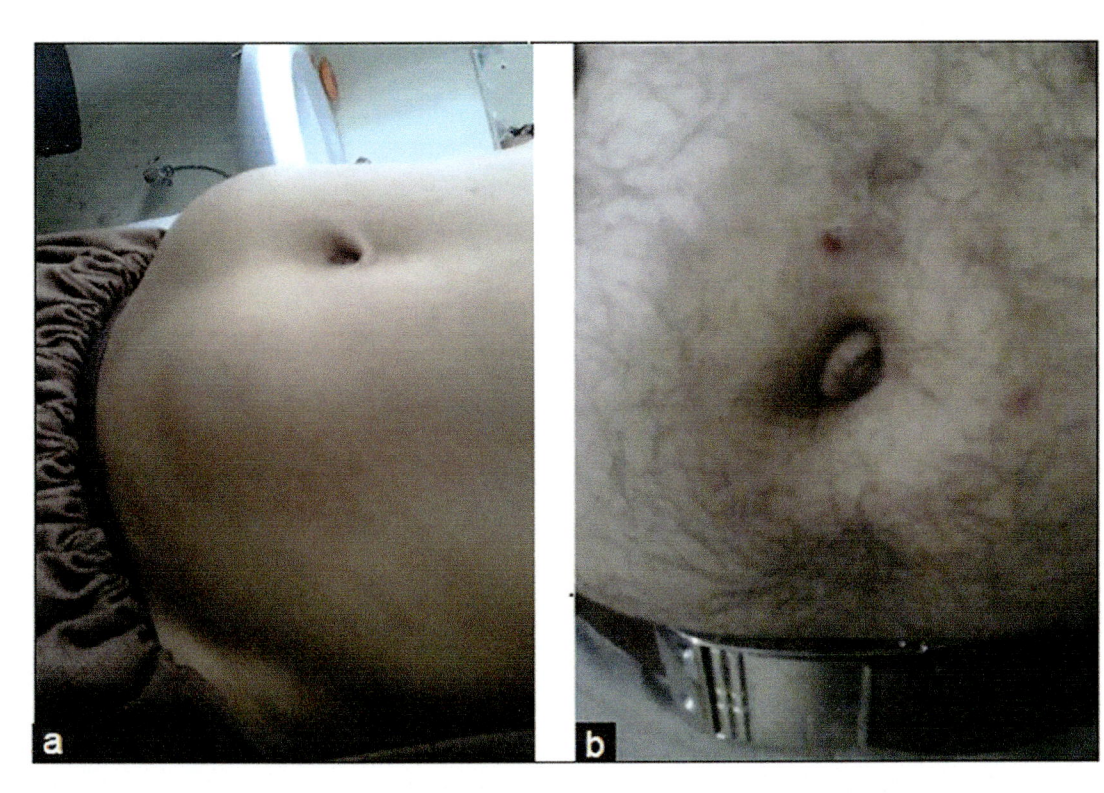

Figure 10.10 Example of lipohypertrophy involving the abdomen around the umbilicus. *From Mokta, Jatinder K et al. Insulin lipodystrophy and lipohypertrophy. Indian journal of endocrinology and metabolism. Vol. 17,4 (2013): 773–4. doi:10.4103/2230-8210.113788.*

♦ With avoidance of the location of lipohypertrophy, it can resolve over a period of months.

Lipoatrophy
♦ This is a much less common lesion in the setting of the creation of purified insulin but can still occur.
♦ The onset of the lesion after exposure to insulin use varies between a few weeks to a couple years.
♦ The insulin elicits an inflammatory response, which causes signaling, inhibiting adipocyte differentiation and leaving a concavity in the skin.
♦ Avoiding injection into sites of lipoatrophy and also utilizing newer analogue insulin typically can help, along with injection of dexamethasone.

Musculoskeletal conditions associated with diabetes

Overview
♦ There are a number of musculoskeletal disorders that are more commonly seen in those with diabetes. While the underlying pathophysiology for a number of these is not entirely clear, the debility caused by the conditions can be significant.
♦ Many of these conditions are felt to be related to abnormal collagen deposition and glycosylation of collagen, which leads to increased cross-linking and thickening. Additionally an abnormal immune response can contribute to a pathologic inflammatory response.
♦ These can be broadly considered to involve the hand, joints, muscle, and skeleton.

Conditions of the hand
Dupuytren's contracture
♦ This is a heritable condition where there is a thickening of the fascia in the palm and base of the fingers which will lead to contracture of the fingers (Figure 10.11).

♦ In those with diabetes, the 3rd and 4th fingers are most limited in mobility.
♦ There is an association with the duration of diabetes, age, and male gender.
♦ Imaging is not a requirement, but ultrasound can be utilized to show thickened fascia and nodules.
♦ Treatment for the condition can range from conservative management if the disease is stable, injections of corticosteroid or needle aponeurotomy, all the way to surgical intervention. Therapy can be utilized to help improve function as well.

Carpal tunnel syndrome
♦ This occurs when the median nerve that passes through the carpal tunnel is compressed by the overlying transverse carpal ligament and surrounding bones. Patients will describe a neuropathy involving the 1st through 3rd fingers of the hand, which worsens in the evening and can be associated with reduced dexterity.
♦ It is more commonly seen in women.
♦ The Phalen and Tinel tests can be performed to confirm the diagnosis (Figure 10.12).
♦ Treatment involves splinting the wrist in a neutral position, particularly overnight. Corticosteroid injections can be used and then surgery in more severe cases.

Flexor tenosynovitis
♦ Otherwise known as "trigger finger", this is an inflammation of the tendon sheaths of the fingers. Swelling proximal to the metacarpophalangeal (MCP) joint of the tendon sheath will cause the flexor tendons to be trapped and leads to locking of the finger in the flexed position (Figure 10.13).
♦ The pain is more common in the evening and then will improve during the day.
♦ On examination, there is often tenderness and swelling proximal to the MCP joint. Imaging is not necessary although ultrasound can be helpful in confirming the diagnosis.

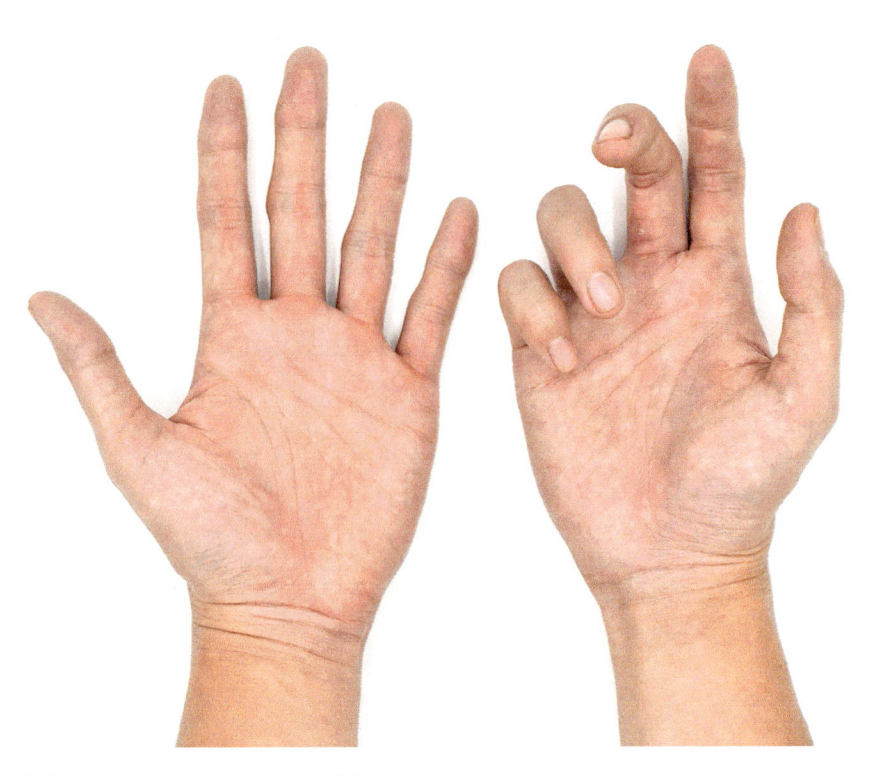

Figure 10.11 Dupuytren's contracture of the right hand.

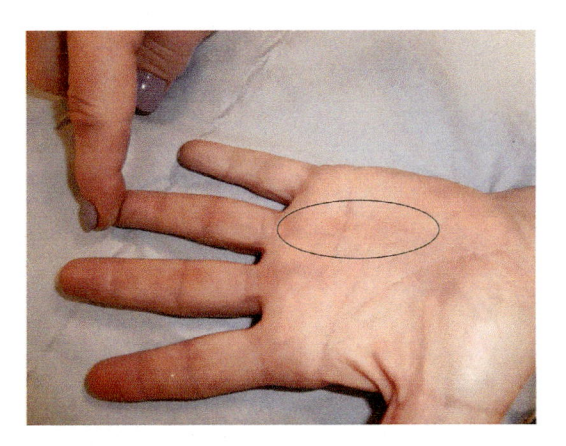

Figure 10.13 Flexor tenosynovitis involving the 4th finger. The area circled shows a thickened tendon. *From M. Merashli, T.A. Chowdhury, A.S.M. Jawad, Musculoskeletal manifestations of diabetes mellitus, QJM: An International Journal of Medicine. Vol. 108, Iss. 11, Nov. 2015, 853–857. https://doi.org/10.1093/qjmed/hcv106.*

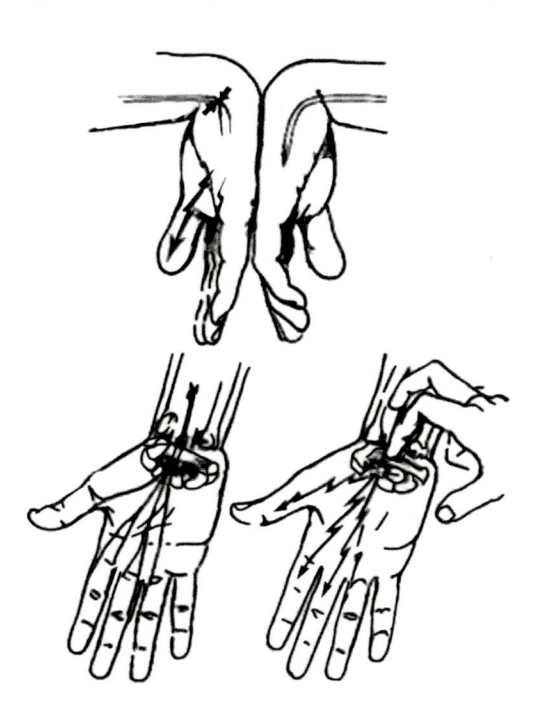

Figure 10.12 Phalen's and Tinel's Tests. Phalen's involves wrist flexion to 90 degrees for up to a minute. Tinel's is where the practitioner taps over the wrist at the point where the median nerve passes through the carpal tunnel. A positive test for each will reproduce the neuropathy associated with the carpal tunnel.

- Treatment typically involves splinting and immobilization of the finger. Corticosteroid injection can be utilized. Surgery is used in more severe cases.

Limited joint mobility
- Otherwise known as diabetic cheiroarthropathy, this is a common complication of diabetes. There is involvement of the MCP and also interphalangeal joints of the hand, typically starting with the 5th finger and then extending to the others.
- There is a thickened, waxy appearance of the dorsum of the hands, particularly along the joints.
- This is more seen with older age and also associated with greater micro- and macrovascular diabetic comorbidities.
- A positive "prayer sign" or "tabletop sign" can be indicative of the condition (Figure 10.14).
- Usually this is asymptomatic and no specific treatments are offered, but symptomatic patients may benefit from improvement glycemic control, stretching of joints, and corticosteroid or anti-inflammatory therapy.

Conditions of the joints
Frozen shoulder
- This is also known as adhesive capsulitis and is one of the most common musculoskeletal conditions affecting those with diabetes. It is seen more with older age and longer duration of diabetes.
- In diabetes, the finding is often bilateral.
- There is reduced range of motion at the glenohumeral joint due to joint capsule contraction (Figure 10.15).
- Usually imaging is normal although can exclude other etiologies of pain at the joint.

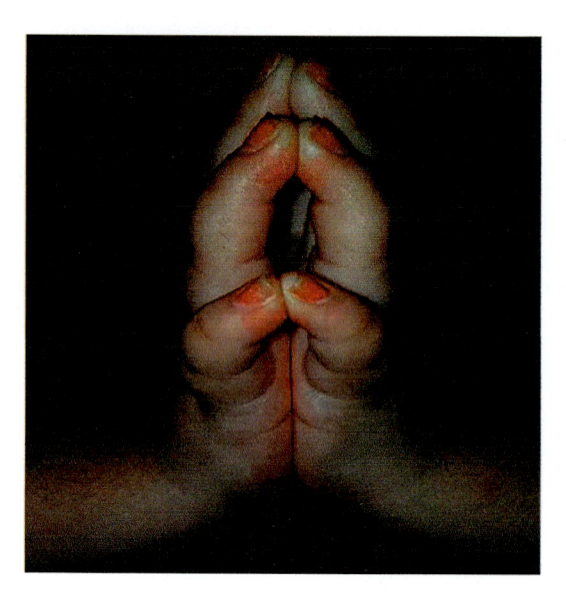

Figure 10.14 A positive "prayer sign" suggestive of limited joint mobility, where the patient cannot place the hands flat together. The "tabletop sign" is similarly where patients cannot place the hand flat on the surface of the table. *From Al-Qahtani, Mohammad H, and Fai A AlQahtani. Limited joint mobility in a child with type 1 diabetes mellitus. Case reports in medicine. Vol. 2021 6397338, 15 Nov. 2021, doi:10.1155/2021/6397338.*

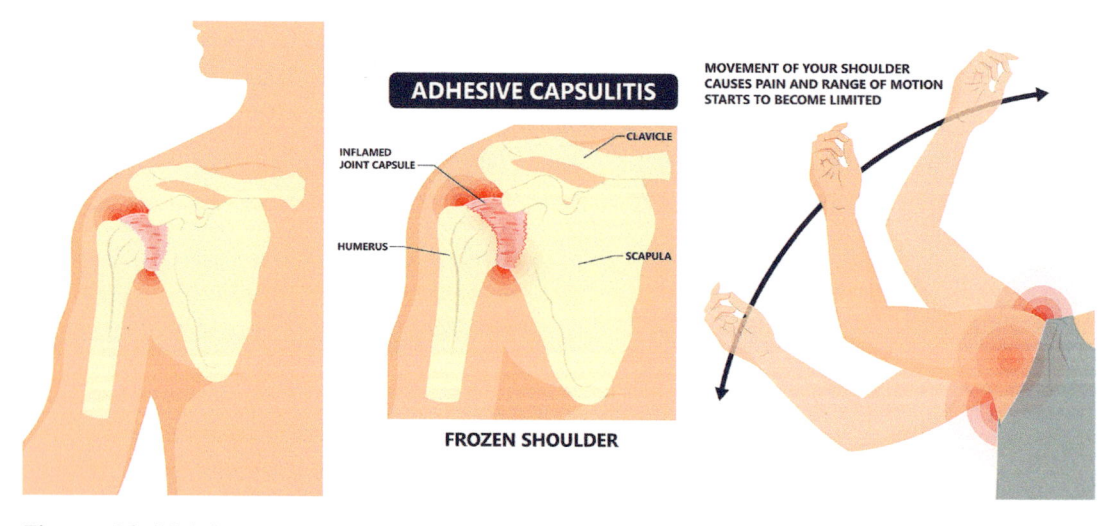

Figure 10.15 Inflammation of the glenohumeral joint capsule underlies frozen shoulder and leads to limited abduction of the shoulder.

- The condition is typically self-limited although it may take months for recovery. Treatment typically involves physical therapy, injections, and sometimes can progress to arthroscopic surgery.

Gout
- This is a deposition of monosodium urate crystals in joints leading to inflammatory arthritis with an incidence as high as 22% in those with diabetes.
- It typically presents affecting a single joint, typically the metatarsophalangeal joint of the foot and MCP, and then wrist.
- In more advanced and poorly controlled gout, tophi can develop which are hardened deposits of urate crystals (Figure 10.16).
- Obesity and male gender along with consumption of alcohol and certain meats and seafoods are known risks.
- Treatment acutely involves use of anti-inflammatory agents, corticosteroids, and colchicine, whereas long-term prophylactic therapy involves the use of urate-lowering agents like allopurinol.

Conditions of the muscles

Diabetic muscle infarction
- This is a very rare complication of poorly controlled diabetes with less than 200 cases reported in the literature. The majority of cases are seen in individuals with multiple microvascular complications of diabetes.
- The pathophysiology is felt to be related to diabetic microangiopathy associated with thromboembolic events leading to ischemia. The subsequent inflammation seen with reperfusion leads to further injury.
- This condition should be suspected in a patient with poorly controlled diabetes without a clear antecedent event for the muscle swelling and pain.
- A deep vein thrombosis should be excluded but otherwise no specific lab findings can rule in the diagnosis.
- Muscle biopsy can be definitive but can delay improvement and is not recommended.
- MRI is the diagnostic modality of choice and typically shows a hyperintense T2-weighted image and an isointense to hypointense T1-weighted image of the affected muscle with edema. Ultrasound can be helpful as well.
- Treatment typically involves pain control, rest, and attention to improved glycemic control. There is a high rate of recurrence of the condition as well.

Diabetic amyotrophy
- Also known as diabetic lumbosacral radiculoplexus neuropathy (DLRPN), this affects less than 1% of individuals with diabetes.
- It is typically seen with type 2 diabetes in men over 50 years of age.
- The presentation is initially pain involving the buttock and thigh of one leg and then spreading within that extremity, followed by involvement of the opposite extremity.
- A few weeks after the neuropathy is muscle weakness and wasting along with general weight loss. The diagnosis is typically based on a careful clinical history and examination of the patient.
- There is typically spontaneous improvement, but it can be slow and incomplete and often there is permanent weakness.

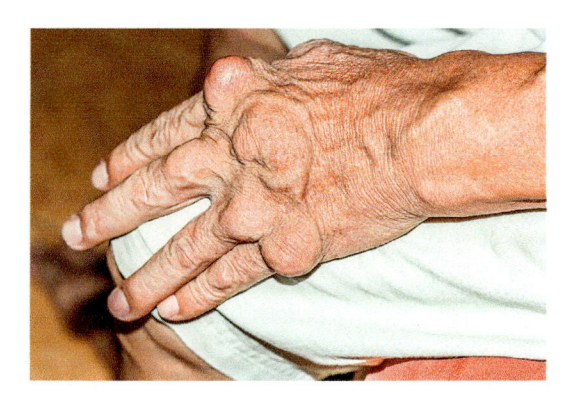

Figure 10.16 Tophi of the hands seen with chronic gout.

Conditions of the skeleton
Diffuse idiopathic skeletal hyperostosis
- DISH is a systemic common condition typically seen in those older than 50 years and has an association with diabetes.
- There is ossification of ligaments and entheses in the joints and axial skeleton.
- It is postulated that the increased insulin and IGF-1 levels seen in diabetes lead to the ossification seen in the condition.
- The diagnostic criteria are made on imaging (plain radiograph or CT which can be more detailed) according to the Resnick criteria (Table 10.2).
- It is unclear how symptomatic patients are, apart from some stiffness of the axial skeleton.
- Treatment is very poorly defined and typically is similar to treatment provided for osteoarthritis. Surgery is typically not needed.

Osteoporosis
- Osteoporosis is more frequently seen in those individuals with diabetes. There appear to be a number of reasons for this, including changes in bone turnover, bone microarchitecture, and strength of the bone matrix.

Table 10.2 The Resnick criteria for DISH, which are based on radiologic findings.

Resnick Criteria for Diffuse Idiopathic Skeletal Hyperostosis Diagnosis (48)
1. Presence of ossifications and calcifications in the anterolateral parts of at least four sequential vertebrae
2. Relatively preserved height of the intervertebral discs and absence of common degenerative disc disease
3. Absence of spondyloarthropathy

- ◇ Diabetes is known to be associated with low bone turnover.
- ◇ There is a reduction in the ability of bone to resist compressive forces in diabetes, perhaps related to a defect in the ability to mineralize bone in the setting of hyperglycemia.
- Microvascular complications of diabetes also predispose to falls (neuropathy and retinopathy).
- Nephropathy can lead to a secondary hyperparathyroidism and worsened bone metabolism.
- Certain medications such as thiazolidinediones can increase fracture risk.
- An important point is that in those with type 2 diabetes, the actual bone density may be increased due to the increased weight but the strength of the bone is typically suboptimal.
- Treatment guidelines for osteoporosis are not significantly altered by the presence of diabetes in a patient.
- Attention should be also paid to reducing risk for falls, which can mean mitigating risk for hypoglycemia among other interventions.

Diabetic foot

Overview
- Diabetic foot problems are responsible for nearly 50% of all diabetes-related hospital bed-days.
- Ten to 15% of diabetic patients develop foot ulcers at some stage in their lives.
- Fifty percent of all lower limb amputations are performed on people with diabetes.
- The risk of amputation is increased 15-fold in diabetes. That risk has declined substantially in the last 30 years but is still particularly high in those on dialysis (about 60 per 1000 person-years) or those with a history of foot ulceration (about 15 per 1000 person-years).
- Conservative management of foot problems has dramatically reduced the risk of

amputation by simple procedures such as good footwear, chiropody, cleanliness, aggressive surgical debridement, and ulcer management. Even that most dramatic of diabetic foot problems, Charcot's arthropathy (see p. 103), no longer means an inevitable progression to amputation.
- Diabetic foot problems are not only an important complication, they are also a preventable complication.

Pathophysiology and risk factors
- The impact of diabetes complications mediated through micro- and macrovascular disease is nowhere better exemplified than by the feet:
  - All the risk factors, especially hyperglycemia, that are important to microvascular disease predispose to peripheral neuropathy and increase the risk of foot problems by disturbing the foot structure, physiology, and immune responses to trauma and infection.
  - Those same risk factors, but especially dyslipidemia, smoking, and hypertension, that predispose to macrovascular disease also increase the risk of foot problems by disturbing the foot physiology, blood supply, and immune responses to trauma and infection.
- The major underlying causes of diabetic foot disease are:
  - Peripheral neuropathy.
  - Peripheral arterial disease.
  - Infection secondary to trauma or ulceration.
  - High plantar pressure.
  - Deformities.

Neuropathy
- *Motor neuropathy.* Loss of neural supply to the intrinsic muscles of the foot leads to an imbalance between the flexor and extensor mechanisms, clawing of the toes, and increased prominence of the metatarsal heads.
- *Autonomic neuropathy.* Loss of sweat gland function leads to dry skin predisposed to skin cracking and infection. Loss of peripheral sympathetic vascular tone increases distal arterial flow and may lead to edema and osteopenia.
- *Sensory neuropathy.* Diminished sensibility to pain means that poorly fitting shoes or early signs of foot deformity or lesions may go unnoticed by the patient and uncorrected. Callus is prevalent in neuropathic ulcers and reduces the healing potential of an ulcer, predisposing to infection.

Diabetic foot problems are preventable.

Peripheral arterial disease
- Reduced blood supply mimics and exacerbates the changes brought about by neuropathy.
- Occlusive arterial disease also results in hypoxia and reduced wound healing with increased infection risk.
- Persistent hyperglycemia results in endothelial cell dysfunction and smooth cell abnormalities in peripheral arteries.
- In Charcot's arthropathy there is an arteriovenous shunt across the foot with distended dorsal veins (Ward's sign) (Figure 10.17, Table 10.3).

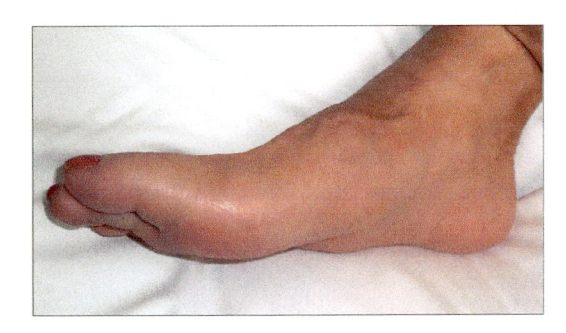

Figure 10.17 Neuropathic foot. Disrupted foot structure associated with Charcot's arthropathy. Note the distended veins associated with arteriovenous shunt.

Skin & musculoskeletal complications

Table 10.3 Evaluating an ulcer in the diabetic foot. Ischemia and neuropathy can be difficult to differentiate; a thorough assessment is important.

Clinical features of neuropathic vs ischemic foot ulcer

NEUROPATHIC ULCER	ISCHEMIC ULCER
Sensory defect	Not necessarily a sensory defect
Pulses present	Pulses absent
Subluxed metatarsal heads (cocked toes)	Foot structure retained
Ulceration of pressure points	Ulceration at points of ischemia, not pressure
Punched-out deep ulcer with surrounding callus	Superficial ulcers without callus

Table 10.4 Ulcer classification. Systematic evaluation and categorization of foot ulcers help guide appropriate treatment. The Wagner system is the most commonly used.

Wagner ulcer classification

GRADE	CLINICAL PRESENTATION
0	No open lesions; may have deformity or cellulitis
1	Superficial ulcer
2	Ulcer extension involving ligaments, tendon, joint capsule or fascia without abscess or osteomyelitis
3	Deep ulcer or osteomyelitis
4	Gangrene to portion of forefoot
5	Extensive gangrene of foot

Infection
- The damage resulting from neuropathy, ischemia, trauma, or all three predisposes to infection. Infection may be bacterial (in association with ulcers) or fungal (especially of toenails).

Pressure
- Repetitive pressure, shear from walking and weight bearing, and/or inappropriate footwear leads to increased plantar pressures, inducing callus formation and skin breakdown.

Clinical presentation and evaluation
- Systematic examination, evaluation, and appropriate categorization of foot ulcers will provide a guide to treatment and prognosis (Table 10.4 and Figure 10.18).

Evaluation
- All patients with diabetes should receive a thorough foot examination at least once a year; those with diabetic foot-related complaints should be evaluated more frequently. Patients are often unaware of serious foot problems because of the masking effect of neuropathy.

Examination
- The following should be inspected/examined:
  ◇ *Footwear:* type; fit; pattern; foreign bodies.
  ◇ *Foot:* structure; distortion, e.g. Charcot's; pressure points; infection or ulcers between the toes; nails (for infection, length and whether ingrowing).
  ◇ *Skin:* whether dry; presence of fissures or calluses.
  ◇ *Vessels:* pulses; venous filling time; color.
  ◇ *Nerves:* examine sensors (reflexes, vibration, temperature, pain); motors (muscle power, muscle atrophy).
- Referral to a podiatrist (chiropodist) or foot clinic is recommended when patients manifest certain foot changes (Table 10.5).
  ◇ In some services, patients with established neuropathy are offered regular monitoring by podiatry; this may be especially important for patients with visual impairment.

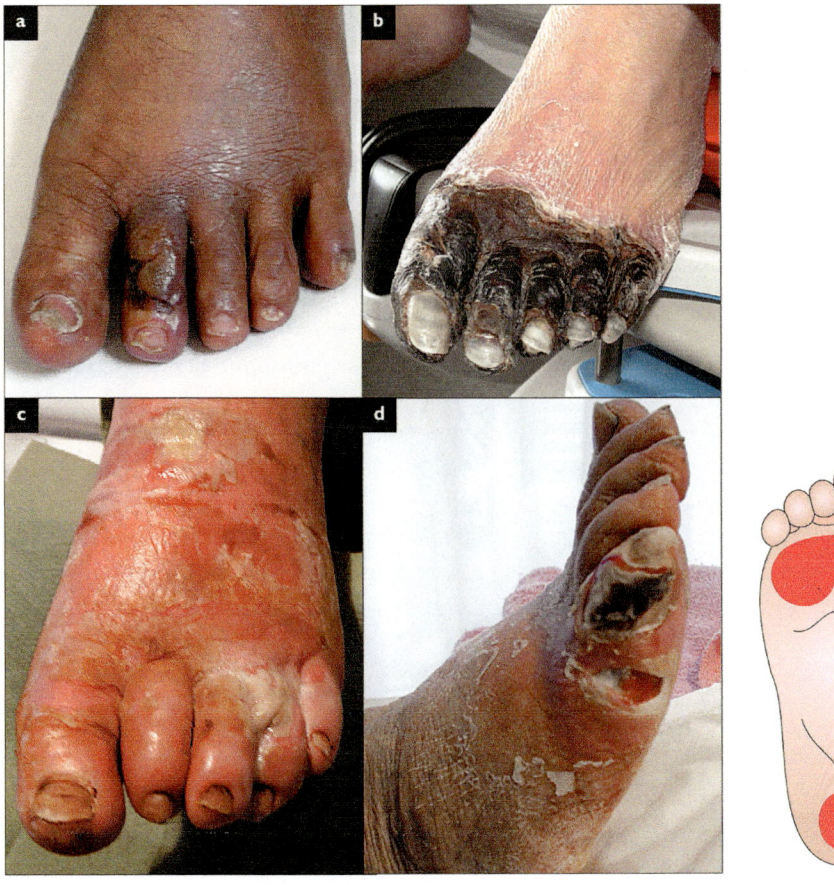

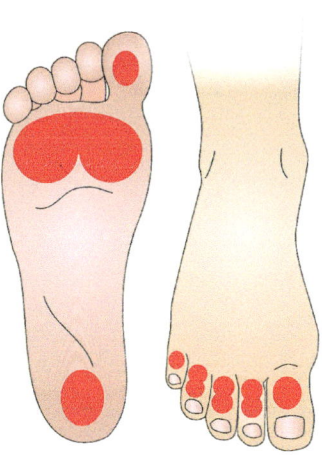

Figure 10.18 Diabetic foot ulcers. (a) Ischemic ulcer: digital ischemia is seen in the second toe. (b) Extensive ischemia affects all toes back to the level of the midfoot. (c) A neuropathic lesion at the base of the fourth toe has been the point of entry of extensive cellulitis of the whole foot. (d) Mixed neuroischemic lesion affecting the small toe. Right: Neuropathic lesions tend to occur on plantar surfaces and ischemic ones over bone prominences.

Table 10.5 Referral criteria. These six features identified by a clinician should prompt referral to an appropriate specialist, e.g. podiatrist (callus, anatomical abnormality) or podiatrist plus specialist foot clinic for all other conditions.

Indications for referral
Callus, corns, or ingrowing toenails
Ulcer
Significant ischemia
Anatomical abnormality
Amputation or previous ulcer
Charcot's arthropathy

Treatment and management

- Since diabetic foot problems are, by and large, preventable, it is important to learn the principles of foot care (Table 10.6).
- Several conditions put the foot at risk of amputation and should be addressed to prevent progression.
  - The five main threats to skin and subcutaneous tissues in the foot are neuropathy, peripheral arterial disease, infection, high plantar pressure, and deformities. Ulcer management centers on these five aspects of care and will typically involve several disciplines, including a physician, a podiatrist, and a surgeon (usually vascular or orthopedic) (Figure 10.19).

Table 10.6 Foot care. Simple management procedures for foot problems dramatically reduce the risk of amputation.

Principles of foot care
Footwear must be carefully measured and checked regularly for foreign objects
Shoes should preferably be lace-up shoes or trainers
Feet should be washed daily and dried well, especially between the toes
Toenails should be cut straight across, carefully and regularly
Feet should be inspected daily, especially on the soles
Moisturizing creams are to be used for calluses or fissures
Refer to podiatrist when appropriate

Infection

- Infections in diabetes should be managed intensively by identifying the relevant organism and using early and aggressive antibiotic treatment.
    ◇ *Streptococcus pyogenes, Staphylococcus aureus*, and anaerobic species are prevalent.
- Since infections may lead to loss of glycemic control, and are a common cause of ketoacidosis, insulin-treated patients need to increase their dose in the face of infection, and noninsulin-treated patients may need insulin therapy when they have an infection.
- Therapy includes ulcer debridement, callus removal, protection of pressure points, and antibiotics.

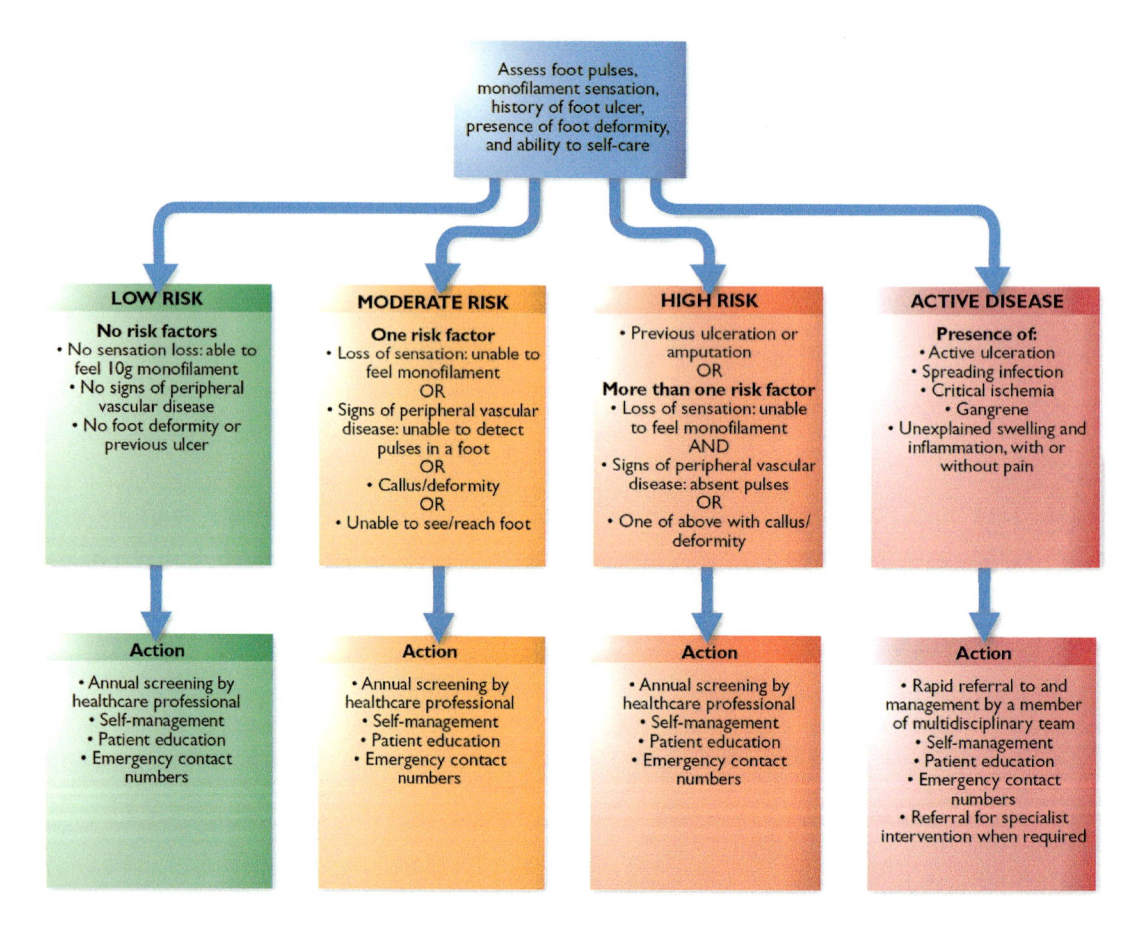

Assess foot pulses, monofilament sensation, history of foot ulcer, presence of foot deformity, and ability to self-care

LOW RISK
No risk factors
- No sensation loss: able to feel 10g monofilament
- No signs of peripheral vascular disease
- No foot deformity or previous ulcer

Action
- Annual screening by healthcare professional
- Self-management
- Patient education
- Emergency contact numbers

MODERATE RISK
One risk factor
- Loss of sensation: unable to feel monofilament
  OR
- Signs of peripheral vascular disease: unable to detect pulses in a foot
  OR
- Callus/deformity
  OR
- Unable to see/reach foot

Action
- Annual screening by healthcare professional
- Self-management
- Patient education
- Emergency contact numbers

HIGH RISK
- Previous ulceration or amputation
  OR
More than one risk factor
- Loss of sensation: unable to feel monofilament
  AND
- Signs of peripheral vascular disease: absent pulses
  OR
- One of above with callus/deformity

Action
- Annual screening by healthcare professional
- Self-management
- Patient education
- Emergency contact numbers

ACTIVE DISEASE
Presence of:
- Active ulceration
- Spreading infection
- Critical ischemia
- Gangrene
- Unexplained swelling and inflammation, with or without pain

Action
- Rapid referral to and management by a member of multidisciplinary team
- Self-management
- Patient education
- Emergency contact numbers
- Referral for specialist intervention when required

Figure 10.19 Risk levels. The risk of diabetic foot can be stratified, and resources prioritized according to need. *From the SCI-DC foot risk stratification tool.*

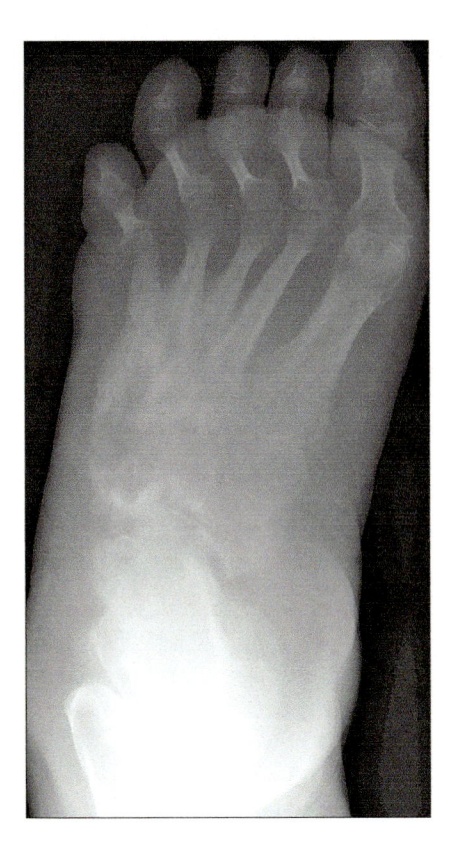

Figure 10.20 Osteomyelitis. Radiograph of a left foot, showing bone destruction and periosteal bone formation, most notably in the 5th metatarsal. *Courtesy Barts and The London Hospital Trust.*

◇ Antibiotics must be broad spectrum, moderately high dosage, and given for prolonged periods, often in excess of 1 month until infection is resolved.

◆ For deep or chronic infections, radiography of the feet may be required to exclude osteomyelitis (Figure 10.20). If doubt remains about osteomyelitis, a magnetic resonance imaging (MRI), computed tomography (CT), or gallium bone scan may provide further evidence.

  ◇ Sequential radiography (e.g. at intervals of 2 weeks apart) may be needed to clarify the situation.
  ◇ Radiological diagnosis of osteomyelitis can be complex given that in an infected diabetic foot, there may be areas of demineralization in bones that are not directly infected, and this topic is beyond the scope of this book.
  ◇ Although the gold standard for diagnosis of osteomyelitis is bone biopsy, this is rarely used due to the hazards of the procedure and concerns about healing subsequently.

◆ Osteomyelitis can be treated with long-term intravenous antibiotics – at least 6 weeks – but may require excision of the infected bone. Arterial revascularization may assist healing.

◆ In patients who decline amputation, antibiotics may contain even osteomyelitis for several months (or even years). However, this is not recommended since chronic infection promotes a systemic catabolic and proinflammatory state that affects the patient's well-being.

Peripheral arterial disease

◆ The blood flow to the feet is assessed clinically, with Doppler ultrasound, or, when severe and surgery is contemplated, by femoral arteriography.

  ◇ Arterial calcification will give false Doppler readings suggesting high blood flow.
  ◇ Localized areas of occlusion as shown on arteriography may be amenable to bypass surgery, stents, or angioplasty, or *in extremis* to amputation.

Ulcer management typically involves several disciplines.

High plantar pressure

◆ Appropriate foot care, removal of callus formation, rest, and, when ulcerated, keeping the ulcerated site non-weight bearing, are essential.

  ◆ A moisturizing cream can be used prophylactically on callus.

- Deep shoes and specially constructed insoles help to move pressure away from critical sites, while lightweight supports (e.g. air-boots or foot casts) limit pressure on the feet.
- Recommence weight bearing gradually, preferably with specially crafted footwear, or, as a less satisfactory alternative, with sports trainers.

Deformities
- Deformities can be managed by appropriate footwear or, if required, surgery.

The wound environment
- Dressings are used both to absorb exudate and to maintain moisture; in addition, they protect the wound from contamination.
- New techniques to promote healing of chronic ulceration are available but there is a paucity of evidence relating to their effectiveness. They are expensive (e.g. hyperbaric oxygen or growth factors) and their role is yet to be established.
  ◇ Hydrogel dressings, hyperbaric oxygen therapy, and larval therapy have some evidence for efficacy.
  ◇ There is perhaps less evidence for alginate-based dressings, platelet-derived growth factors, negative pressure wound therapy, dimethyl sulfoxide dressings, and cultured dermis; the latter is like a skin graft but constructed from neonatal fibroblasts embedded in a synthetic matrix.

The key components of ulcer management include avoiding pressure, treating infection, improving circulation, and promoting healing.

Surgery
- Amputations need to be undertaken at the appropriate time. They are the definitive treatment of osteomyelitis, but a trial of antibiotics (with or without soft-tissue debridement) will usually precede amputation.
  ◇ Amputation should be avoided, where possible, as it has long-term implications for the patient, both physiological and psychological.
- Amputations can be:
  ◇ Local, involving a ray excision of the second, third, or fourth toe and the associated metatarsal.
  ◇ More radical, including above- or below-knee amputations of the limb.
- Sometimes an angioplasty will be required to improve blood supply before amputation is attempted.
  ◇ When multiple levels of occlusion are present, revascularization at each point is necessary to restore arterial blood flow.
  ◇ Transluminal angioplasty of the iliac arteries allied to surgical bypass in the distal extremity may be valuable.
- Amputation inevitably changes the biomechanics of the limb(s) that remain and will necessitate a review of footwear after recovery from the procedure.
  ◇ The effort required to walk with a prosthesis is high and may be too much for the elderly, who are then confined to a wheelchair.
  ◇ The shift in weight can promote ulceration in the contralateral limb.

Amputation has long-term implications and should be avoided if possible.

Charcot's arthropathy

- Charcot's arthropathy results from a dense peripheral sensory neuropathy. It was originally described as a feature of syphilis and leprosy, but the most common cause today is diabetes. The structure of the foot (though any large joint can be affected) is lost, accompanied by bone thinning and small fractures. Subsequently, the joints of the feet are disrupted and disorganized and the abnormal structure is subject to further distortion, pressure points, ulceration, and joint instability (Figures 10.21–10.23).

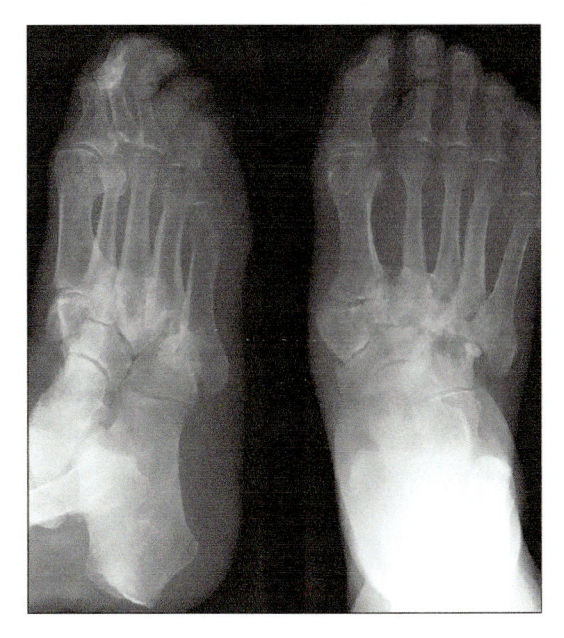

Figure 10.21 Charcot's arthropathy. Radiograph showing destruction and coalescence of the tarsometatarsal region (where the process usually starts) of the right foot. *Photo courtesy Barts and The London Hospital Trust.*

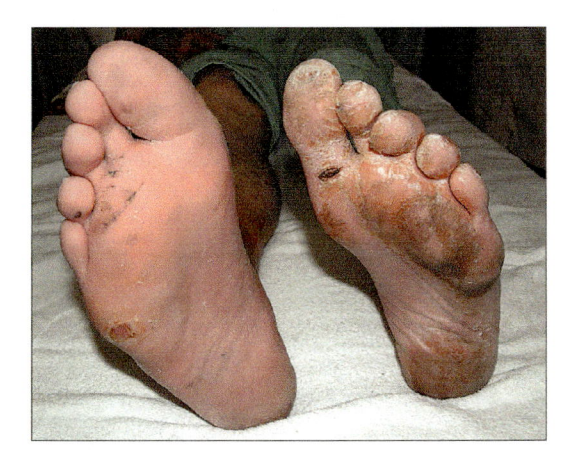

Figure 10.22 Charcot's arthropathy. A patient with neuropathic feet bilaterally; the right foot showing changes of Charcot's arthropathy along its lateral border, with an overlying ulcer. The left foot shows callus formation.

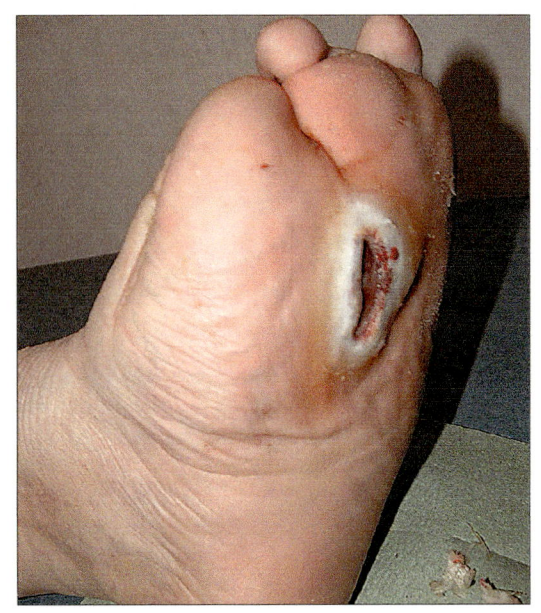

Figure 10.23 Charcot's arthropathy. An 'end-stage' Charcot's foot with previous amputations and a severely distorted foot structure with marked callus around a neuropathic ulcer.

- There are two main classifications of Charcot neuroarthropathy (Eichenholz and Brodsky), which describe disease progress and distribution, respectively.
- The Eichenholz classification describes the evolution of the condition over time:
  - Stage 1: destruction.
  - Stage 2: coalescence.
  - Stage 3: consolidation.
- A 'stage 0' has also come into use to classify the swollen, hot, usually rather painful foot in which plain foot radiograph is normal but MRI shows bone edema and stress fractures.
- Management of Charcot's arthropathy includes:
  - Immobilization.
  - Custom-made footwear.
  - Reconstruction (including realignment of unstable joints).
  - Intravenous bisphosphonates (which suppress osteoclast activity).
- The key to management is early diagnosis and reduction of pressure.

CHAPTER 11

Infections and diabetes

Overview

- Both type 1 and type 2 diabetes are associated with a significantly higher risk of infection.
- Upwards of 50% of individuals with diabetes will have a claim for an infectious disease within a year.
- Diabetes accounts for 6% of infection-related hospitalization and 12% of infection-related hospitalizations.
- When presenting in the emergency room, there is a 2-fold increased risk of admission to the hospital compared with those without diabetes.
- Association between diabetes and infection strongest for musculoskeletal infections and skin infections.
- Diabetes results in deficits in both innate and adaptive immunity, leading to an increase in infections.
- Diabetes can result in much more rapidly progressive and severe infections, associated with greater morbidity and mortality as well. As such, a decision may be made for more aggressive therapy earlier in the course of treatment.

Pathophysiology

- There are a number of changes in immunity that occur in diabetes (Table 11.1).
- The first layer of protection lost is at the skin level.
- Peripheral neuropathy can make a patient more susceptible to lesions that penetrate the barrier of the skin.
- Subsequent poor vascular flow will lead to further compromise of the immune response.
- There is also a change in the microbes that inhabit the tissues of patients with diabetes. This can lead to more opportunistic infections.

Change in innate immunity

- The innate immune system refers to the initial defense that is mounted by the body in response to a pathogen.
- *Complement System:* There appears to be a reduction in the levels of complement in diabetes. Glycosylation of complements has been suggested to also reduce their function. The complement system plays an important role in the phagocytosis of pathogens. Studies have demonstrated that in the presence of hyperglycemia, there is reduced phagocytosis of pathogens.
- *Cellular Recruitment:* It has been well described that there is reduced chemotaxis of polymorphonuclear (PMN) leukocytes in those with diabetes that is inversely proportional to the degree of hyperglycemia the cells are exposed to. There is also reduced ability of PMN leukocytes to move across the endothelium to the site of the pathogen.
- *Cellular Dysfunction:* There is reduced bactericidal activity of phagocytes. There is also reduced activity of natural killer cells.
- *Cytokine Signaling Dysfunction:* Cytokine signaling plays a vital role in both innate and adaptive immunity and serves to

Table 11.1 Changes seen in the immune system in the setting of infection in an individual with diabetes or hyperglycemia.

Skin and Mucosal Barrier	Neuropathy predisposes to penetration of the skin Poor vascular flow can inhibit an appropriate immune response Change in the microbial makeup leads to more opportunistic infection
Innate Immunity Complement System Cellular Recruitment Cellular Dysfunction Cytokine Signaling	Reduction in levels of complement Glycosylation-reduced function of complement secreted Reduced chemotaxis and transendothelial migration of PMN Reduced bactericidal activity of phagocytes Reduced bactericidal activity of NK cells Lower levels of cytokines seen
Adaptive Immunity T Cell Dysfunction	Aberrant increase in T cell activation Reduced numbers of regulatory T cells

allow cross-talk between the two systems. In the setting of hyperglycemia, there are lower levels of cytokines secreted in the setting of infection.

Change in adaptive immunity

- *T Cell Dysfunction*. There is ultimately an aberrant increase in T cell activation but reduced regulatory T cell function, which can lead to an inappropriate inflammatory response.
- Notably, those with diabetes appear to have a normal response to the hepatitis B and influenza vaccinations, which suggests that the adaptive humoral immune response is largely intact.

Infections

- Many infectious processes are impacted by diabetes.
- There are also specific infections that those with diabetes are more prone to (Figure 11.1).
- A number of infectious processes themselves are potentially associated with the development of diabetes.

Head and neck infections

- *Malignant otitis externa*, also referred to as necrotizing otitis externa, is a rare infection involving the external auditory canal, temporal bone, and the skull base.

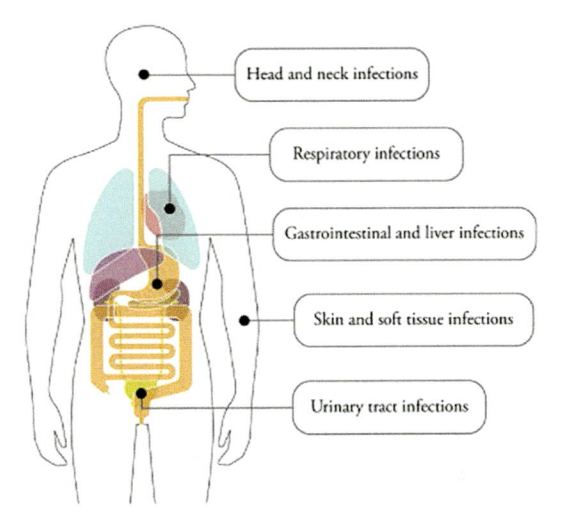

Figure 11.1 Depiction of common systems with higher rates of infection in those with diabetes. *From Suheda Erener, Diabetes, infection risk and COVID-19, Molecular Metabolism. Volume 39, 2020, 101044, ISSN 2212–8778. https://doi.org/10.1016/j.molmet.2020.101044.*

- ◇ It carries with it a high morbidity and mortality as well.
- ◇ Patient will describe an earache and often drainage associated with headache along with sometimes cranial nerve involvement, most commonly the facial nerve on the side impacted.
- ◇ It is typically seen in elderly patients with diabetes.

Table 11.2 Diagnostic criteria for malignant otitis externa. All of the major criteria must be met.

MAJOR CRITERIA (OBLIGATORY)	MINOR CRITERIA (OCCASIONAL)
Pain	Pseudomonas in culture
Exudate	Diabetes mellitus
Edema	Old age
Granulations	Cranial nerve involvement
Microabscesses (when operated)	Positive radiograph
Positive Technetium-99 (99Tc) bone scan of failure of local treatment after more than 1 week	Debilitating conditions

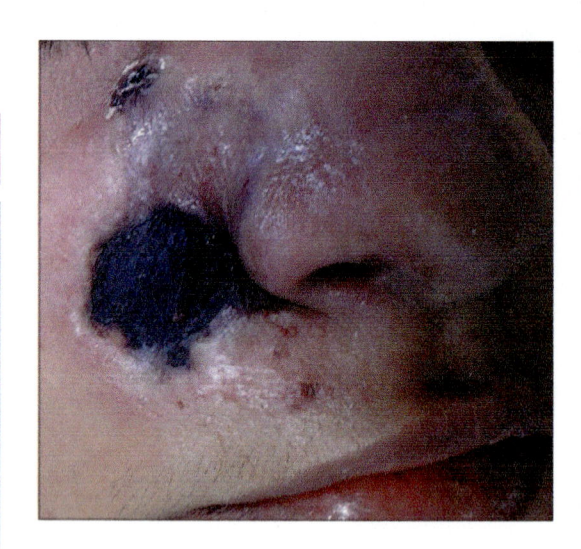

Figure 11.2 Rhinocerebral mucormycosis with black eschar noted on the face. *From Lunge, Snehal Balvant, et al. Rhinocerebrocutaneous mucormycosis caused by Mucor species: A rare causation.* Indian dermatology online journal. Vol. 6,3 (2015): 189-92. doi:10.4103/2229-5178.156393.

- ◇ The most common organism which causes this is *Pseudomonas aeruginosa*.
- ◇ Diagnosis is made clinically, along with radiologic findings on CT and/or MRI (Table 11.2).
- ◇ Treatment typically is IV or oral antimicrobial agents, depending on the infectious etiology. Surgery is typically not utilized. Often higher doses are required due to compromised vascularization of the area.
- ◆ *Mucormycosis* references infections that are caused by a group of molds.
   - ◇ It is rare but more common in those with poorly controlled diabetes.
   - ◇ The most common infection is ***rhinocerebral mucormycosis***, which refers to an infection involving the sinuses, orbits, and brain.
   - ◇ Typically there is headache, fever, swelling, sinus congestion and a black eschar can form around the nasal and oral cavities (Figure 11.2).
   - ◇ There is a high mortality rate which can be up to 57%.
   - ◇ Blindness is common after infection.
   - ◇ The mucormycetes can also infect other locations, with the second and third most common locations being the respiratory tract and the skin.
   - ◇ Diagnosis is made via imaging with CT and/or MRI.
   - ◇ Treatment involves use of IV antifungal therapy, surgical debridement, and hyperbaric oxygen.

Respiratory Infections
- ◆ In the setting of acute respiratory failure and respiratory distress syndrome in the ICU, there has been some data which suggests that the presence of diabetes can actually be protective.
- ◆ It is felt that this might be related to reduced inflammation and immune-related injury, which is a key component of the pathogenesis of these conditions.
- ◆ *Pneumonia* is more commonly seen in those with diabetes and is associated with greater morbidity and mortality in those with diabetes than those without (15.2% vs 13.5% in a hospitalized cohort).
   - ◇ Presentation typically is more severe with altered mentation and vital instability, such as hypotension, more likely to be present.

NATURAL HISTORY AND TREATMENT OUTCOMES

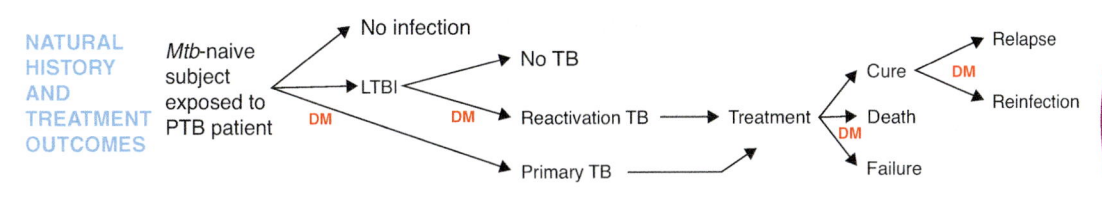

Mtb-naive subject exposed to PTB patient → No infection / LTBI (DM) → No TB / Reactivation TB (DM) → Treatment / Primary TB → Treatment → Cure (DM) → Relapse / Reinfection; Death (DM); Failure

Figure 11.3 Patients with diabetes infected by TB have a more aggressive course of disease and poorer response to therapy as noted in this timeline, starting with exposure. The bolded lines identified with DM reflect the path that most with diabetes will take after exposure to an individual with TB.

- The most common causative organism is *Streptococcus pneumoniae*.
- Treatment is with combination antibiotics so as to have broader coverage.

♦ *Influenza* severity is heightened in those with diabetes. This became apparent in the setting of the 2009 H1N1 virus where the presence of diabetes would quadruple a patient's risk of ending up in the ICU and double their risk of dying.
- In addition to the immune cellular dysfunction seen in diabetes, hyperglycemia is associated with reductions in forced vital capacity and forced expiratory volume, which are deleterious to pulmonary function reserve in times of illness.
- Furthermore, there is data to suggest that glycemic variability will negatively impact the integrity of the endothelial lining, which is the major site which the virus attacks.

♦ *Tuberculosis (TB)* is seen much more commonly in those with diabetes, with patients with diabetes having a 3-fold risk of developing TB.
- Patients with diabetes who have TB are less likely to have the traditional risk factors associated with contracting the disease state, so a greater level of suspicion needs to be present.
- They are also more likely to present with pulmonary, cavitary, and sputum-smear positive TB at the time of diagnosis and have infection with drug-resistant TB.
- Treatment is more challenging, with a longer time to response and a higher risk of relapse and re-infection in those with diabetes (Figure 11.3).
- Some specific recommendations have been provided for TB therapy in those with diabetes:
  - DM screening should be expanded in those newly diagnosed with TB.
  - Vitamin B6 should be provided with isoniazid due to risk of neuropathy.
  - A longer course of therapy to 9 months should be completed.
  - Drug concentration monitoring should be considered.
  - Optimization of glucose levels is imperative.

Gastrointestinal and Liver Infections

♦ *Hepatitis* infections are more commonly seen in those with diabetes, particularly hepatitis C.
- In the US, there is almost a 3-fold increase in prevalence of hepatitis C among those with diabetes compared with those without.
- Cirrhosis, part of the natural history of hepatitis, can itself lead to impaired glucose metabolism and type 2 diabetes.
- Interferon alpha, historically commonly used in the treatment of hepatitis, appears to also be able to induce type 1 diabetes through unclear mechanisms.
- There is an association between presence of diabetes and risk of developing hepatocellular carcinoma in those with chronic hepatitis C infection.
- Treatment outcomes appear to be worse in those with diabetes, hence

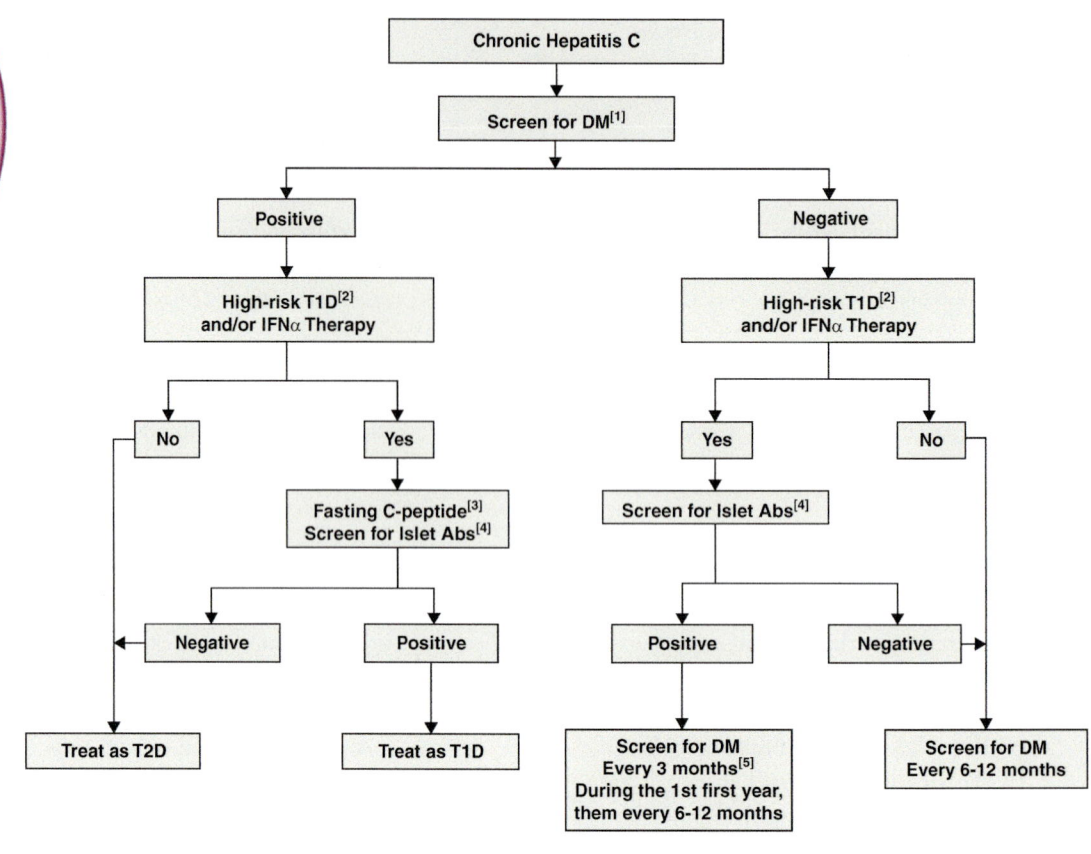

```
Chronic Hepatitis C
        │
        ▼
   Screen for DM[1]
   ┌────┴────┐
Positive   Negative
   │          │
   ▼          ▼
High-risk T1D[2]      High-risk T1D[2]
and/or IFNα Therapy   and/or IFNα Therapy
   │                      │
 ┌─┴─┐                  ┌──┴──┐
 No  Yes               Yes   No
      │                 │
      ▼                 ▼
Fasting C-peptide[3]   Screen for Islet Abs[4]
Screen for Islet Abs[4]
   ┌──┴──┐              ┌──┴──┐
Negative Positive    Positive Negative
   │        │           │        │
   ▼        ▼           ▼        ▼
Treat as  Treat as   Screen for DM    Screen for DM
T2D       T1D        Every 3 months[5] Every 6-12 months
                     During the 1st first year,
                     them every 6-12 months
```

Figure 11.4 Screening for diabetes in those with hepatitis C is strongly encouraged. There is an association with both hepatitis C itself and the therapy for hepatitis C with development of diabetes, both in type 1 and type 2. *From Hammerstad, Sara Salehi et al.* Diabetes and Hepatitis C: A Two-Way Association. Frontiers in endocrinology. Vol. 6 134. 14 Sep. 2015. doi:10.3389/fendo.2015.00134.

the recommendation is to screen all patients for diabetes. Screening for islet autoantibodies is also recommended prior to the initiation of interferon therapy.
- ◇ During treatment, regular screening for diabetes is also needed (Figure 11.4).
- ◇ Metformin should not be avoided as there may be reduced risk for hepatocellular carcinoma and death or need for transplant with its use in those with diabetes and hepatitis C.
- ◆ *Helicobacter pylori* (*H. pylori*) is a microbe that is found more commonly in the gastric antrum of those with diabetes.
  - ◇ Worsening glycemic control appears to increase the incidence of active and symptomatic infection, potentially being up to 50% more prevalent in those with diabetes.
  - ◇ The interaction is not unidirectional as there is increasing evidence that the infection itself causes insulin resistance and development of type 2 diabetes (Figure 11.5).
  - ◇ Clearance of *H. pylori* is more challenging in those with diabetes, especially where there is evidence of microvascular complications such as retinopathy and neuropathy.
- ◆ *Emphysematous cholecystitis* is a rare form of acute cholecystitis that most commonly impacts individuals between 50–70 years of age, of whom around 50% will have diabetes.
  - ◇ Ischemia of the gallbladder is felt to play an important role in the

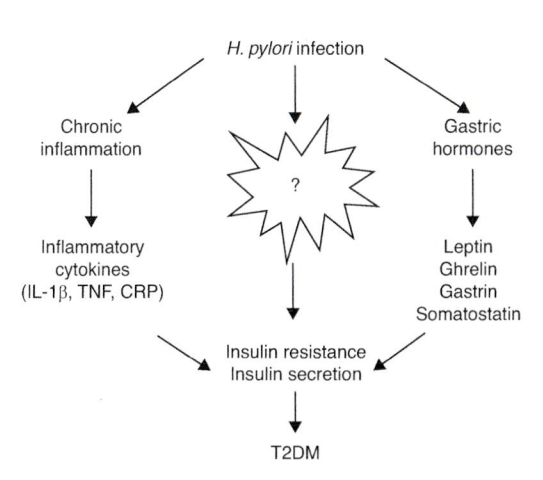

Figure 11.5 Depiction of mediators of the development of type 2 diabetes in an infection with *H. pylori*.

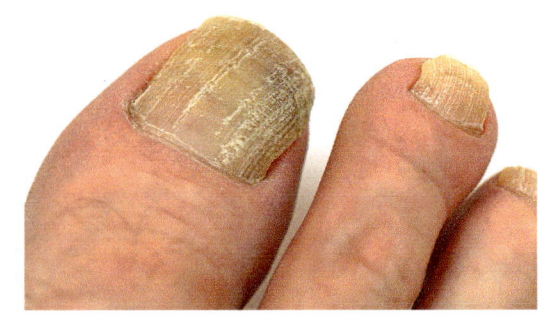

Figure 11.6 Onchomycosis of toenails, showing hyperkeratosis and discoloration.

development of this condition. Since vascular disease is more commonly seen in those with diabetes, this is felt to be one of the mechanisms for the association.
- ◇ The symptoms commonly resemble that of acute cholecystitis, although they can be more severe.
- ◇ It is diagnosed by finding gas in the gallbladder wall or around the gallbladder on imaging, which can be done via x-ray, ultrasound, or CT typically.
- ◇ Because of the high rate of mortality in those with diabetes who have this condition (up to 15%), rapid treatment with cholecystectomy and broad-spectrum antibiotic coverage is needed

Skin and soft tissue infections
- ◆ Diabetic neuropathy and vascular disease greatly increase the risk for a skin and soft tissue infection in diabetes.
- ◆ Diabetic foot infections are the most common soft tissue infection and are covered separately in Chapter 10.
- ◆ *Onychomycosis* is a fungal infection of the nails that is very common in those with diabetes, potentially present in up to 1/3 of individuals (Figure 11.6).
  - ◇ A positive fungal culture is needed.
  - ◇ Oral antifungals are the most effective, but topicals can be utilized.
- ◆ *Cellulitis* is a common cutaneous infectious process seen in diabetes that involves the deeper dermis.
  - ◇ Worsened glycemic control is correlated with an increased risk for cellulitis, with a 1.12-fold risk of cellulitis for every 1% increase in HbA1c.
  - ◇ There has been a dramatic increase in the prevalence of methicillin-resistant *Staphylococcus aureus* (MRSA) which along with streptococcus species represent 2 of the most important organisms involved in cellulitis in those with diabetes. However, there is an increase in the presence of gram-negative bacilli as well.
  - ◇ Broad-spectrum coverage is often required, particularly in the hospital setting.
- ◆ *Necrotizing fasciitis* is a more severe infection causing necrosis of subcutaneous tissue and fascia, typically not involving the muscle (Figure 11.7).
  - ◇ There is a high fatality rate, up to 34%.
  - ◇ Diabetes is the most common underlying condition seen in more than 50% of patients with necrotizing fasciitis.

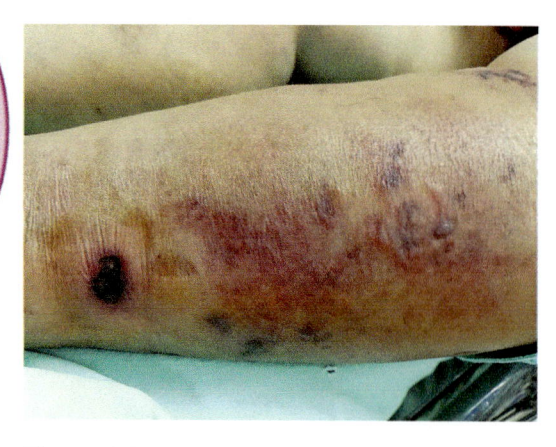

Figure 11.7 Necrotizing fasciitis involving the left leg.

- In those with diabetes, *Klebsiella pneumoniae* is more commonly seen as a causative organism.
- Given the often polymicrobial nature of necrotizing fasciitis, antibiotic coverage should be broad.
- In those with diabetes, amputation is commonly seen during the treatment course and surgical debridement is needed.
- Without early treatment, death can occur within 1–4 days.
- *Fournier gangrene* is a very rare form of necrotizing fasciitis involving the external genital organs and perianal regions, typically seen in men.
    - In the presence of treatment delay, there can be up to 90% mortality.
    - The most common risk factor appears to be diabetes.
    - Diagnosis is made via radiology.
    - Treatment is a combination of broad-spectrum antibiotics along with surgical debridement.

Genitourinary infections

- *Urinary tract infections (UTIs)* are more common in those with type 2 diabetes, and various population studies have suggested almost a 2-fold increased risk of UTI in the setting of diabetes versus without diabetes.
    - In theory, the increase in glucosuria in the setting of diabetes should make urinary tract infections more common, but there is not a clear link between the level of glycemic control and frequency of UTI.
    - The mechanism for the increase in UTI appears to be related more to impairment in the immune system response and autonomic neuropathy that results in urinary retention.
    - There is also dysfunction of the uro-epithelial cells, leading to increased ability of bacteria to adhere.
    - The most common organisms appears to be *Escherichia coli*, *Enterobacteriaceae*, and enterococci species. There is also increased risk of fungal UTI.
    - Diagnosis should be made by urinalysis, with urine culture for the organism at fault (Figure 11.8).
    - Treatment should not be initiated until an organism is identified unless there this is an uncomplicated acute cystitis case, which does not represent a recurrence.
    - When choosing a regimen, attention should be paid to the increased prevalence of drug-resistant organisms in those with diabetes.
    - Notably, there is no need to treat asymptomatic bacteriuria in patients with diabetes.
    - Outcomes are worse with a higher rate of treatment failure, relapse, and reinfection in those with diabetes compared to those without. Acute cystitis represents the most common form. However, there is also often progression to complicated forms of UTI:
        - *Emphysematous cystitis* represents an infection with gas-forming organism of the bladder wall. While rare, over 50% of patients have concurrent diabetes. Radiologic confirmation is required and CT is the best modality.
        - *Pyelonephritis* and *emphysematous pyelonephritis* are infections

```
                    ┌─────────────────────┐
                    │ Presence of symptoms? │
                    └──────────┬──────────┘
                         ┌─────┴─────┐
                         ▼           ▼
                       ┌────┐      ┌────┐
                       │ No │      │ Yes│
                       └─┬──┘      └─┬──┘
                         ▼           ▼
```

Urine culture
≥10^5 cfu/mL of same uropathogen in two separate clean voided mis-stream urine specimens
OR
≥10^2 cfu/mL from sterile in-and-out urinary catheter

Urine culture
Mid-stream urine
Women: ≥10^5 cfu/mL of uropathogen
Men: ≥10^6 cfu/mL of uropathogen

OR
≥10^2 cfu/mL for uropathogen with clear symptoms and no alternative diagnosis

In-and-out sterile urinary catheter
≥10^2 cfu/mL of uropathogen

Long-term indwelling catheter or intermittent catheterization
≥10^2 cfu/mL from a new catheter urine specimen and no alternative diagnosis

Asymptomatic

Yes → Frequency, urgency, dysuria, or suprapubic pain → Cystitis

Costovertebral angle pain, tenderness, fever, or chills ± lower UTI symptoms → Pyelonephritis/urosepsis

No → No urinary tract infection

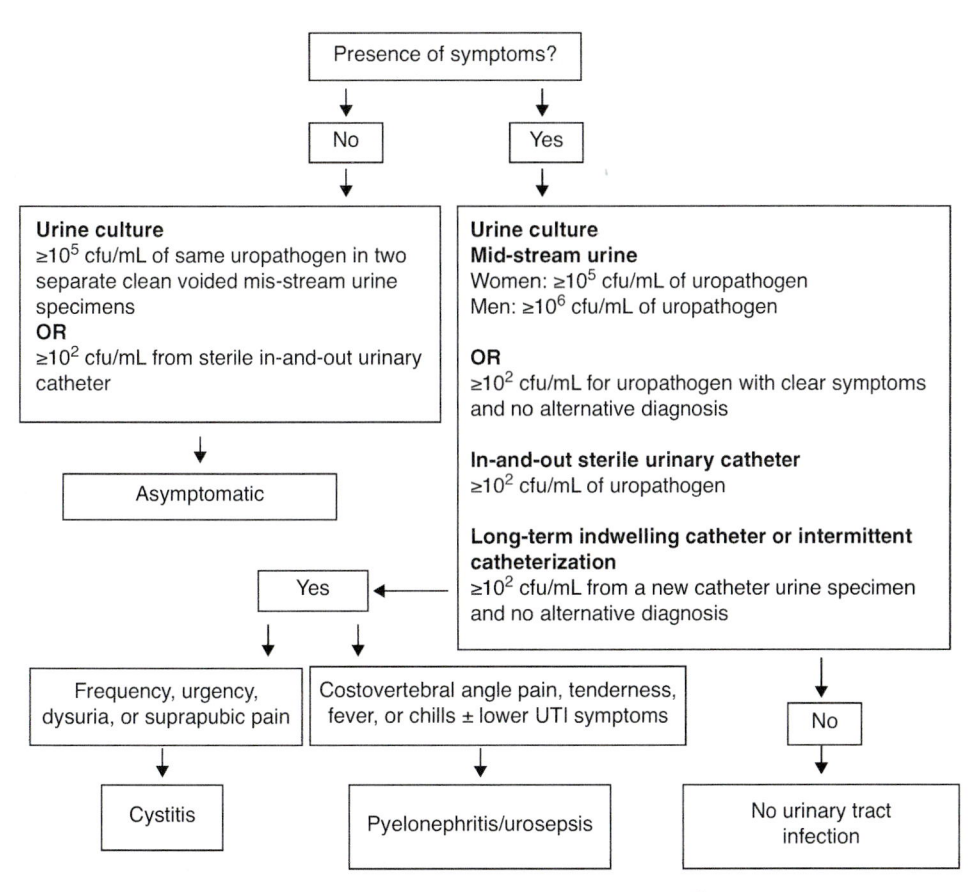

Figure 11.8 Flowchart showing how to make diagnosis of urinary tract infection. This utilizes common symptoms to help distinguish the location of the urinary tract infection and describes the different collection methods for the urine sample. Emphysematous forms of UTIs and abscesses will require imaging modalities for confirmation of their presence.

of the renal parenchyma, the difference being that in the emphysematous form there is gas present. These are 4–5 times more common in those with diabetes. In pyelonephritis in the setting of diabetes, there is often bilateral involvement. Emphysematous pyelonephritis requires imaging confirmation via ultrasound and/or CT.

- *Renal* and *perinephric abscess* are collections of purulent material in and around the kidneys respectively. Diabetes is concurrent in up to 40% of cases. The best modality for diagnosis is ultrasound and/or CT. Often with diabetes present, the presentation is insidious, and this should be considered in cases of acute pyelonephritis that is not improving with use of antibiotic therapy.
  ◇ For complicated UTIs, aggressive antibiotic therapy is needed quickly.
  ◇ Appropriate urinary drainage must be established and often percutaneous or surgical interventions will be needed.
- *Mycotic genital infections* are driven by candida species in both men and women.
  ◇ Women with a candida infection of the genital area have vulvovaginal candidiasis while in men an infection

of the genitalia with candida is called balanitis.
◇ Diagnosis is made based on symptoms, along with microscopy confirmation or culture respectively.
◇ Topical antifungals are the mainstay of therapy.

The impact of SGLT2 inhibitors
◆ There appears to be an increased risk with use of the class of SGLT2 inhibitors and development of genital infections due to the presence of glucosuria.
◆ The association with UTI is less clear and there is no known association with upper UTIs such as pyelonephritis.
◆ There have also been cases of Fournier's gangrene that have been described in the setting of SGLT2 inhibitors use as well. This led to the publication of a 2018 Food and Drug Administration warning about a potential association.

COVID-19 and diabetes

Overview
◆ Coronavirus disease-2019 (COVID-19) is caused by severe acute respiratory syndrome coronavirus-2 (SARS-CoV-2). Increasingly, it is becoming apparent that diabetes is a significant risk factor for contracting COVID-19, a more severe disease course, and increased mortality.
◆ Compared with COVID-19 without diabetes:
   ◇ Diabetes carries with it a 2-fold increase in risk of being in the ICU.
   ◇ Diabetes carries with it a 3-fold increased risk of death from COVID-19.
◆ In those with diabetes:
   ◇ Up to 40% will require hospitalization.
   ◇ Between 21-43% will require intensive care with a ¼ fatality rate.
   ◇ Those with poorer glycemic control in the antecedent months will have a higher risk of poor outcomes.
◆ There are indirect ways in which the COVID-19 pandemic has impacted health of those with diabetes:
   ◇ Reducing both access to the health care system and deferred care.
   ◇ Changes in lifestyle, including a more sedentary behavior, worse sleep, and increased food intake.

Mechanisms for Infection and Severe Disease
◆ There are a number of mechanisms for the association between diabetes and increased risk of infection and worse disease course (Figure 11.9):
   ◇ SARS-CoV-2 enters cells via the angiotensin-converting enzyme 2 (ACE2) receptor in the respiratory system. In diabetes, there are increased levels of receptors.
   ◇ Medications commonly used in diabetes such as ACE inhibitors and GLP-1 receptor agonists are able to upregulate the levels of expression of the ACE2 receptor as well.
   ◇ A reduced initial immune response that is followed by a dysregulated excessive inflammatory response seen in those with diabetes.
   ◇ Reduction in baseline pulmonary function seen in both type 1 and type 2 diabetes.
      ▪ This includes alveolar dysfunction, specifically reduced permeability and O_2 uptake
◆ In COVID-19, there is a propensity towards a hypercoagulable state. Diabetes and hyperglycemia predisposes to a hypercoagulable state as well.

Impact of therapy
◆ Improved glycemic control appears to reduce the risk of mortality.
◆ There has been an association with the use of metformin and SGLT2 inhibitors with lower mortality, while there has been some suggestion of higher mortality with insulin therapy and DPP4 inhibitors.

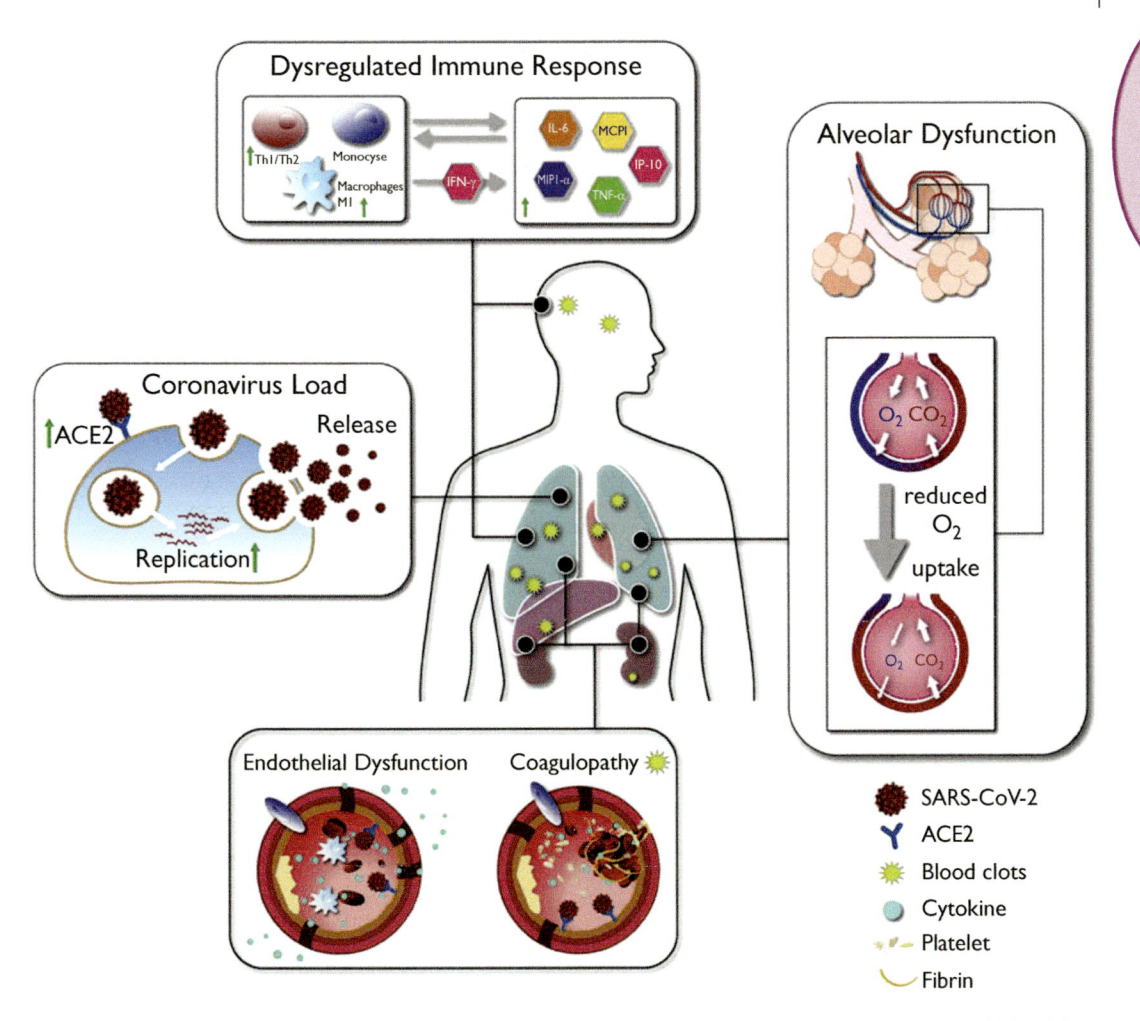

Figure 11.9 Various mechanisms for increased infection risk and worse clinical course in individuals with diabetes for COVID-19. *From Erener, Suheda. Diabetes, infection risk and COVID-19. Molecular metabolism. Vol. 39 (2020): 101044. doi:10.1016/j.molmet.2020.101044.*

Glycemic control and infection outcomes

- Although there have been a large number of studies showing a strong association between level of glycemic control and likelihood of infection, fewer prospective studies have been done assessing the impact of lowering glucose on infection outcomes.
- In vivo, chemotaxis of PMN appears to be restored in the setting of insulin.
- After cardiothoracic surgery, postoperative control of glucose to keep sugars <11.1 mmol/L (<200 mmol/L) was associated with a decrease in deep wound infection from 2.4% to 1.5%. Other post-cardiac surgery studies have found a similar reduction in sternal wound infections in the setting of improved glycemic control.
- Metformin appears to have an ability to improve production of carious cytokines and levels of T cells.

CHAPTER 12

Severe diabetic metabolic disturbances

Metabolic disturbances in diabetes can have extremely serious consequences. If unrecognized, they may result in coma. There are two major forms of such disturbances – diabetic ketoacidosis (DKA) and hyperosmolar hyperglycemic state (HHS) (also known as hyperosmolar nonketotic coma or HONK). The two generally differ based on the absence or relative lack of insulin to counteract the processes that lead to hyperglycemia, and subsequent production of ketones and an acidic milieu (more pronounced in DKA).

Table 12.1 Features of DKA and HHS. The main distinguishing feature of DKA is the presence of significant ketoacidosis.

Comparison of DKA and HONK	
DKA	HONK
Hyperketonemia	No hyperketonemia
Metabolic acidosis	Metabolic acidosis in some cases
Severe hyperglycemia	Severe hyperglycemia

Diabetic ketoacidosis

- DKA is a life-threatening condition that can be reversed if there is early recognition and prompt treatment.
- The underlying pathology is insulin deficiency, leading to blood glucose generally >13.9 mmol/L (250 mg/dL), pH <7.3, and a bicarbonate of usually <15 mmol/L (15 mEq/L).
- Most of the time it is easy to differentiate between DKA and HHS but in some situations features may overlap.
- Diabetic ketoacidosis is often precipitated by:
  - ◇ Omission of insulin.
  - ◇ Stress such as infection, myocardial infarction, or trauma (Table 12.1).
- DKA in younger people is often from noncompliance, e.g. stopping insulin, excess alcohol, or recreational drug use, while DKA in older people is often precipitated by infection or acute cardiovascular events.
- Ketoacidosis is predominantly seen in type 1 diabetes.
  - ◇ It can also occur in type 2 diabetes under stressful conditions such as infections, myocardial infarction, or trauma; it may be induced by atypical antipsychotic agents such as risperidone and olanzapine, and the class of diabetes medications called SGLT2 (sodium-glucose linked transporter 2) inhibitors.
- DKA is the presentation at diagnosis in 20–25% of type 1 diabetes patients.
  - ◇ The majority of DKA episodes occur in previously known rather than newly diagnosed diabetes.
  - ◇ About 20% of patients who have had DKA have multiple episodes in a year.
- The majority of cases reaching hospital are preventable because the metabolic disturbances take a while to develop and often result from the patient being unaware of how to manage insulin therapy. Important components of prevention therefore include:

- ◇ Earlier detection.
- ◇ Proper education.
- ◇ Good communication between patient and physician.
- ◇ The capacity to self-manage insulin injections at home even when sick. Sick-day rules should be part of the education given to patients so that they may give themselves bolus doses of insulin while awaiting further instructions from their physician.
- ◆ For patients on an insulin pump, detachment and malfunction of the pump and delivery system can be readily suspected with rising glucose levels on frequent capillary blood glucose checks or use of a continuous glucose monitor, thereby alerting the patient to take steps to avert DKA. It is important to realize that DKA will develop rapidly, within several hours, in a patient treated with a subcutaneous insulin infusion pump in the event of pump failure, due to the lack of any depot of long-acting insulin.
- ◆ In many cases of DKA, the patients reduced or omitted their insulin doses because they were not eating due to nausea or vomiting. In this situation insulin actually needs to be increased, not reduced, but a source of glucose needs to be provided to avoid hypoglycemia. This strengthens the case that continued education needs to be provided to patients, their family, and friends. Insulin should never be stopped without medical advice.

Education about managing insulin therapy is essential in the prevention of DKA.

Pathogenesis
- ◆ Ketoacidosis is the primary manifestation, and results from a deficiency of insulin and the resulting uncontrolled catabolism from excess counter-regulatory hormones – glucagon, epinephrine, cortisol, and growth hormone.
  - ◇ Only modest insulin levels are needed to inhibit hepatic ketogenesis, so when there is absolute or relative insulin deficiency, ketogenesis ensues.
  - ◇ As ketoacids are produced, bicarbonate and other buffers are lost, and metabolic acidosis follows.
  - ◇ With insulin deficiency, glucagon stimulates gluconeogenesis and ketogenesis. As the other counter-regulatory hormones come into play, peripheral glucose utilization is inhibited, and lipolysis takes place (Figure 12.1).

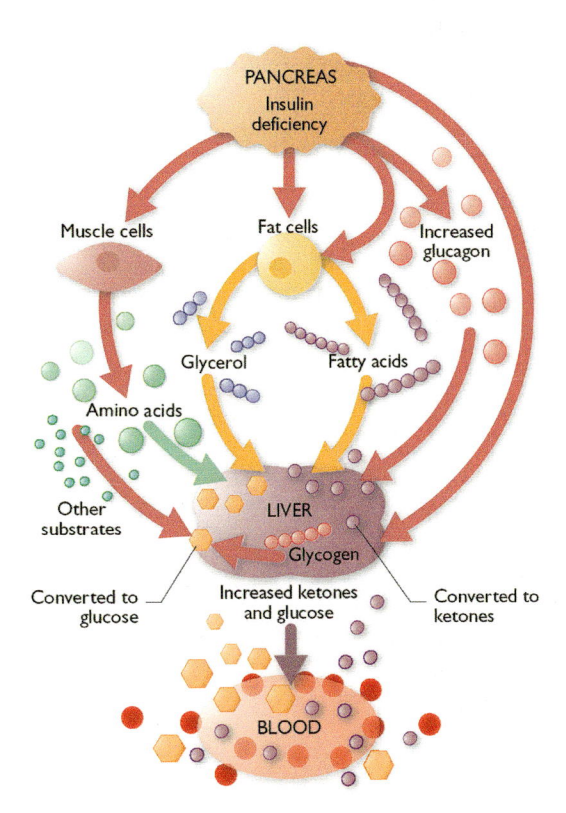

Figure 12.1 Pathogenesis of diabetic ketoacidosis. Insulin deficiency and the concomitant increase in glucagon lead to increased breakdown of triglycerides into free fatty acids, and increased hepatic glycogenolysis, gluconeogenesis, and ketogenesis.

Diabetic metabolic disturbances

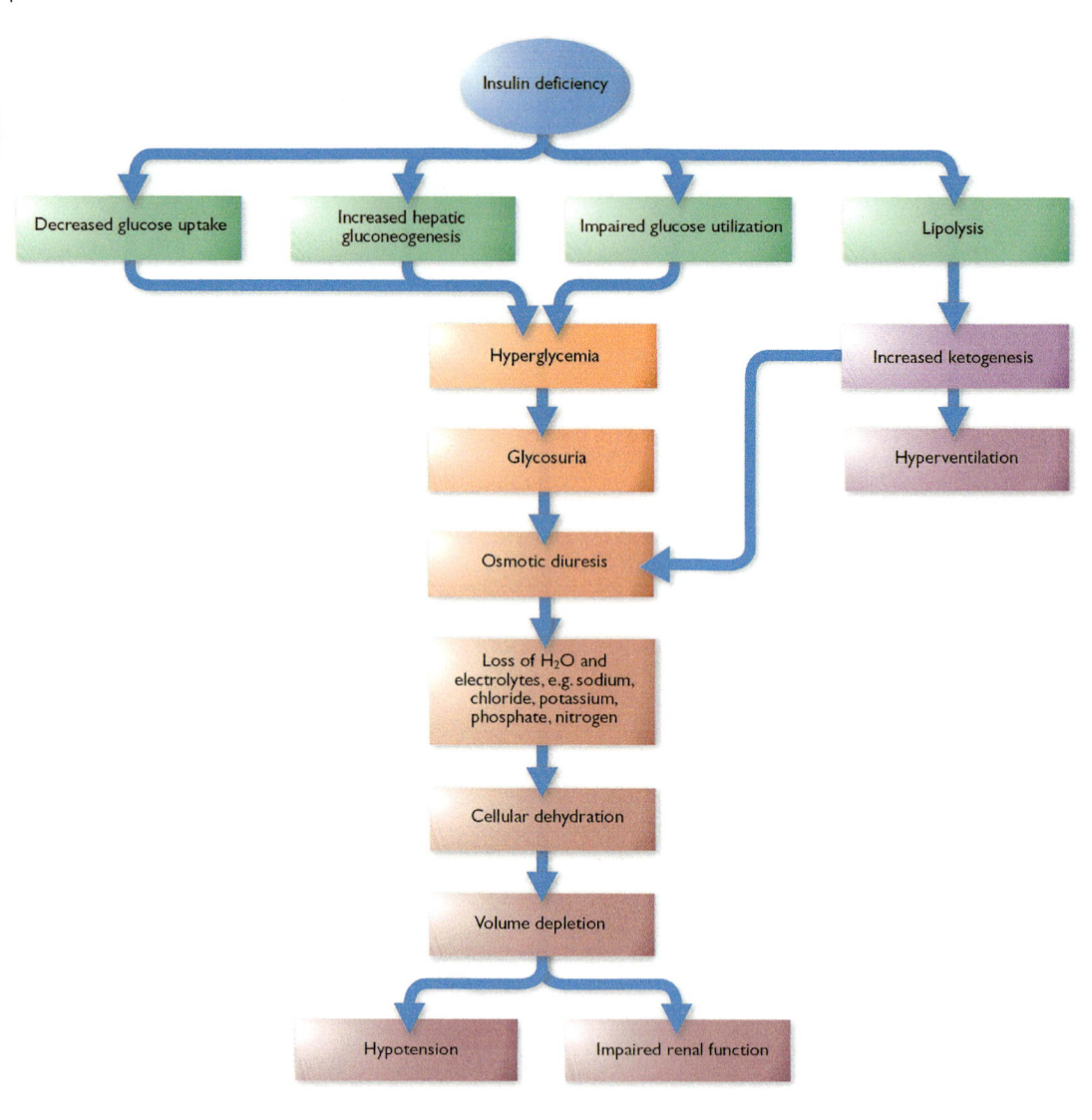

Figure 12.2 Physiological disturbances in DKA. Insulin deficiency can lead to hepatic glucose production and decreased glucose uptake, resulting in hyperglycemia, and can also stimulate lipolysis and ketone body production, resulting in ketoacidosis. Both hyperglycemia and hyperketonemia will induce osmotic diuresis and fluid and electrolyte depletion.

- After ketoacidosis, the second important feature is fluid depletion resulting from diuresis (Figure 12.2).
    ◇ The blood glucose may be 10–20 mmol/L (180–360 mg/dL) in some cases, particularly in children, but often in excess of 20 mmol/L (360 mg/dL).
    ◇ Glycosuria results as blood glucose levels exceed the renal threshold. Hyperglycemia causes an osmotic diuresis, with loss of both water and electrolytes.
- Ketoacidosis and fluid depletion occurring together exacerbate the condition through a fall in muscle and renal perfusion. The excess of glucagon and epinephrine exacerbates the insulin deficiency and results in additional metabolic derangement, e.g. increased lipolysis and ketone

body production, the latter predisposing to vomiting.
- Rapid lipolysis occurs, leading to elevated circulating free fatty acid levels. The free fatty acids are broken down to fatty acyl-CoA within the liver cells, and this in turn is converted to ketone bodies within the mitochondria.
  - Accumulation of ketone bodies leads to metabolic acidosis.

DKA is fatal if untreated.

- Vomiting exacerbates loss of fluid and electrolytes.
- The excess ketones are excreted in the urine but also appear in the breath, producing a distinctive smell similar to that of acetone.
- Respiratory compensation for the acidosis leads to hyperventilation, described as 'air hunger'.
- Progressive dehydration impairs renal excretion of hydrogen ions and ketones, which are retained, aggravating the acidosis.
- As the pH falls below 7.0 ([H+] >100 nmol/L), pH-dependent enzyme systems in many cells function less effectively.
- Untreated DKA is invariably fatal.
  - In tertiary centers, the mortality rate is <5%.
  - The highest mortality occurs in patients aged 75 years or older.
  - In children, cerebral edema is a complication that increases the risk of mortality.
  - Coma as a presenting sign also carries a high risk of mortality.

Clinical features

- Clinically a patient with diabetic ketoacidosis is very unwell, even comatose, with marked weight loss, thirst, and polyuria. They may be gasping for air or vomiting (Figure 12.3).

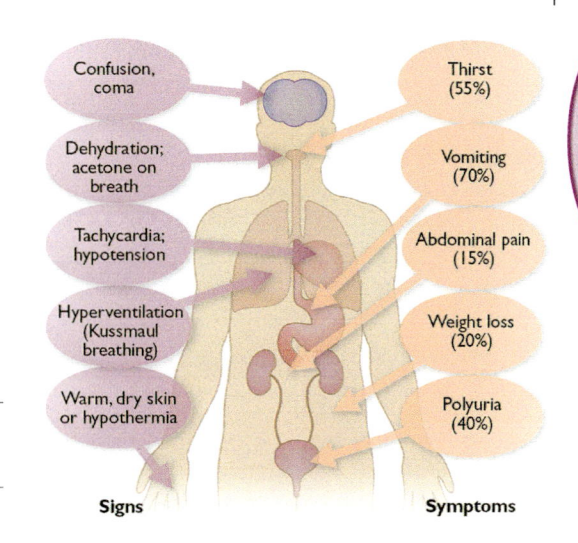

Figure 12.3 Clinical features of ketoacidosis.
Normally DKA has a rapid onset, but some symptoms, such as weight loss and lethargy, may develop several weeks before presentation.

Investigations

- The initial investigations to be done in suspected DKA include taking a good history of insulin doses missed, medications that might precipitate DKA, blood and urine tests, bacteriology, ECG, and imaging (Table 12.2).
  - It is important to differentiate DKA from other causes of coma or altered consciousness (Table 12.3).
- DKA often results in high anion gap acidosis, with the 'gap' being the unmeasured anions in the plasma, primarily albumin and phosphate.
  - Anion gap (in mEq/L or mmol/L) is measured as:
    Measured (or uncorrected) serum sodium – (chloride + bicarbonate).
  - A value of 12 mmol/L (mEq/L) is usually taken as the cut-off to determine if the anion gap is increased.
- Other causes of high anion gap acidosis are usually easy to distinguish from DKA, but should be kept in mind if the presentation is not straightforward.
  - Salicylate poisoning can be tested by plasma salicylate levels in the toxic range.

Table 12.2 Investigations. Glucose and blood gas measurements should be obtained without delay.

Initial investigations in ketoacidosis	
Blood	Glucose, creatinine and electrolytes, full blood count, arterial blood gases including pH, blood ketones, beta-hydroxybutyrate, blood culture
Urine	Dipstick analysis for ketones, pyuria, blood, protein, and urine culture
Bacteriology	Swab any infection and as above do blood and urine cultures
ECG	To detect peaked T waves (hyperkalemia), flat T waves (hypokalemia), or undetected arrhythmia or infarction
Chest radiography	To detect infection or cardiac failure
CT or MRI scan	If cerebral edema is suspected or cause of coma unclear
Other investigations	Directed at finding the precipitating cause

Table 12.3 Coma and impaired consciousness. A decrease in the level of consciousness may be attributable to causes other than DKA.

Other causes of coma or impaired consciousness
Hyperosmolar nonketotic coma
Hypoglycemia
Other electrolyte disorders such as hyponatremia, hypernatremia, hypercalcemia
Head trauma
Toxins, drugs
Uremia
Lactic acidosis
Hepatic encephalopathy
Hypoxemia
CNS infections
Intracranial lesions such as hemorrhage, stroke, hematoma, abscess

◇ Ethylene glycol or methanol poisoning is suspected if there is an 'osmolal gap', i.e. the measured plasma osmolality is greater than the calculated plasma osmolality.
◇ Alcoholic acidosis and starvation acidosis also present with increased anion gap.

Acute management

◆ Different hospitals and societies have developed their own protocols for managing DKA. The general principles include fluid replacement, administration of insulin, and attention to acid-base and electrolyte status. The general management in adult patients are given below. Children will require different proportions and volumes.
◆ *Fluid*. Fluid replacement must be started immediately.
  ◇ Normal saline is given at an initial rate of 1 L/hour, or 15–20 ml/kg/hour for the first 1–2 hour. Careful monitoring should be done when treating patients at risk of cardiovascular disease and cardiac or renal dysfunction.
  ◇ Thereafter, fluids can be reduced to 4–14 ml/kg/hour using normal saline or 0.45% saline, depending on the patient's sodium level and state of hydration.
◆ *Insulin deficiency*. An initial dose of regular insulin, 0.1 unit/kg, can be given as an intravenous bolus. Afterwards, regular insulin intravenous infusion is given at 0.1 unit/kg/hour.
  ◇ This lowers blood glucose by suppressing hepatic glucose output.

- ◇ Regular insulin, 50 units, can be added to 500 ml of normal saline to make a 1:10 concentration. Some of the solution is then flushed to prime the tubing.
- ◇ During the COVID-19 pandemic, several hospitals had to resort to subcutaneous administration of rapid-acting (fast-acting) insulin every 2 hours in pediatric and adult populations.
- ◆ *Electrolytes*. Potassium levels must be monitored both with blood tests and by ECG.
  - ◇ Although there is a total body potassium deficit, initially potassium in the blood may be high.
  - ◇ If initial serum K+ is greater than 5.2 mmol/L (mEq/L), replacement is not given and K+ levels are checked every 2 hour.
  - ◇ When K+ is in the normal range (3.3–5.2 mmol/L [mEq/L]), 20–30 mmol/L [mEq] K+ is given in each liter of intravenous fluid.
  - ◇ If K+ is less than 3.3 mmol/L (mEq/L), insulin is withheld until K+ is above 3.3 mmol/L (mEq/L) and K+ is given at 20-30 mmol/L/hour (mEq/L/hour).
- ◆ *Acid–base balance*. Both fluid replacement and insulin therapy will usually restore acid-base imbalance.
  - ◇ Administration of bicarbonate is controversial and seldom necessary and is only considered if the pH is below 6.9.
  - ◇ Prospective studies have not shown either a benefit or an increased morbidity or mortality in patients where pH is 6.9–7.1. Below a pH of 6.9, even in the absence of solid data, it seems reasonable to administer bicarbonate since severe acidosis can also lead to vascular derangements.
- ◆ Successful management of DKA depends upon fluid resuscitation, insulin therapy, and correcting metabolic acidosis and electrolyte imbalances. Frequent monitoring of these parameters is necessary (Table 12.4). Figure 12.4 presents a treatment algorithm.

Table 12.4 Monitoring. Regular, frequent monitoring is required to assess progress and avoid complications.

Initial monitoring interval for DKA parameters	
Vital signs and mental status	Every hour
Glucose	Every hour
Potassium	Every 2 hours
Other electrolytes, blood urea nitrogen (BUN), creatinine	Every 4 hours

- ◆ *Seek the underlying cause*. Physical examination, chest radiography, and urine tests may reveal a source of infection.
  - ◇ As fever may be absent even in the presence of infection, and polymorphonuclear leukocytosiscan be present even in the absence of infection, a search for other causes can be directed by the patient's clinical features.
  - ◇ For example, a 65-year-old male with hypertension and positive smoking history would lead you to obtain an ECG to exclude a silent myocardial infarction, which can present with ketoacidosis.
- ◆ *Other problems*. These can include:
  - ◇ Altered sensorium. For patients in coma, the insertion of a nasogastric tube can help reduce the risk of aspiration pneumonia.
  - ◇ Hypotension. Intravenous fluid resuscitation should be administered. If hypotension continues, plasma expanders or whole blood may be considered, as well as insertion of a central venous pressure line.
  - ◇ Hypothermia. Mortality rate is high, about 30–60%, in patients with DKA and hypothermia.
  - ◇ Cerebral edema. This is most often seen in children and adolescents. The cause is thought to be very rapid correction of hyperglycemia and the use of excessive hypotonic fluids. Though rare, it can be fatal.

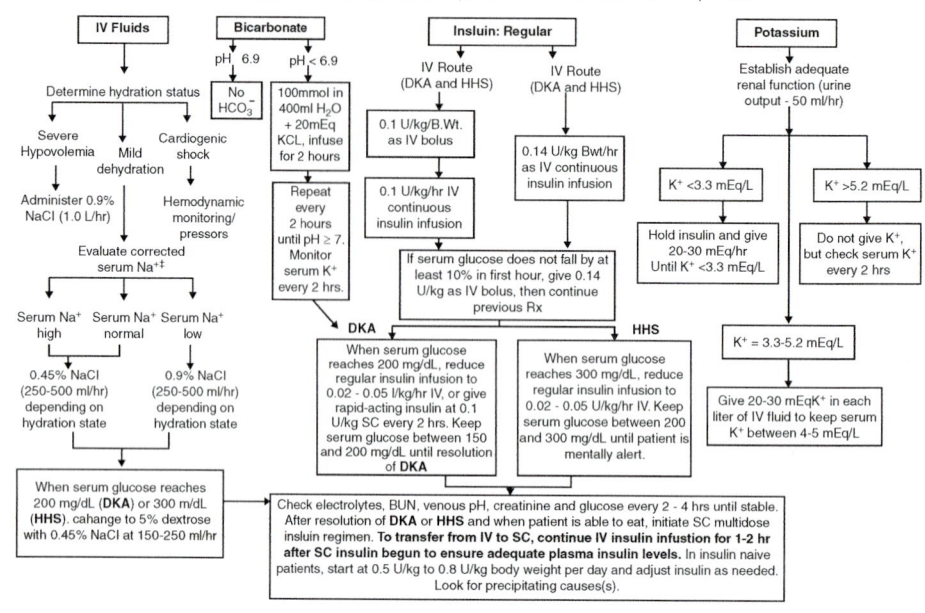

Figure 12.4 Treatment algorithm for DKA and HHS in adults. The cornerstones of acute management are fluid resuscitation, insulin therapy, correction of metabolic acidosis and electrolyte abnormalities, as well as treatment of precipitating factors. *From Kitabchi, Abbas E, et al.* Hyperglycemic crises in adult patients with diabetes. *Diabetes Care.* Vol. 32,7 (2009): 1335–43. doi:10.2337/dc09-9032.

- Deep venous thrombosis can be prevented by prophylactic measures such as subcutaneous heparin.
- Complications of therapy. With excess insulin infusion, hypoglycemia and hypokalemia can develop, hence the need for close monitoring of these parameters. Excess fluid replacement can cause cardiac dysfunction; in patients with cardiac compromise, monitoring of central venous pressure is recommended.

Subsequent management

- Once glucose reaches 11 mmol/L (200 mg/dL), the infusion is changed to 5% dextrose in 0.45% NaCl at 150–250 ml/hour until acidosis is corrected. The addition of dextrose allows continued infusion of insulin without hypoglycemia, since it takes longer to clear the acidosis than to lower the blood glucose.
- When the acidosis has been corrected, insulin is then given through the subcutaneous route.
  - The intravenous insulin infusion is turned off 2–4 hours after the first subcutaneous dose of insulin is given, depending on the kind of subcutaneous insulin used. The insulin infusion is not discontinued right away since the half-life of intravenous insulin is just a few minutes.
- Once the patient is able to eat, the dextrose infusion can be taken down.
- One subcutaneous insulin regimen that closely mimics the physiological secretion of insulin by the pancreas is the administration of long-acting insulin such as glargine once a day (occasionally even twice daily) or detemir, with rapid-acting insulin such as lispro or aspart or glulisine before meals.
- The total daily dose of subcutaneous insulin can be determined in three ways.

Using a combination of these methods is helpful to make sure an appropriate dose is arrived at:
  ◇ Estimation of the dose required via the intravenous insulin infusion (calculate requirements from the past 6 or 8 hours and multiply by 4 or 3, respectively, to come up with a 24-hour dose).
  ◇ Basing it on total body weight. 0.3 Unit/kg/day is usually a good dose for newly diagnosed patients with diabetes; the dose increases if the duration of diabetes is longer, or if the patient has features of insulin resistance.
  ◇ Basing it on home insulin doses and adjusting for degree of control prior to the episode of DKA.

Monitoring of glucose, potassium, and fluid levels is essential in order to avoid complications of therapy.

- Sliding scale regimens (rapid-acting or regular insulin doses given based on glucose levels alone, without regard for meal intake or basal needs) have been popularized, but these reflect lack of familiarity with insulin dosage and may delay the establishment of stable blood glucose levels.
  ◇ Sliding scales are reactive and not proactive; rapid-acting or short-acting insulin is usually just given when blood glucoses are elevated, and insulin is omitted when blood glucoses are within the normal range. Basal insulin is not provided. Unfortunately, sliding scales have permeated the medical culture, for they ensure that the house staff get called only when blood glucose levels are too high or too low.
  ◇ Re-education of medical providers is needed so that basal and prandial insulin are administered.

- For patients who were on an insulin pump prior to the episode of DKA, proper functioning of the entire pump system has to be ascertained prior to resuming its use, since clogging and failure of insulin delivery are potential causes of DKA.
- Confirmation of the cause of DKA with a review of the history and investigations is important so that patients can be advised on how to avoid its recurrence.

A thorough search for the precipitating cause of HHS is essential.

Hyperosmolar hyperglycemic state or hyperosmolar nonketotic state

- Hyperosmolar hyperglycemic state is also known as hyperosmolar nonketotic hyperglycemia (hyperosmolar nonketotic state, and hyperosmolar nonketotic coma (HONK)).
- HHS is characterized by severe hyperglycemia, dehydration, hyperosmolality, and absence of significant ketoacidosis.
- These patients usually have type 2 diabetes, so patients are often adults; however it can also occur in patients with type 1 diabetes.
- Blood glucose is generally higher than in DKA, reaching levels of 33 mmol/L (600 mg/dL) or more, and sometimes greater than 83 mmol/L (1500 mg/dL), with a serum osmolality greater than 320 mmol/L (mOsm/kg).
- High anion gap acidosis is not normally found, but patients can have acidosis from poor tissue perfusion (lactic acidosis), uremia, and from ketone formation.
- As with DKA, an underlying illness must be sought. Common precipitating factors (Figure 12.5) causing HONK include
  ◇ Intercurrent illness (such as infection, trauma, myocardial infarction).

Diabetic metabolic disturbances

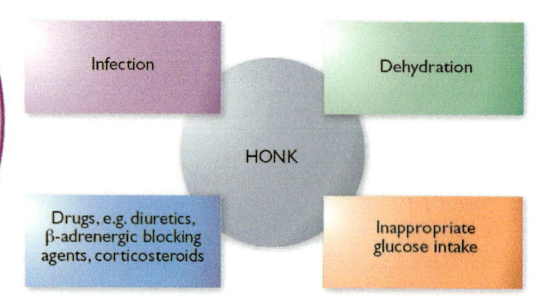

Figure 12.5 HHS: precipitating factors. Common precipitating factors are infection and inadequate insulin therapy. Underlying medical conditions, particularly in the elderly, can lead to reduced water intake and the development of severe dehydration.

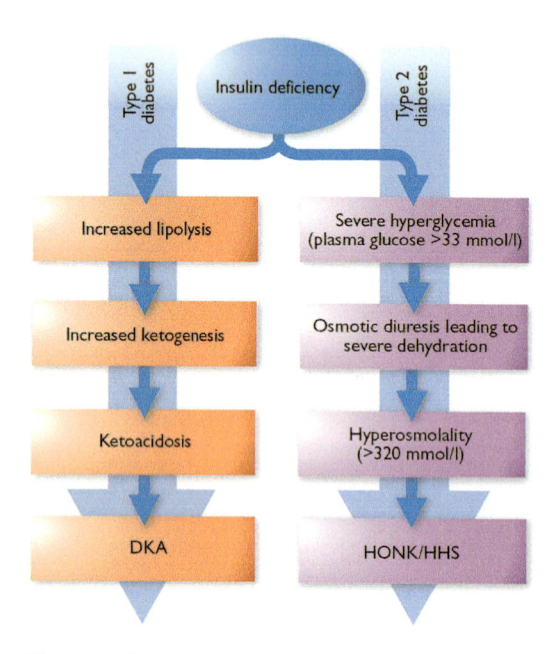

Figure 12.6 HHS and DKA. HHS differs clinically from DKA by an absence of ketoacidosis and a higher degree of hyperglycemia. It is further characterized by high osmolality and dehydration. HHS will often present in a patient with previously undiagnosed type 2 diabetes.

- ◇ Medications such as glucocorticoids.
- ◇ Drinking glucose-rich or 'energy' drinks. In patients who are not able to achieve adequate hydration, osmotic diuresis from the glucosuria and impaired concentrating ability of the kidneys lead to further rises in glucose levels.

- ◆ HHS and DKA represent two ends of a common spectrum (Figure 12.6). Severe cases are easily distinguishable from each other, but milder cases may be less distinct. The biochemical differences between the two conditions are due to:
  - ◇ *Age*. Severe dehydration seen in HHS may be due to altered thirst (caused by an impaired cerebral thirst center) leading to less impetus to access fluids. The same problem can arise from restricted access to fluids (e.g. from physical disability, mental deficiency).
  - ◇ *Degree of insulin deficiency*. In type 2 diabetes, though there is relative lack of insulin, there is often enough endogenous insulin to inhibit ketogenesis.

Clinical features
- ◆ Typically patients are over 60 years of age, often with previously undiagnosed type 2 diabetes. A history of diuretic or steroid therapy is an additional risk factor.
- ◆ The history often is that of days to weeks of increasing thirst and polyuria, with weight loss and weakness.
- ◆ On presentation, patients have severe dehydration and altered mentation. Impairment of consciousness is related to the degree of hyperosmolality.
  - ◇ Abdominal complaints such as nausea and vomiting are not as common as in DKA.
- ◆ On examination, patients have poor skin turgor, hypotension, and tachycardia. Kussmaul breathing is uncommon.

Investigations
- ◆ Serum osmolality is usually greater than 320 mmol/L (mOsm/kg), and glucose greater than 33 mmol/L (600 mg/dL). Serum osmolality is measured as:

$$2\,[Na + K\ (\text{in mmol/L or mEq/L})] + \text{blood glucose (divided by 1 when using mmol/L, or by 18 when using glucose in mg/dL)}.$$

- Monitoring of serum osmolality and electrolytes is key to management, and should be checked every 2–4 hours.
- The measured serum sodium is often falsely low because of the osmotic effect of glucose. To calculate for corrected serum sodium, 1.6 mmol/L (mEq) of Na+ is added for each 5.5 mmol/L (100 mg/dL) of glucose above 5.5 mmol/L (100 mg/dL) or:
  - Corrected serum Na in mEq/L = measured Na in mEq/L + (1.6 [glucose in mg/dL – 100] divided by 100). If using glucose in mmol/L, multiply glucose by 18 first.
- Blood glucose should be checked hourly.
- HHS patients are usually older than patients who have DKA and mortality is higher, so a thorough search for the precipitating cause is important and will direct further management.
  - Chest radiography, urinalysis and cultures to look for infection, and an ECG to rule out myocardial infarction are reasonable screening tests, especially if a good history is unobtainable and physical findings are lacking.
  - In patients presenting with altered mental status, a stroke or an intracranial bleed should be considered.

Complications

- Vascular occlusions are important complications of HHS.
  - Arterial thrombosis is said to cause one third of the deaths in diabetic coma. Arterial thrombosis leads to cerebrovascular accidents, myocardial infarction, or arterial insufficiency in the lower limbs.
  - Mesenteric artery occlusion and disseminated intravascular coagulation may also occur.

Patients with HHS are particularly prone to arterial thrombosis.

Treatment

- The general principles of management are similar to those for DKA. However, the following are the differences or points of emphasis:
  - Plasma osmolality is often very high. This should be monitored as treatment progresses. Normal osmolality is between 280 and 295 mmol/L or mOsm/kg.
  - Normal saline is recommended for fluid replacement. Half-normal saline (0.45%) may result in rapid hemodilution and subsequent cerebral damage.
  - Patients can be sensitive to insulin. With a brisk fall in glucose, smaller insulin doses (e.g. 3 unit/hour not 6 unit/hour) are appropriate. Otherwise, a rapid fall in glucose may result in cerebral edema. When glucose level reaches 300 mg/dL, intravenous fluids should be changed to 5% dextrose with 0.45%NaCl at a rate of 150–250 mL/hour.
  - Anticoagulant prophylaxis is particularly important.

Prognosis

- Mortality in HHS is seen in 10–50% of cases, on the higher end for the elderly.
- For patients who recover, however, many can be treated with diet and oral agents alone.

Brittle diabetes mellitus

- This term is used to describe patients with recurrent ketoacidosis and/or recurrent hypoglycemic coma, but there is no precise definition. Most patients are those who experience recurrent severe hypoglycemia.
- Once underlying causes and improvements in management have been implemented, attention should focus on psychosocial issues.

A combination of chaotic food intake and insulin omission is the primary cause of recurrent ketoacidosis.

Recurrent ketoacidosis

- This usually occurs in adolescents or young adults, particularly girls. Metabolic decompensation may develop very rapidly.
- A combination of chaotic food intake and insulin omission, whether consciously or unconsciously, is now regarded as the primary cause of this problem. It almost always occurs in the context of considerable psychosocial problems, particularly eating disorders. This area needs careful and sympathetic exploration in any patient with recurrent ketoacidosis. It is perhaps not surprising that in an illness where much of one's life is spent thinking of and controlling food intake, 30% of women with diabetes have had some features of an eating disorder at some time.
- Other causes include:
  - Iatrogenic. Inappropriate insulin combinations may be a cause of swinging glycemic control. For example, a once-daily regimen may cause hypoglycemia during the afternoon or evening and pre-breakfast hyperglycemia due to insulin deficiency.
  - Intercurrent illness. Unsuspected infections, including urinary tract infections and tuberculosis, may be present. Thyrotoxicosis can also manifest as unstable glycemic control.

Lactic acidosis

- The topic of lactic acidosis is beyond the scope of this book.
- It is important to know that lactic acidosis was associated with the biguanide phenformin in the past, and can occur with the use of the biguanide metformin. Though the risk of developing lactic acidosis with the use of metformin is low, the mortality rate is about 45%.
- Symptoms of lactic acidosis include anorexia, nausea, vomiting, and lethargy.
- Predisposing factors in the setting of metformin use include renal dysfunction and liver disease.
- The use of bicarbonate for treatment is controversial, and management is mainly through hemodialysis.

CHAPTER 13

Long-term management of hyperglycemia

Overview

- Long-term management of hyperglycemia is aimed both at risk factors for complications, and at identification and treatment of complications. The broad approach includes education, diet, exercise, oral antihyperglycemic therapy, non-insulin injectables, and insulin.
- Patients with type 1 diabetes will generally require lifelong insulin treatment, often from the time of diagnosis.
    - ◇ Autoimmune diabetes diagnosed later in life may masquerade as type 2 and respond, at least temporarily, to non-insulin therapy.
- In type 2 diabetes the traditional approach had been to start with diet and exercise, then adding oral therapy, first as monotherapy followed by combination therapy as appropriate, with insulin being reserved until oral therapy proves insufficient, often late in the course of the disease.
- This traditional treatment paradigm had been challenged and a movement was made towards more aggressive and rapidly instituted early treatment because of:
    - ◇ results of clinical trials.
    - ◇ the fact that doctors and other healthcare providers respond much too slowly to continuing inadequate glycemic control.
    - ◇ the development of new classes of drugs for diabetes.
- The European Association for the Study of Diabetes (EASD) and the American Diabetes Association (ADA) have jointly sponsored consensus conferences on this issue, resulting in the publication of a treatment algorithm for the management of hyperglycemia in type 2 diabetes (Figure 13.1).
    - ◇ This suggests that, unless there is a specific contraindication, oral antihyperglycemic therapy with metformin should be initiated, in most cases, along with lifestyle modification, as soon as diabetes has been diagnosed.
    - ◇ The rationale for this is that lifestyle modification – essentially diet and exercise – on its own will inevitably be insufficient.
- This issue is bound to remain under constant scrutiny as a less didactic, more personalized approach is widely employed.
    - ◇ For example, a randomized trial of temporary intensive insulin therapy versus the more traditional oral therapy at the onset of type 2 diabetes showed that both approaches will induce relatively normal blood glucose levels in the majority of patients, but the former appears to give a more sustained improvement in β-cell function and normoglycemia (Figure 13.2).

Long-term adherence to any diet plan is notoriously difficult.

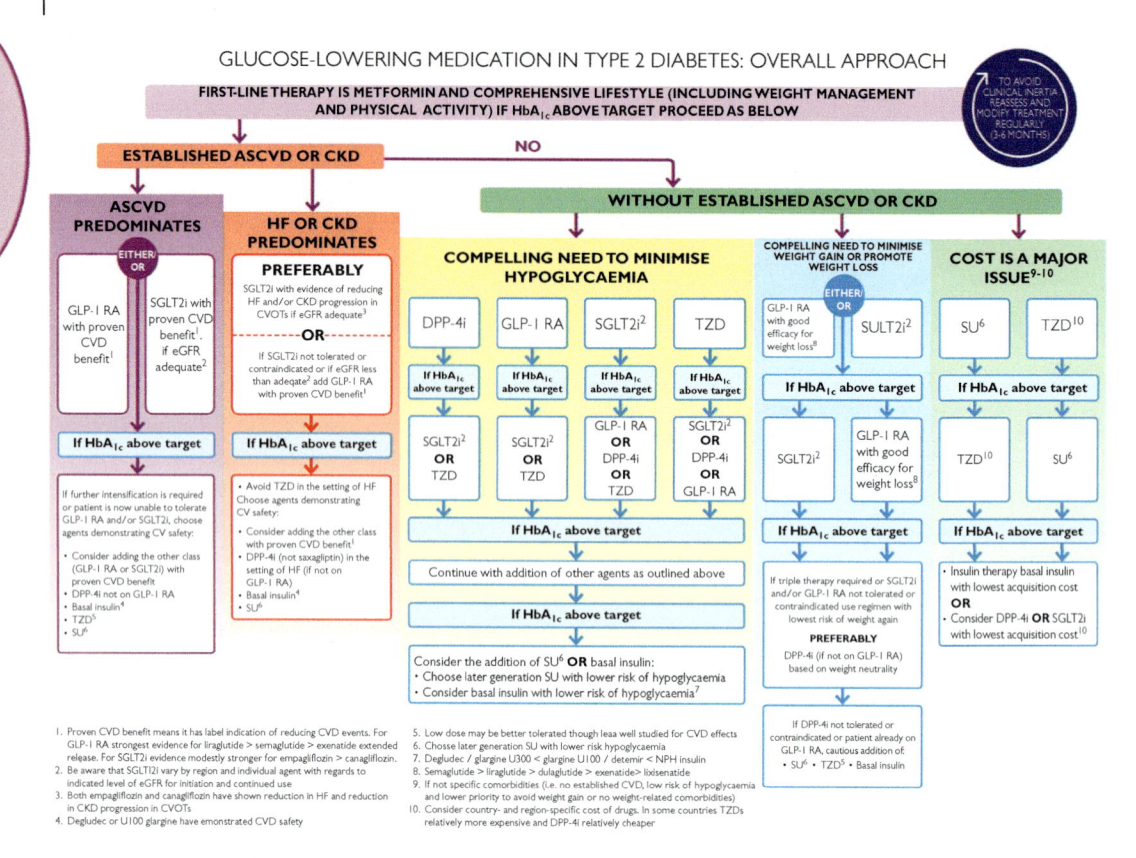

Figure 13.1 Treatment algorithm. The ADA/EASD guidelines for management of Type 2 diabetes. *From Buse, JB, Wexler, DJ, Tsapas, A, et al. 2019 update to: Management of hyperglycaemia in type 2 diabetes, 2018. A consensus report by the American Diabetes Association (ADA) and the European Association for the Study of Diabetes (EASD). Diabetologia 63, 221–228 (2020). https://doi.org/10.1007/s00125-019-05039-w.*

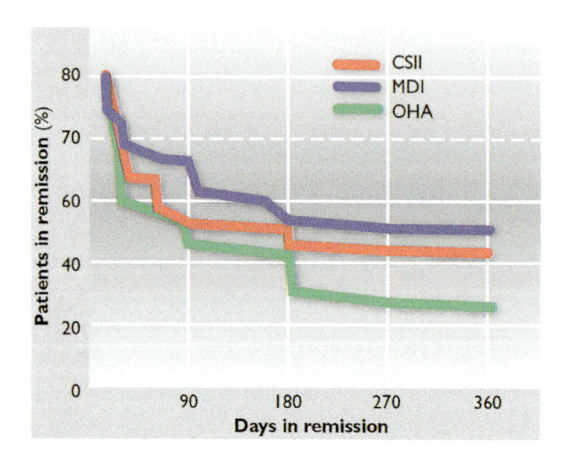

Figure 13.2 Intensive insulin therapy. A trial to compare the effects of continuous subcutaneous insulin infusion (CSII) or multiple daily insulin injections (MDI) with oral hypoglycemic agents (OHA) demonstrated that intensive insulin therapy in patients with newly diagnosed type 2 diabetes improves β-cell function and remission rates compared with treatment with oral hypoglycemic agents. *From Weng, J. et al., 2008.*

Targets of treatment

- Targets may be set for patients to achieve weight loss, lower blood pressure and glucose levels, or improved blood lipid profile (Table 13.1 and Figure 13.3).
- Glucose targets are usually estimated by HbA1c levels, and these targets will vary with age, diabetes duration, and complication risk, including risk of hypoglycemia.
  ◇ The younger the patient, the lower the HbA1c; the older the patient, the higher the HbA1c (except for those under 12 years of age when recommended levels are <8.0% [64 mmol/mol] or when under 6 years of age <8.5% [69 mmol/mol]).
  ◇ Self-monitored blood glucose (SMBG) can improve glycemic control,

Table 13.1 Therapeutic targets. These should be agreed between the patient and the healthcare team.

Therapeutic targets	
Weight	Body mass index <25
	Waist:hip ratio men <0.95; women <0.8
Glucose	HbA1c <7.0% (53 mmol/mol) (but depends on age, diabetes duration, complication risk)
Lipid profile	Cholesterol <4.0 mmol/L (155 mg/dL)
	LDL cholesterol <2.6 mmol/L (100 mg/dL) (lower if overt vascular disease i.e. <2.0 mmol/L [70 mg/dL])
	Triglycerides <1.7 mmol/L (150 mg/dL)
Blood pressure	130/80 mmHg (but depends on age, diabetes duration, complication risk)
Smoking	Nil

Table 13.2 Self-monitored blood glucose. Glycemic goals should be individualized based on age, history, and self-management capabilities.

Plasma glucose goals for SMBG	
AACE Fasting	<110 mg/dL (6.1 mmol/L)
2-hour postprandial	<140 mg/dL (7.8 mmol/L)
ADA and EASD Preprandial	70–130 mg/dL (3.9–7.2 mmol/L)
1–2 hour peak postprandial	<180 mg/dL (10 mmol/L)
IDF Fasting	<115 mg/dL (6.4 mmol/L)
Postprandial	<160 mg/dL (8.9 mmol/L)

AACE: American Association of Clinical Endocrinologists

ADA: American Diabetes Association

EASD: European Association for the Study of Diabetes

IDF: International Diabetes Federation

- Separate AACE from IDF
- AACE goals stay as above
- IDF goals:International Diabetes Federation Clinical Guidelines Task Force. Global guideline for type 2 diabetes. IDF-Guideline-for-Type-2-Diabetes.pdf accessed December 2021
- Fasting <115
- Postprandial <160 mg/dL]

Source: International Diabetes Federation Clinical Guidelines Task Force. Global guideline for type 2 diabetes. IDF-Guideline-for-Type-2-Diabetes.pdf accessed December 2021.

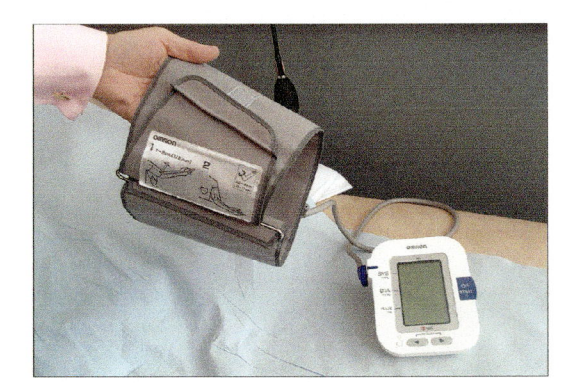

Figure 13.3 A large BP cuff, suitable for patients with obesity. Blood pressure levels are one of the clinical parameters that are used to monitor the effectiveness of diabetes management.

particularly if it forms part of a program of patient education and staff training that promotes management adjustments according to the ensuing blood glucose values (Table 13.2).

Lately, continuous glucose monitors (CGMs) have been made more accessible for use by patients, and can similarly be part of a management program while minimizing the pain of doing frequent fingersticks. Generally accepted glucose level goals are outlined in Table 13.3).

Dietary management

- ◆ The incidence of type 2 diabetes has risen in parallel with a massive increase in obesity, and it is clear that the two are causally linked.
  - ◇ Obesity greatly increases the likelihood that a susceptible individual

Table 13.3 Commonly used glucose level goals using continuous glucose monitoring in non-pregnant adult patients with diabetes. Goals should be modified based on age, history, and co-morbidities.

	Percentage of glucose readings in this range
Above 250 mg/dL	<5
Above 180 mg/dL	<25
70-180 mg/dL	>70
Less than 70 mg/dL	<4
Less than 54 mg/dL	<1

will develop diabetes, and failure to address the problem once diabetes has been diagnosed hampers attempts to achieve glycemic control.
- The main dietary issue in type 2 diabetes is that of excessive calorie intake. This problem is also becoming more prevalent in type 1 diabetes.
- Despite the fact that diet has long been recognized as an important issue in both type 1 and type 2 diabetes, little of the dietary advice given to patients, other than the proven benefit of calorie restriction, is truly evidence-based. It is important to observe that:
  ◇ Long-term adherence to any dietary plan is notoriously difficult, and this is a major stumbling block both in performing the appropriate studies and in applying the results of short-term studies.
  ◇ Dietary advice to patients with diabetes is largely empirical and owes much to the consensus views of 'nutritional experts' and to prevailing fashions.
- It seems reasonable to suggest that the diet of a patient with diabetes should, in principle, be no different from that considered healthy for the population as a whole, perhaps with special emphasis on the avoidance of refined sugar.
  ◇ Diet and exercise should be regarded as the cornerstone of treatment for type 2 diabetes.

Calorie intake

- Calorie intake should be tailored to individual patients, taking into account their weight at the time they come to medical attention.
  ◇ At diagnosis, type 1 diabetic patients will typically have lost weight and are likely to be below ideal body weight.
  ◇ Patients with type 2 diabetes will likely have had weight gain for several years, but then start losing weight in the weeks to months leading up to the diagnosis of diabetes; most remain overweight, sometimes substantially so, when diabetes is diagnosed.
  ◇ Those patients with latent autoimmune diabetes of adults (LADA), who are often initially misdiagnosed as having type 2 diabetes, will *generally* have had more weight loss and been more symptomatic than true type 2 patients. However, the overlap between the two groups in respect of these features is considerable.
- A reasonable goal is to try to achieve and maintain a weight close to ideal body weight.
- While there are usually advantages to a 'slow and steady' approach to weight loss, others advocate using a newly diagnosed patient's high motivation to aim for more rapid loss.
- When considering a dietary strategy that will help achieve this it is useful to think in terms of overall calorie intake, and composition of the diet in terms of carbohydrate, protein, and fat content.
  ◇ An overweight patient (BMI 25–30 kg/m^2) should be started on a reducing diet of approximately 4–6J (1000–1500 kcal) daily.
  ◇ Opinions vary as to whether obese individuals, BMI >30 kg/m^2, should be advised on even greater calorie restriction; a target of 3.2–4 J (800–1000 kcal) daily is ideal, although many patients will have difficulty complying with this.

- Patients who have lost weight because of untreated diabetes may require energy supplementation.
- Successful weight loss soon after diagnosis of type 2 diabetes was associated in one study with a reduced subsequent mortality.

Most people with type 2 diabetes will benefit from an overall reduction in calorie intake.

Carbohydrates

- In the past, a meal plan consisting of 50–55% carbohydrates was appropriate for patients with diabetes. However, meal plans with less than this have been found to be helpful for glucose control without compromising cardiovascular health if adhering to other principles of healthy lifestyle.
  Diabetes diets or food plans should include unrefined carbohydrate rather than simple sugars such as sucrose.
- Carbohydrate is absorbed relatively slowly from fiber-rich foods, but when refined sugar is eaten the blood glucose may rise rapidly. For example, the glucose peak seen in the blood after eating an apple is much flatter than that seen after drinking the same amount of carbohydrate as apple juice (Figure 13.4).
- The glycemic index (GI) ranks carbohydrates according to the extent to which they raise blood sugar levels. Foods with a high GI are those which are rapidly absorbed and result in marked fluctuations in blood sugar levels. Low-GI foods, which are slow acting, produce gradual rises.
  ◇ Low-GI diets have been shown to improve glucose, lipid, and insulin levels in people with diabetes. They can also aid weight control by delaying hunger.

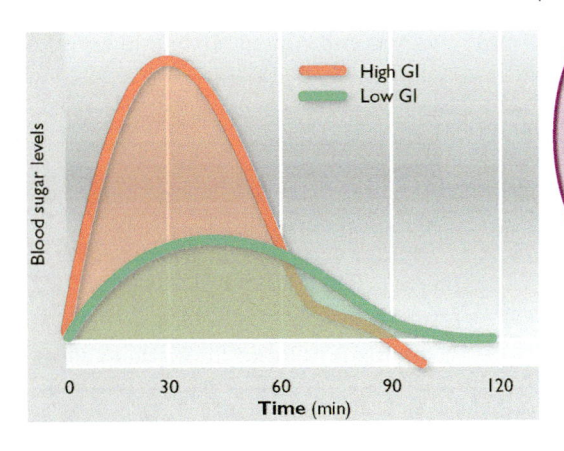

Figure 13.4 Glycemic index. The GI rating of a food is calculated by dividing the area under the blood glucose curve (AUC) for the test food by the AUC for the reference food (the same amount of glucose) and multiplying by 100.

  ◇ For insulin-treated patients, estimating the carbohydrate content and GI of a meal may be useful in estimating the insulin requirement.
  ◇ This requires that patients receive education in estimating the carbohydrate content of meals.
- The glycemic index is not universally accepted among endocrinologists, since when you take in carbohydrate, it is usually in combination with fat and protein, which often negates the value of the GI, and GI is highly dependent upon the way the food is cooked.

Fats

Attention should be given to reducing intake of saturated fats, and choosing foods with monounsaturated (such as avocados) and polyunsaturated fats. Examples of polyunsaturated fats are docosahexaenoic acid (DHA) and eicosapentaenoic acid (EPA) found in fatty fish, and alpha linolenic acid (ALA) found in nuts, seeds, and seed oils.

Protein

Several meal plans have promoted a higher proportion of protein in the diet (20–30% rather than the previous 15–20%) to help with satiety and glucose control. It should be noted that protein intake might increase the insulin response to carbohydrates.

Prescribing a diet

◆ For most people changing the dietary habits of a lifetime is challenging, so one needs to take a sympathetic approach.
  ◇ The main point to be made to most people with type 2 diabetes is that an overall reduction in calorie intake is appropriate and will be beneficial. This needs to be emphasized, even – or especially – to those patients who, despite their excess weight, insist that they do not overeat. Equivocation on the part of medical carers on this issue does a disservice to patients.
◆ A diet history should be taken, and review of a complete 3-day diet diary, including all snacks, can lead many patients to recognize previously unappreciated sources of excess calories. Soft drinks ('sodas' in the US) and fruit juices are particularly rich 'hidden' sources of calories, particularly among younger patients.
◆ Another aspect of concern to many is alcohol. The American Diabetes Association recommends a daily limit of one drink per day for women, and two drinks per day for men (examples of one drink would be a 12-oz beer, a 5-oz glass of wine, or 1.5 oz of distilled spirits).
◆ Patients on insulin should be warned to avoid alcoholic binges since these may precipitate severe hypoglycemia, and late-evening alcohol will increase the risk of nocturnal hypoglycemia.

The topic on Ramadan is discussed briefly under Screening and Patient Care in Chapter 5.

Aim for at least 30 minutes of exercise a day.

Exercise

◆ Along with dietary change there must be an emphasis on overall lifestyle change, particularly in respect of exercise. It is useful to point out that small changes in everyday activities can be useful, for example:
  ◇ Using stairs instead of lifts (elevators) to go up two or three floors.
  ◇ Parking at the point furthest from one's place of work or the supermarket rather than as close as possible.
  ◇ Doing small local errands on foot rather than always jumping into the car.
  ◇ Getting off the bus a stop early.
  ◇ Walking faster; walking a dog.
◆ Regular scheduled exercise, even if only walking, should be encouraged, perhaps even prescribed, the aim being at least a half-hour each day on average (Table 13.4).

Table 13.4 Exercise guidelines. All levels of physical activity can be undertaken by people with type 1 diabetes who do not have complications and have good glycemic control. Therapeutic regimens can be adjusted to allow safe participation consistent with an individual's goals and abilities.

Exercise guidelines in type 1 diabetes
GENERAL ADVICE
Exercise regularly; even walking has metabolic benefits
Tailor exercise regime to fit individual needs and physical fitness
Avoid hypoglycemia during exercise by: • Taking 20–40 g extra carbohydrate before and hourly during exercise • Reduce pre-exercising insulin doses by 30–50%, if necessary • Use nonexercising sites for injections • Avoid heavy exercise during peak from insulin injection
CONTRAINDICATIONS
For those taking insulin, sports where hypoglycemia could be dangerous (e.g. climbing, motor racing, diving, single-handed sailing)

(Continued)

Table 13.4 (Continued)

Exercise guidelines in type 1 diabetes

In those with proliferative retinopathy, strenuous exercise (due to the risk of possible hemorrhage)

CAUTIONS

Take care if cardiovascular comorbidities are present

Those with peripheral neuropathy need to be aware of the potential for damage to the feet

---

Aerobic exercise improves insulin sensitivity and reduces cardiovascular risk.

- It is important to point out that even vigorous exercise uses up fewer calories than most people realize, and that a large soft drink or a snack can quickly cancel out the calories expended.
- Another point to be emphasized is that perhaps the greatest value of regular exercise, even when there is disappointingly little weight loss, is that it reduces insulin resistance and improves cardiovascular risk (Figures 13.5 and 13.6). Exercise is therefore a cornerstone of diabetes therapy.

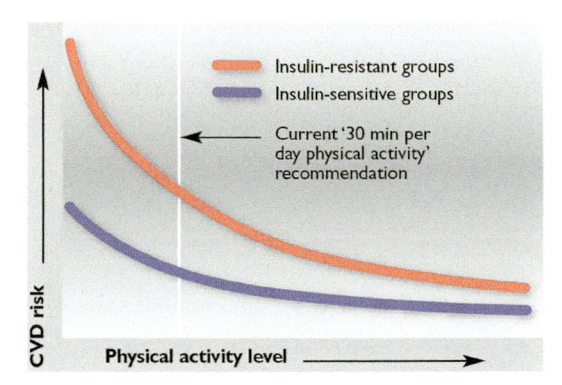

Figure 13.5 Physical activity and cardiovascular disease. Dose-response relationship between physical activity level and CVD risk in normal weight nondiabetic individuals with no family history of diabetes (insulin-sensitive) and in individuals who are insulin resistant or with a predisposition to insulin resistance. Those most at risk are most likely to benefit from exercise. *From Gill JMR, Malkova D, 2006.*

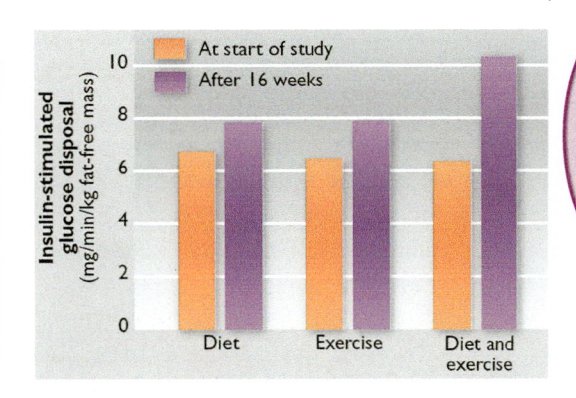

Figure 13.6 Exercise and insulin sensitivity. A study of 25 nondiabetic obese individuals demonstrated greater improvement in insulin sensitivity through diet and exercise combined, compared with either diet or exercise alone – possibly as a result of improved fatty acid metabolism. *From Goodpaster BH, et al, 2003.*

Table 13.5 Glycemic response. The glycemic response to exercise in people with type 1 diabetes varies between individuals and according to the intensity and duration of the exercise.

Glycemic response to acute exercise in type 1 diabetes	
BLOOD GLUCOSE LEVEL	EXERCISE CONDITIONS
Decreases	Hyperinsulinemia exists during exercise
	Exercise is intensive or prolonged (>30–60 min in duration)
	<3 h have elapsed since the preceding meal
	No extra snacks are taken before or during the exercise
Generally remains unchanged	Plasma insulin concentration is normal during exercise
	Exercise is brief
	Appropriate snacks are taken before and during exercise
Increases	Hypoinsulinemia exists during exercise
	Exercise is marked, but not prolonged
	Excessive carbohydrates are taken before and/or during exercise

- When planning an exercise regime it is important to:
  - Assess contraindications and limitations.
  - Be realistic – people will only continue to do what they enjoy.
  - Build up the amount of exercise gradually.
  - Advise about the risk of hypoglycemia.
  - Remember, any exercise is better than none.

Remission of type 2 diabetes

Pharmacologic approaches to glycemic management are tackled in Chapters 14 and 15. However, it should be noted that glycemic control can be achieved in type 2 diabetes with dietary changes, and in those where the benefits outweigh the risks, bariatric surgery.

Dietary intervention

The Diabetes Remission Clinical Trial (DiRECT) randomized patients to control or intervention (where diabetes and blood pressure medications were withdrawn and patients were given total diet replacement of 825–853 kcal/day formula diet for 3–5 months, stepped food reintroduction for 2–8 weeks, and structured support for long-term weight loss maintenance. After one year, weight loss was achieved in varying degrees in the intervention group, with 46% of them achieving diabetes remission, compared to 4% remission in the control group. At 24 months, 36% in the intervention group and 3% in the control group had sustained remission of diabetes.

Bariatric surgery

- Weight loss is the cornerstone of the management of overweight and obese subjects with type 2 diabetes.
- Increasingly, patients are coming to bariatric surgery after exhausting other methods of weight control. Bariatric surgery should be considered for adults with BMI >35 kg/m², but data are insufficient to make a broad-based recommendation for surgery at lesser weights.
- There are two general types of bariatric surgery, depending on their mechanism of inducing weight loss: malabsorptive and restrictive. The following are some examples (Figure 13.7).
  - *Laparoscopic adjustable gastric banding (restrictive)*. A band is placed around the stomach, limiting its size and producing early satiety. The size of the stomach can be adjusted by injecting saline into the band.
  - *Sleeve gastrectomy (restrictive)*. The stomach is resected parallel to its greater curvature.
  - *Jejunoileal bypass (malabsorptive)*. The jejunum is divided and then connected to the ileum just proximal to the ileocecal valve. This method is not commonly performed.
  - *Roux-en-Y gastric bypass (malabsorptive and restrictive)*. This is one of the most common procedures. A gastric pouch of around 30 ml is created and the small intestine is divided. Food drains into the distal (Roux) limb, which is connected to the gastric pouch, while the proximal limb drains secretions from the stomach remnant, liver, and pancreas. The two limbs are connected in the distal jejunum by a 'Y'-shaped anastomosis.
- Malabsorptive procedures show faster and more durable weight loss and improvement in glycemic control than restrictive procedures.
- For operations that physically limit food intake, the time course and degree of improvement in diabetes are more or less in line with predictions based on the degree of postoperative weight loss.
- For bypass procedures, improvements in glycemia have been reported well before weight loss becomes apparent.
  - Increased secretion of a number of gut peptides with insulinotropic actions, such as GLP-1 and GIP, and decreased secretion of orexigenic peptides, such as ghrelin, imply gastro-endocrine effect.

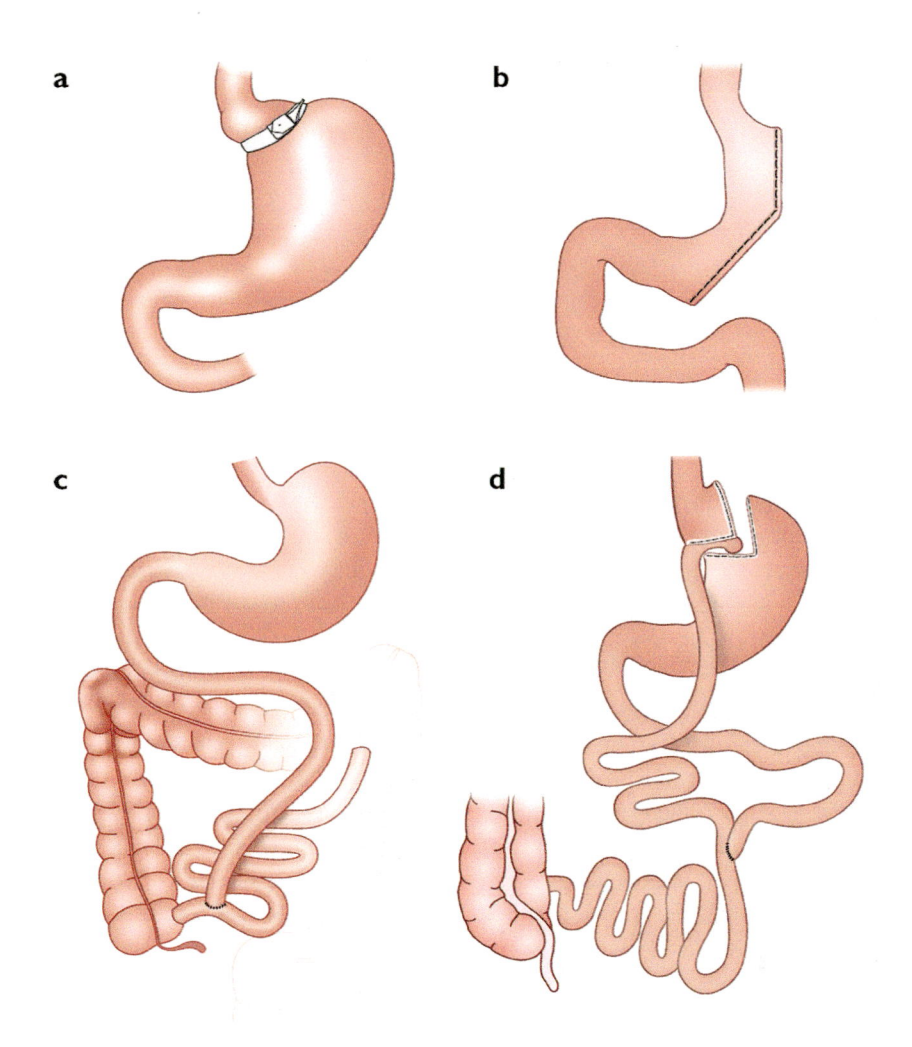

Figure 13.7 Types of bariatric surgery. Illustrated are (a) the laparoscopic band, (b) sleeve gastrectomy, (c) jejunoileal bypass, and (d) Roux-en-Y gastric bypass.

- The Surgical Treatment and Medications Potentially Eradicate Diabetes Efficiently (STAMPEDE) trial showed that gastric bypass and sleeve gastrectomy plus intensive medical therapy were superior to intensive medical therapy alone in sustaining lower hemoglobin A1c levels, body mass index, and reductions in diabetes medication use through at least 5 years from randomization.

Bariatric surgery may be considered for adults who have not succeeded with other methods of weight control.

Management of hyperglycemia

CHAPTER 14

Noninsulin therapies

Overview

- Diet and lifestyle changes are the key to successful treatment of type 2 diabetes. If there can be satisfactory metabolic control by these means then oral anti-diabetes agents (OADs) and non-insulin injectables may not be required.
  - ◇ The UKPDS showed, however, that an initial favorable response in most patients is transient, so additional therapy is almost always necessary within 6 months. However, as discussed in the previous chapter, glycemic control with diet and weight loss is possible and can be sustainable with a structured program.
  - ◇ Structured programs can be inaccessible and costly, however, and most patients will probably barely be able to join an educational session on diabetes and lifestyle changes, if at all. Nevertheless, there may be patients who could undertake an initial period (up to 3–6 months) of diet and lifestyle change; this would impress on them that this is the cornerstone of treatment, and it would identify those for whom it is sufficiently successful. It is then important to guard against 'clinical inertia,' with patient and medical adviser too slow to accept the need for progressive treatment decisions.
- Given these limitations, the European Association for the Study of Diabetes and the American Diabetes Association consensus report in 2018 (updated in 2019) supports the use of the OAD metformin along with lifestyle modification as the first step in treatment (Figure 14.1). The UKPDS group trial found that metformin appeared to decrease the risk of diabetes-related endpoints and was associated with less weight gain and fewer hypoglycemic attacks than insulin and sulfonylureas (glibenclamide and chlorpropamide). Initial responses to all agents were similar but sulfonylureas demonstrated less later benefit.
- Since then, many newer classes of OADs and non-insulin injectables have been studied, not just for glycemic control but for cardiovascular and renal outcomes, resulting in a more personalized algorithm for patients with type 2 diabetes depending on comorbidities such as obesity, heart failure, and kidney disease. The HbA1c level at the start of treatment is another variable determining the likely magnitude of HbA1c fall; so a drug may be able to cause a reduction in HbA1c from 10% (86 mmol/mol) to 8% (64 mmol/mol), but would be unlikely to cause a reduction from 8% (64 mmol/mol) to 6% (42 mmol/mol).

The natural history of type 2 diabetes suggests that insulin secretory capacity is already decreased by 50% or more on average at the time of diagnosis and it can be expected to continue decreasing for at least 6 years after that (Figure 14.2). Apart from the insulin secretagogues (sulfonylureas and glinides), most other medications developed for type 2 diabetes demonstrate a favorable effect on insulin resistance, with some also improving insulin secretion.

Noninsulin therapies

GLUCOSE-LOWERING MEDICATION IN TYPE 2 DIABETES: OVERALL APPROACH

FIRST-LINE THERAPY IS METFORMIN AND COMPREHENSIVE LIFESTYLE (INCLUDING WEIGHT MANAGEMENT AND PHYSICAL ACTIVITY) IF HbA₁c ABOVE TARGET PROCEED AS BELOW

TO AVOID CLINICAL INERTIA REASSESS AND MODIFY TREATMENT REGULARLY (3-6 MONTHS)

ESTABLISHED ASCVD OR CKD — NO — **WITHOUT ESTABLISHED ASCVD OR CKD**

ASCVD PREDOMINATES
EITHER/OR
- GLP-1 RA with proven CVD benefit[1]
- SGLT2i with proven CVD benefit[1], if eGFR adequate[2]

If HbA₁c above target

If further intensification is required or patient is now unable to tolerate GLP-1 RA and/or SGLT2i, choose agents demonstrating CV safety:
- Consider adding the other class (GLP-1 RA or SGLT2i) with proven CVD benefit
- DPP-4i if not on GLP-1 RA
- Basal insulin[4]
- TZD[5]
- SU[6]

HF OR CKD PREDOMINATES
PREFERABLY
SGLT2i with evidence of reducing HF and/or CKD progression in CVOTs if eGFR adequate[3]
OR
If SGLT2i not tolerated or contraindicated or if eGFR less than adequate[2] add GLP-1 RA with proven CVD benefit[1]

If HbA₁c above target

- Avoid TZD in the setting of HF
- Choose agents demonstrating CV safety:
  - Consider adding the other class with proven CVD benefit[1]
  - DPP-4i (not saxagliptin) in the setting of HF (if not on GLP-1 RA)
  - Basal insulin[4]
  - SU[6]

COMPELLING NEED TO MINIMISE HYPOGLYCAEMIA

DPP-4i	GLP-1 RA	SGLT2i[2]	TZD

If HbA₁c above target (each column):

| SGLT2i[2] OR TZD | SGLT2i[2] OR TZD | GLP-1 RA OR DPP-4i OR TZD | SGLT2i[2] OR DPP-4i OR GLP-1 RA |

If HbA₁c above target

Continue with addition of other agents as outlined above

If HbA₁c above target

Consider the addition of SU[6] OR basal insulin:
- Choose later generation SU with lower risk of hypoglycaemia
- Consider basal insulin with lower risk of hypoglycaemia[7]

COMPELLING NEED TO MINIMISE WEIGHT GAIN OR PROMOTE WEIGHT LOSS
EITHER/OR
- GLP-1 RA with good efficacy for weight loss[8]
- SGLT2i[2]

If HbA₁c above target

SGLT2i[2] | GLP-1 RA with good efficacy for weight loss[8]

If HbA₁c above target

If triple therapy required or SGLT2i and/or GLP-1 RA not tolerated or contraindicated use regimen with lowest risk of weight again
PREFERABLY
DPP-4i (if not on GLP-1 RA) based on weight neutrality

If DPP-4i not tolerated or contraindicated or patient already on GLP-1 RA, cautious addition of:
- SU[6]
- TZD[5]
- Basal insulin

COST IS A MAJOR ISSUE[9-10]

| SU[6] | TZD[10] |

If HbA₁c above target

| TZD[10] | SU[6] |

If HbA₁c above target

- Insulin therapy basal insulin with lowest acquisition cost
OR
- Consider DPP-4i OR SGLT2i with lowest acquisition cost[10]

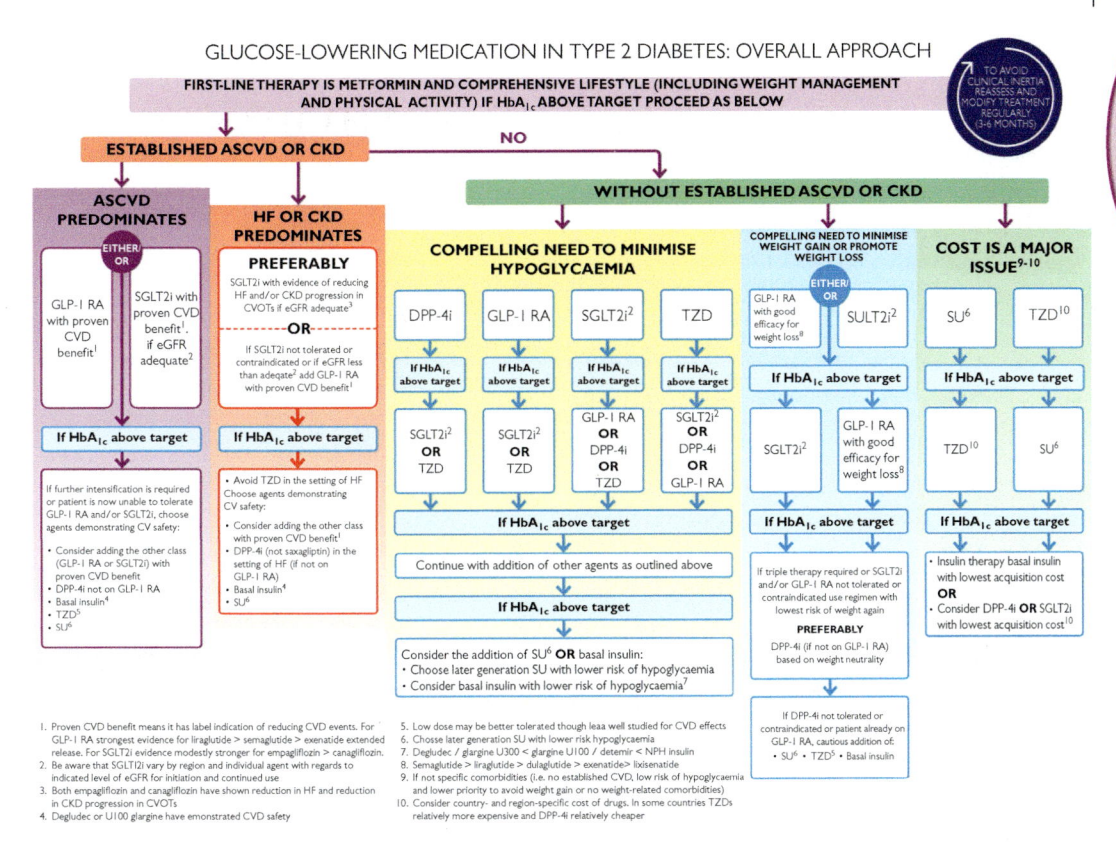

1. Proven CVD benefit means it has label indication of reducing CVD events. For GLP-1 RA strongest evidence for liraglutide > semaglutide > exenatide extended release. For SGLT2i evidence modestly stronger for empagliflozin > canagliflozin.
2. Be aware that SGLT2i vary by region and individual agent with regards to indicated level of eGFR for initiation and continued use
3. Both empagliflozin and canagliflozin have shown reduction in HF and reduction in CKD progression in CVOTs
4. Degludec or U100 glargine have emonstrated CVD safety
5. Low dose may be better tolerated though leaa well studied for CVD effects
6. Chosse later generation SU with lower risk hypoglycaemia
7. Degludec / glargine U300 < glargine U100 / detemir < NPH insulin
8. Semaglutide > liraglutide > dulaglutide > exenatide> lixisenatide
9. If not specific comorbidities (i.e. no established CVD, low risk of hypoglycaemia and lower priority to avoid weight gain or no weight-related comorbidities)
10. Consider country- and region-specific cost of drugs. In some countries TZDs relatively more expensive and DPP-4i relatively cheaper

Figure 14.1 The ADA/EASD guidelines for management of type 2 diabetes. *From Buse, JB, Wexler, DJ, Tsapas, A, et al. 2019 update to: Management of hyperglycaemia in type 2 diabetes, 2018. A consensus report by the American Diabetes Association (ADA) and the European Association for the Study of Diabetes (EASD). Diabetologia 63, 221–228 (2020). https://doi.org/10.1007/s00125-019-05039-w.*

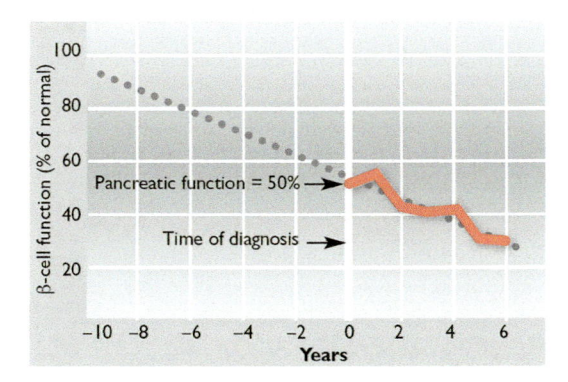

Figure 14.2 Decline in β-cell function. The UKPDS showed that newly diagnosed people with type 2 diabetes had, on average, only about 50% of normal β-cell insulin-secretory function, with a further progressive fall in the years of follow-up. By extrapolating backward (dotted line), it was estimated that this β-cell defect had begun 5–10 years before diagnosis (Table 14.1).

Oral agents

Metformin

- Metformin is a biguanide. Its mechanism of action is still not completely clear, but it decreases gluconeogenesis and hence hepatic glucose output and fasting blood glucose. It increases glucose uptake in skeletal muscle. These effects are mediated, at least in part, by AMPK activation.
- Metformin is the initial drug of preference for patients with type 2 diabetes, together with lifestyle intervention.
  ◇ It is associated with reduced cardiovascular risk in overweight patients, especially as monotherapy.
  ◇ Metformin is associated with some weight loss.

Table 14.1 Oral anti-diabetes agents and non-insulin injectables. The benefits and risks of the types of glucose-lowering agents are summarized.

Non-insulin diabetes medications		
DRUG	BENEFITS	RISKS
Oral therapies		
Metformin	Weight gain not common; might result in weight loss; low risk of hypoglycemia; inexpensive; may reduce HbA1c by 1.5–2%	Contraindicated in renal dysfunction, acute heart failure, or other conditions that predispose to lactic acidosis; gastrointestinal side effects are common
Insulin secretagogues; sulfonylureas	Inexpensive: may reduce HbA1c by 1.5–2%	Hypoglycemia is common; may cause weight gain
Insulin secretagogues; nateglinide, repaglinide	Weight gain seems to be less than with sulfonylureas	Hypoglycemia may occur
Thiazolidinedione	Reduces insulin resistance; low risk of hypoglycemia when used alone	May cause weight gain and fluid retention; mild anemia; increased risk of limb fracture and microfracture; contraindicated in heart failure and in patients with bladder cancer
Alpha-glucosidase inhibitors	Weight gain not common	Gastrointestinal side effects are common
DPP-4 inhibitors	Low risk of hypoglycemia; weight gain not common	Rare cases of angioedema and Stevens–Johnson syndrome have been reported
SGLT-2 inhibitors	Low risk of hypoglycemia; some weight loss might occur; may reduce progression of heart failure and chronic kidney disease	Dizziness, genitourinary infections are common; diabetic ketoacidosis may occur, especially if insulin doses are reduced rapidly
Colesevelam	Lowers cholesterol and glucose levels (though HbA1c reduction only 0.5–0.6% on average)	Gastrointestinal side effects are common
Bromocriptine	Low risk of hypoglycemia	Nausea and dizziness are common
Injectables		
GLP-1 analogs	Weight loss is common; may reduce cardiovascular event	Nausea is common; possibly associated with pancreatitis; contraindicated if with medullary thyroid carcinoma history or family history, and in medullary thyroid carcinoma
Combined GLP-1 and GIP agonist	weight loss is common; as of press time, being investigated for cardiovascular outcomes	Nausea is common; same contraindication as GLP-1 agonist
Pramlintide	Might result in weight loss	Nausea is common at first; contraindicated in confirmed gastroparesis and hypoglycemia unawareness

- DPP-4 inhibitors – modify second column to just say: low risk of hypoglycemia; weight gain not common
- Add SGLT-2 inhibitors right below DPP-4 inhibitors—low risk of hypoglycemia, some weight loss might occur, may reduce progression of heart failure and chronic kidney disease – Dizziness, genitourinary infections are common; diabetic ketoacidosis may occur especially if insulin doses are reduced rapidly
- GLP-1 analogs – remove exenatide and liraglutide; for second column, add: may reduce cardiovascular event; third column: remove the word liraglutide]

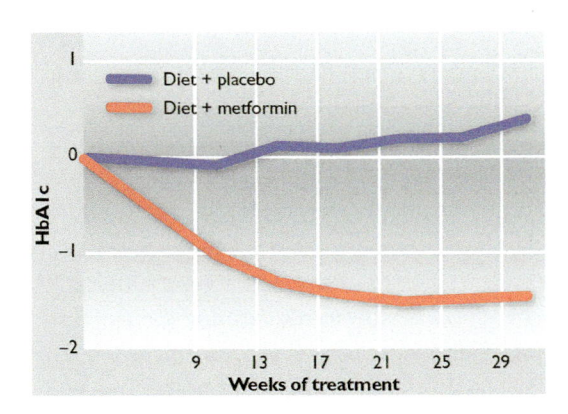

Figure 14.3 Efficacy of metformin. Mean changes in HbA1c in treatment-naive noninsulin-dependent diabetes patients treated with metformin or placebo. *From DeFronzo RA, et al. 1995.*

- As monotherapy it typically reduces HbA1c by 1.5–2% depending on baseline level, and in patients with type 2 diabetes on insulin treatment it reduces HbA1c by about 1% (Figure 14.3).
- Metformin can be used in combination with all other diabetes drugs.
   ◇ Even obese patients with type 1 diabetes may benefit in terms of reduced HbA1c from using metformin.
- Its dose-response relationship is linear up to a dose of 2000 mg per day, usually given as 1000 mg morning and evening.
   ◇ In Europe (but not in the US) doses up to 3000 mg per day are sometimes prescribed; at levels above 2000 mg per day there is little further hypoglycemic effect, though there may be an effect on lipids, particularly triglycerides.
- The ability of metformin to prevent or delay the onset of diabetes in subjects at increased risk (with impaired glucose tolerance) was suggested in the Diabetes Prevention Program, in which over 3000 subjects with prediabetes – defined as elevated fasting and post-glucose-load plasma glucose – were randomly assigned to lifestyle intervention, metformin, or placebo (no intervention), and the incidence of diabetes was observed over 4 years (Figure 14.4).

◇ The drug did reduce the risk of diabetes being diagnosed by 31% over a 4-year period when compared with placebo, but was not as effective as a supervised program of lifestyle change (diet and exercise), which reduced the likelihood of diabetes by 58% compared with placebo.
◇ As yet, the prescription of metformin in this situation is not necessarily approved or agreed upon, but off-label prescription is common.

Side effects
- The major side effects are abdominal discomfort, nausea, and diarrhea.
   ◇ These problems are idiosyncratic and often dose-related; they can be limited by initiating therapy at a low dose (500 mg daily), taking the drug with food, and then titrating gradually to the maximally tolerated dose, or by using a modified-release formulation.
- Because its mode of action does not involve increased insulin secretion, hypoglycemia is rarely a problem when metformin is used as monotherapy. In combination with insulin or insulin secretagogues the risk is greater, and in those circumstances it makes sense to adjust the

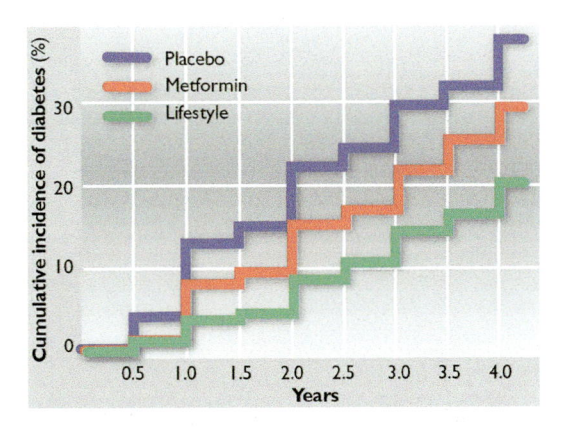

Figure 14.4 Metformin vs lifestyle intervention. In the DPP study the cumulative incidence of diabetes was lower in the metformin and lifestyle-intervention groups than in the placebo group throughout the follow-up period. *From Knowler WC, et al. 2002.*

dosage of the other drug rather than to give metformin at less than optimal levels.
◆ A rare complication of biguanide therapy is the development of lactic acidosis, which can be fatal. This was seen more commonly with phenformin, another biguanide with metabolic effects significantly different from those of metformin. The risk of precipitating lactic acidosis is extremely low in otherwise healthy individuals.

Sulfonylureas
◆ Sulfonylureas are insulin secretagogues. They increase insulin secretion from the pancreatic β cell by closing ATP-sensitive potassium (KATP) channels, depolarizing the β-cell plasma membrane, and increasing intracellular calcium concentration (Figure 14.5).
◆ Sulfonylureas are effective in decreasing both fasting blood glucose and postprandial hyperglycemia.
◆ About 20% of patients have little or no glycemic response to sulfonylureas.
◆ It has been said that some patients (perhaps 30%) eventually cease to respond to these drugs, leading to the concept of 'sulfonylurea failure'. Evidence for this is marginal at best, and studies in patients treated long term who then discontinue treatment invariably show a rise in HbA1c, indicating that the drug was still having an effect.
  ◇ The term 'sulfonylurea failure' really relates to failure of the drug, either on its own or in combination with another agent, to achieve the desired degree of glycemic control; this is not a reason to discontinue the drug.
◆ Sulfonylureas typically cause HbA1c levels to drop by 1.5–2% as monotherapy, with smaller decreases when added to other agents.
◆ With all sulfonylureas most of the hypoglycemic effect is achieved at low doses; addition of a drug from another class will usually produce a greater fall in HbA1c than increasing the dose of sulfonylurea from minimum starting dose to the maximum approved.
◆ Because sulfonylureas stimulate insulin release it is tempting to think that they would be most appropriate when insulin deficiency is the predominant factor, and that they would be less effective in patients with insulin resistance.
  ◇ Measurement of the extent of these dual impairments is imprecise even under controlled research conditions, and is simply beyond the scope of day-to-day practice; since both are

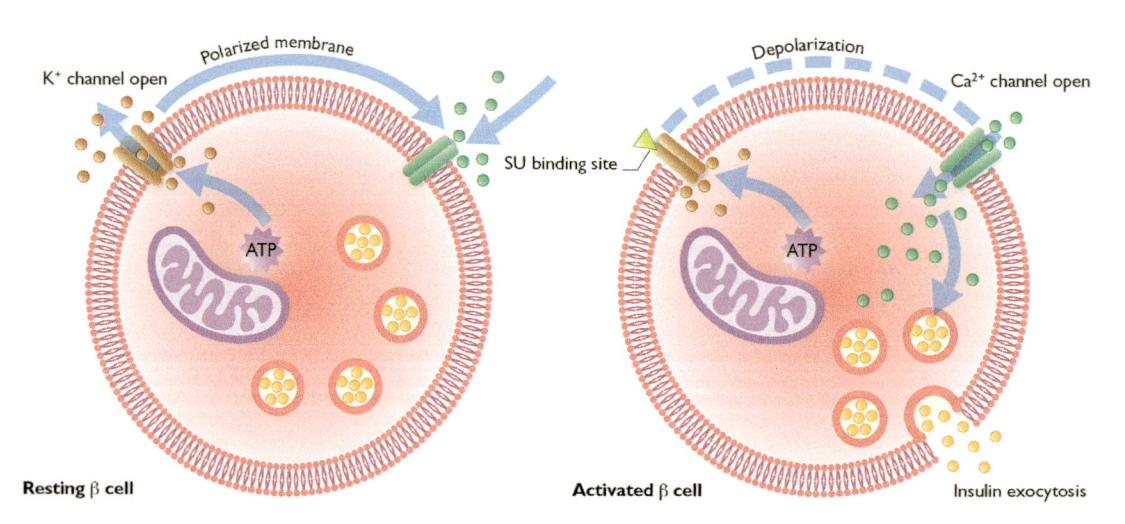

Figure 14.5 Sulfonylurea action. Sulfonylureas inhibit the outflow of potassium from the K_{ATP} channels, leading to the depolarization of the cell membrane, the opening of the Ca^{2+} channels, and an increased secretion of insulin.

present to some degree in most type 2 diabetes patients, a sulfonylurea represents a reasonable treatment option.
- One rare indication for sulfonylureas is for patients with neonatal diabetes due to potassium channel gene mutations; in these children, sulfonylureas can circumvent the defect in stimulus-secretion coupling, so that insulin secretion can be restored and insulin therapy stopped.
  ◇ Glibenclamide (glyburide in the US), glipizide, glimepiride, and gliclazide all have the advantage of being effective on a once-daily dosage though they are often prescribed in split doses when using the maximum dosage.

Drug interactions and side effects
- Sulfonylureas bind to circulating albumin, and they may be displaced by other drugs that compete for their binding sites, e.g. warfarin.
- Hypoglycemia, particularly during the late postprandial period or at night, is the most common and dangerous side effect and, despite the relatively poor dose-response relationship mentioned above, tends to be dose-dependent.
  ◇ Impaired renal and hepatic function increase the risk of hypoglycemia, especially with glibenclamide, so sulfonylureas should be used with care in patients with renal and liver disease. Gliclazide is the preferred sulfonylurea in patients with impaired renal function, and glyburide should definitely be avoided.
  ◇ The elderly are also at greater risk of hypoglycemia, probably due to decreased renal function and slower clearance of most sulfonylureas; glibenclamide, in particular, has been associated with severe hypoglycemia in the elderly with impaired renal function.
- Many patients will gain weight with sulfonylurea treatment.
  ◇ In large part this is due to decreased urine glucose wasting as blood glucose levels fall to below the renal threshold for glycosuria.
  ◇ It may also occur because subclinical hypoglycemia, which can occur with all sulfonylureas, may stimulate appetite.
- Rash can occur, though it is not common, and it is dose-independent.
- Patients who have had allergy to sulfonamides should avoid sulfonylureas.

Sulfonylureas are generally inexpensive and are thus commonly used. However, the risk of hypoglycemia, weight gain, and lack of cardiovascular or renal benefit do not make them an ideal second-line agent.

Hypoglycemia is the most common and dangerous side effect of sulfonylureas.

Glinides
- Glinides are the other class of OADs that are insulin secretagogues. Two drugs in this category, repaglinide and nateglinide (Figure 14.6) belong to two similar,

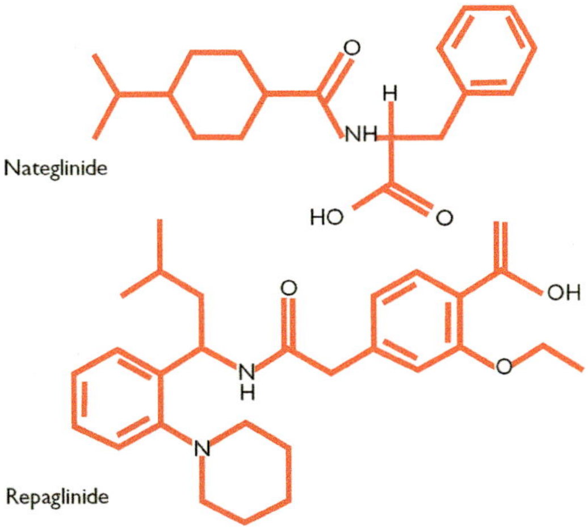

Figure 14.6 Chemical structure of repaglinide and nateglinide. Both these agents have a benzamido group that binds to the sulfonylurea receptor on the β-cell membrane.

though not identical, classes of drugs, but are often grouped together as meglitinides or 'glinides'.
◆ They work by closing the KATP channels on the β-cell membrane and stimulating glucose-dependent insulin secretion, which is quickly reversed when glucose levels fall.
  ◇ This action is more rapid in onset than that of the sulfonylureas, significantly decreasing postprandial hyperglycemia when taken shortly before each meal.
  ◇ However, because of their relatively short duration of action, these drugs have less effect on fasting glucose. This may explain why, despite their effect on postprandial insulin secretion, they have no greater ability to lower HbA1c than do the sulfonylureas. In fact, in a head-to-head trial, nateglinide as monotherapy lowered HbA1c less than glibenclamide.

Side effects
◆ Weight gain may be less than with sulfonylureas although full comparative studies are not yet available.
◆ As with any drug that stimulates the KATP channels, hypoglycemia is possible. It was initially hoped that their rapid onset and shorter duration of action would eliminate the risk of nocturnal hypoglycemia, but this can occur, at least with repaglinide.

◆ There is evidence that patients with the most common form of MODY (HNF-1α mutations) (see p. 18) suffer less from hypoglycemia on these agents than they do with sulfonylureas, and therefore they may be the treatment of choice for this condition.

Thiazolidinediones
◆ The thiazolidinediones (also known as 'glitazones' or TZDs) act on the peroxisome proliferator-activated receptors (PPARs), particularly PPAR-γ. These nuclear receptors regulate DNA expression including genes involved in lipid metabolism (Table 14.2).
◆ Two different heterozygous mutations that damage the function of PPAR-γ have been identified in patients with severe insulin resistance, type 2 diabetes, and hypertension at an unusually early age. These loss-of-function mutations provide genetic evidence that this receptor is important in the control of insulin sensitivity and blood pressure.
◆ The precise mechanism by which TZDs increase insulin sensitivity in the peripheral tissues is unclear.
  ◇ It is known that they promote the development of mature adipocytes.
  ◇ Subcutaneous fat is increased in comparison to visceral adiposity, although whether glitazones actually decrease visceral fat mass is less clear.

Table 14.2 PPARs. These are a group of receptor proteins found in the cell nucleus; three types (α, γ, and δ) have been identified. PPAR-γ is linked to type 2 diabetes.

Peroxisome proliferator-activated receptors (PPARs)			
	PPAR-α	PPAR-δ	PPAR-γ
Tissue expression profile	Liver, kidney, skeletal muscle, brown adipose tissue	Ubiquitous	Adipose tissues, skeletal muscle, heart, liver, kidney, gut, macrophages, vascular smooth muscle cells (VSMCs)
Isoforms	α	δ	γ_1, γ_2
Pharmacologic activators	Fibrates, hypolipidemics	Thiazolidinediones	

- ◇ Concomitant with these changes is a rise in serum adiponectin levels, which are usually decreased in type 2 diabetes and insulin resistance compared with the levels seen in nondiabetic subjects and the nonobese.
- ◆ TZDs (Figure 14.7) were introduced in the late 1990s, but troglitazone was withdrawn in the UK in 1997 and the USA in 2000, due to adverse liver effects. Rosiglitazone was withdrawn in the UK in 2010 over concerns about its cardiovascular safety; in 2011 it was removed from the market in New Zealand and its use in the USA has been severely restricted. Pioglitazone is still available.
- ◆ TZDs improve glycemic control in patients with insulin resistance when used either as monotherapy or in combination with other antidiabetic agents in type 2 diabetes.
- ◆ As monotherapy their glucose-lowering effect is similar to that of other oral agents. In type 2 diabetes the addition of a glitazone to insulin treatment can further reduce the HbA1c by about 1%; in this situation particular care should be exercised because of fluid retention (see below), weight gain, and potential for increase in risk of heart failure.
- ◆ TZDs have a slower onset of action than other antihyperglycemic agents, taking several weeks to achieve their full effect, but it is possible the effect may be more durable than is the case with other oral agents (Figure 14.8).
- ◆ TZDs have a synergistic effect with metformin, showing that they act by a different mechanism.
- ◆ As with metformin, there has been speculation that, because of their mode of action, TZDs might prevent or delay the onset of diabetes.
  - ◇ The TRIPOD (Troglitazone in the Prevention of Diabetes) study recruited Hispanic women who had had gestational diabetes, but who subsequently were shown not to be diabetic after the index pregnancy; compared with placebo, troglitazone led to a 58% reduction in the incidence of diabetes over a 2.4-year mean treatment period (Figure 14.9).
  - ◇ A similar protective effect against the development of type 2 diabetes has been observed for pioglitazone.
- ◆ Patients with more insulin resistance may be expected to get the greatest benefit.
  - ◇ The precise assessment of insulin resistance (and insulin secretion) is not done in routine clinical practice, but simple observations such as degree of obesity (particularly central), dyslipidemia, and acanthosis

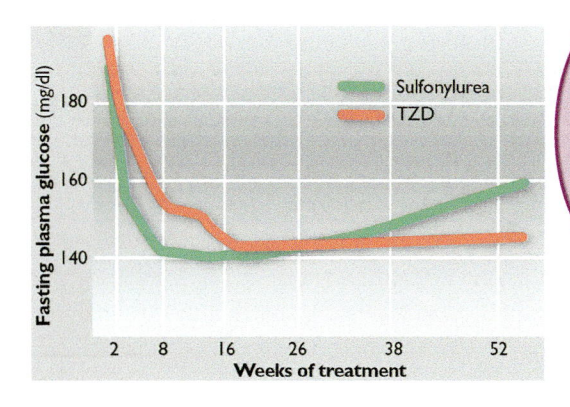

Figure 14.8 TZDs and blood glucose. As monotherapy, the TZDs have been shown to reduce fasting plasma glucose levels by around 3.3 mmol/L (60 mg/dL), with a longer-lasting effect than sulfonylureas.

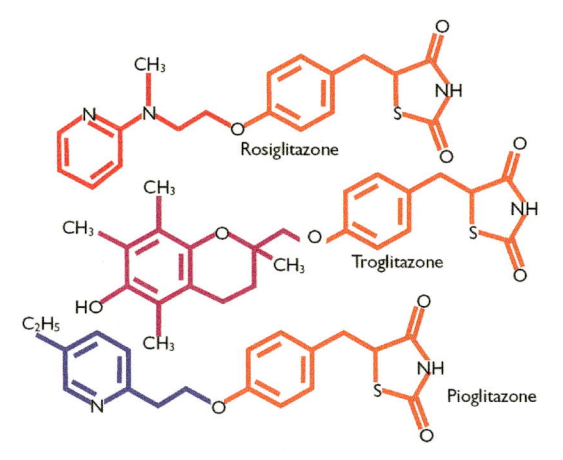

Figure 14.7 Chemical structure of TZDs. All the members of this class of drugs are derived from the parent compound thiazolidinedione.

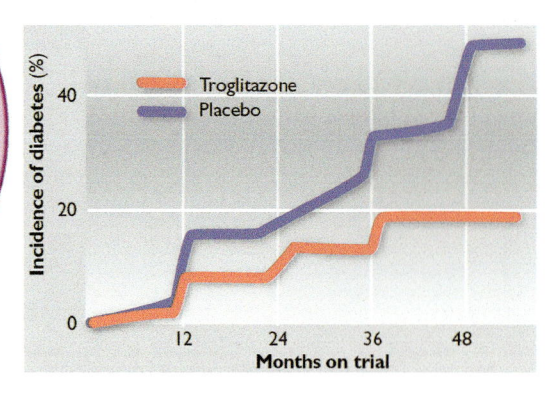

Figure 14.9 TRIPOD study. Cumulative incidence rates of type 2 diabetes in high-risk Hispanic women randomized to either placebo or troglitazone were significantly lower in the troglitazone group. *From Buchanan TA, et al, 2002.*

nigricans can serve as surrogate markers of increased insulin resistance.

Side effects
- TZDs often cause weight gain, due to a combination of increased adipose tissue and fluid retention. Co-prescription with metformin may limit the weight gain, but it is a significant problem for many, who are already overweight to begin with.
  - The increased adiposity is distributed mainly subcutaneously
  - Fluid retention may be seen, and the precise cause of this is uncertain, but it can be severe enough to precipitate heart failure, as confirmed by the PROactive study (see below), particularly in patients already on insulin treatment.
- Mild anemia may also occur, and it is hypothesized that this is at least partly due to hemodilution associated with fluid retention.
- Studies have shown an increased risk of limb fracture in women treated with TZDs, as a result of bone loss.
  - The precise pathophysiology is uncertain, but it may relate to the TZDs leading precursor cells to develop preferentially into adipocytes rather than osteocytes.

- Data suggest that pioglitazone is associated with an increased risk of bladder cancer, and hence is contraindicated in at-risk patients. The etiology is not yet clear.

TZDs and cardiovascular disease
- A completed study of pioglitazone compared with placebo showed that it reduced cardiovascular events in patients with type 2 diabetes who already had documented vascular disease (the PROactive study). There was no significant difference in outcome so far as the primary endpoint was concerned, though pioglitazone treatment was associated with a significant decrease in a composite of cardiovascular death, stroke, and nonfatal myocardial infarction. This was offset, however, by an increase in the incidence of, and hospitalization for, heart failure.
- Set against these observations has been a controversial meta-analysis suggesting that rosiglitazone can increase not only the risk of heart failure but also of cardiovascular mortality.

Alpha-glucosidase inhibitors
- Acarbose and miglitol are the two currently available drugs in this class.
- Alpha-glucosidase inhibitors can reduce postprandial hyperglycemia by inhibiting breakdown and digestion of complex carbohydrates in the small bowel (Figure 14.10). Because of their mode of action they are generally ineffective in patients eating either very high or very low amounts of monosaccharides.
- The reduction in HbA1c levels is modest compared with other oral agents, limiting their use.
- These drugs may have potential to reduce the risk of diabetes.
  - In the STOP-NIDDM trial, treatment of people with IGT with the drug acarbose reduced the risk of developing diabetes by 25% over 3 years (Figure 14.11).

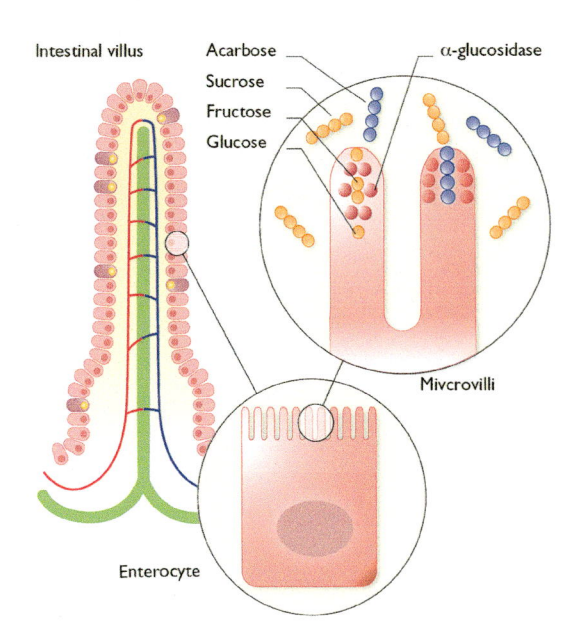

Figure 14.10 Action of alpha-glucosidase inhibitors. Acarbose competitively inhibits alpha-glucosidases, enzymes found in the brush border (microvilli) of the enterocytes that break down complex carbohydrates into simpler sugars. This leads to delayed absorption of carbohydrates in the intestine.

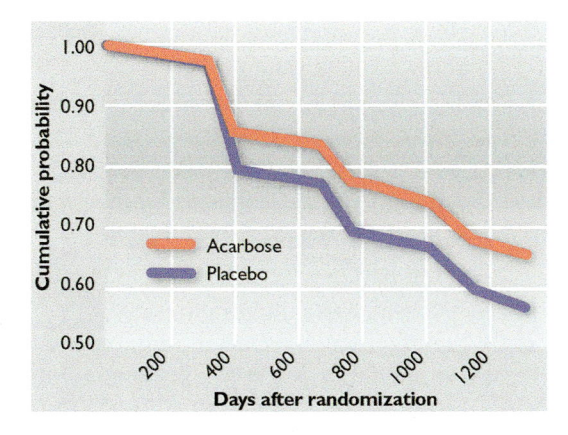

Figure 14.11 Alpha-glucosidase inhibitors. Patients with impaired glucose tolerance assigned to acarbose in the STOP-NIDDM randomized trial were 25% less likely to develop diabetes than those on placebo. This effect was noted at 1 year and continued throughout the study. *From Chiasson et al, 2002.*

Side effects

- Side effects also tend to restrict their clinical usefulness.
- Undigested starch enters the large intestine, where it is broken down by fermentation causing abdominal discomfort, flatulence, and diarrhea.
  ◇ Dosage needs careful adjustment to avoid these side effects.
- As little or no acarbose enters the circulation – it is mainly inactivated in the gut – other side effects are rare, but liver dysfunction may occasionally occur with high doses.

Alpha-glucosidase inhibitors are of potential value in limiting progression to diabetes.

Dipeptidyl peptidase-4 inhibitors

The class of OADs called dipeptidyl peptidase-4 (DPP-4) inhibitors and the non-insulin injectables called glucagon-like peptide-1 (GLP-1) agonists capitalize on the effects of incretins on plasma glucose levels.

- Incretins – notably glucose-dependent insulinotropic peptide (GIP) and glucagon-like peptide-1 (GLP-1), secreted respectively from the K and L cells of the small and large intestines – are gut hormones that enhance insulin secretion in a glucose-dependent fashion in response to ingested food (Figure 14.12).

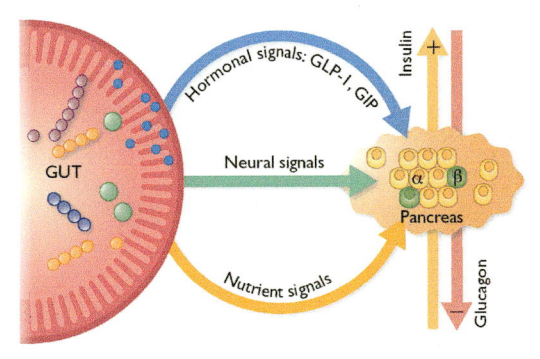

Figure 14.12 The enteroinsular axis. Metabolic, neural, and hormonal signals are transmitted postprandially from the small intestine to the endocrine pancreas. These gut hormones – incretins – stimulate the production of insulin and inhibit that of glucagon.

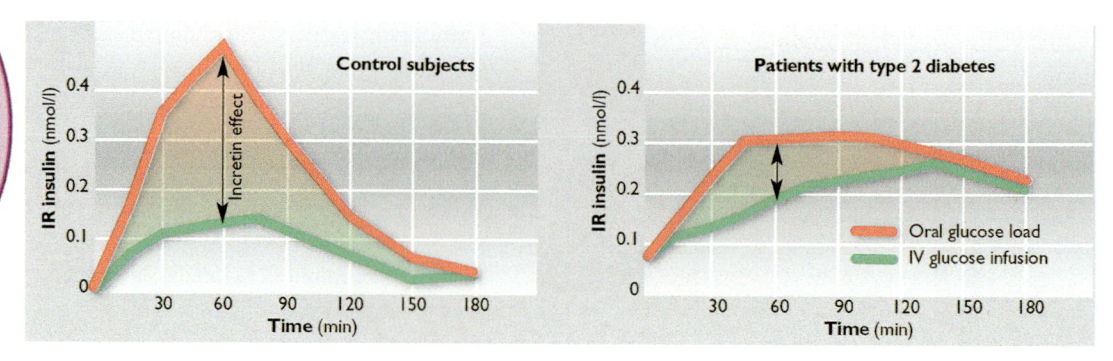

Figure 14.13 The incretin effect. Orally administered glucose has a greater effect on insulin secretion than when it is given intravenously, owing to the action of glucose on gut hormones. This augmented insulin secretion – the incretin effect – comprises up to 60% of postprandial insulin secretion and is diminished in type 2 diabetes.

- GIP and GLP-1 are rapidly (within minutes) inactivated in vivo by the enzyme DPP-4.
- Up to approximately 60% of postprandial insulin secretion is due to the incretin effect (Figure 14.13). This accounts for the long-established observation that insulin secretion is greater after ingestion of an oral glucose load than after intravenous injection of an equivalent glucose load.
  - ◇ This effect is present, but diminished, in patients with type 2 diabetes.

Since GLP-1 is rapidly degraded by DPP-4, giving it a half-life of less than 2 minutes, blocking the action of DPP-4 prolongs and optimizes the physiological action of GLP-1 (Figure 14.14).

- Examples of gliptins approved for therapeutic use include sitagliptin, vildagliptin, saxagliptin, linagliptin, and alogliptin.
- In patients with type 2 diabetes, gliptins – either as monotherapy or as add-on therapy to metformin or TZD – will reduce HbA1c by, on average, 0.6–1.0% over a 3–6-month period.
- When given as monotherapy at full dose gliptins are almost as effective as metformin monotherapy at a dose of 500 mg twice a day, but have a lesser effect on HbA1c than metformin at 1000 mg twice a day.
- When the two drugs are used in combination at maximal doses as initial oral therapy, HbA1c will often be lowered by more than 2% (Figure 14.15).
- As might be predicted, there is a greater effect on postprandial than on fasting glucose.
- Gliptins in combination with sulfonylureas will reduce HbA1c, but less effectively than in combination with metformin.
  - ◇ There is renal-dosing for these agents, and in the case of linagliptin, the same dose is given whether or not patients have chronic kidney disease.

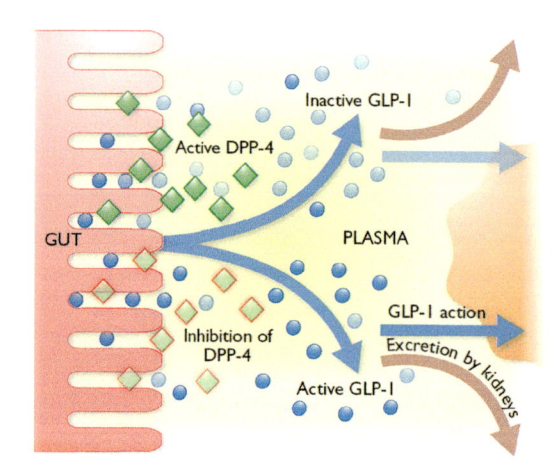

Figure 14.14 Action of DPP-4 inhibitors. The DPP-4 enzyme rapidly inactivates and degrades GLP-1. Gliptins bind to DPP-4, allowing the GLP-1 to remain active for longer and enhancing the endogenous incretin effect.

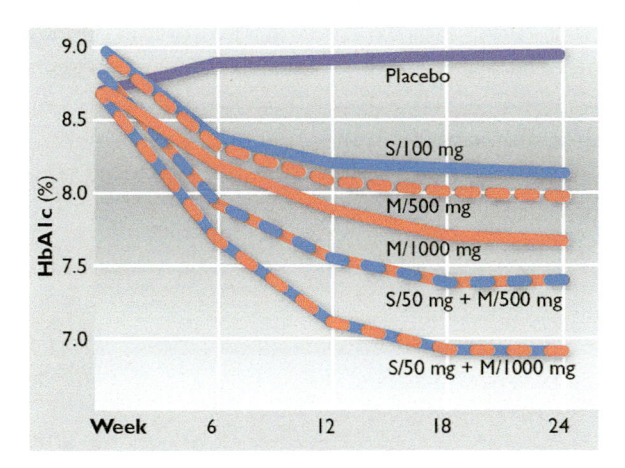

Figure 14.15 Effectiveness of DPP-4 inhibitors. This 24-week study found that a combination of sitagliptin (S) with metformin (M) therapy significantly improved glycemic control in type 2 diabetes patients. *From Goldstein BJ, et al. 2013.*

Side effects
- Sitagliptin was the first marketed and was well tolerated by patients in the pivotal clinical trials leading to its approval for general prescription.

The absence of an increased occurrence of hypoglycemia with DPP-4 inhibitor monotherapy reflects the glucose-dependent nature of incretin activity.

- Hypoglycemia may occur with concomitant sulfonylurea treatment.
- Gliptins do not seem to cause significant gastrointestinal side effects, unlike GLP-1 agonists, discussed later.
    ◇ The difference is likely due to the fact that gliptins enhance the physiological incretin effect, whereas GLP-1 agonists result in a pharmacological supranormal GLP-1-like action.
- Postmarketing surveillance suggests that mild headache may be the commonest side effect.
- There have been several reports of hypersensitivity reactions including angioedema and Stevens-Johnson syndrome; the frequency seems rare, though precise figures are not available.

Saxagliptin and alogliptin were reported to have some association with heart failure, prompting the US FDA to add warning to this effect.

Oral glucagon-like peptide 1 (GLP-1) agonist

Oral semaglutide falls under this category, and is discussed together with the other GLP-1 agonists (which are injectables) later in this chapter.

Sodium–glucose linked transporter 2 or sodium-glucose cotransporter 2 (SGLT2) inhibitors

- Plasma glucose is normally filtered in the renal glomeruli and then reabsorbed via sodium-glucose cotransporters (SGLTs) in the proximal tubules, mostly through SGLT type 2. By inhibiting SGLT2, glucose reabsorption is decreased, glucosuria is promoted, and plasma glucose levels are decreased.
- Dapagliflozin, canagliflozin, empagliflozin, and ertugliflozin belong to this class of medications. HbA1c reduction is generally around 0.5–0.8%.

The risk of hypoglycemia is low on monotherapy. Reductions in systolic blood pressure of 2–4 mmHg, diastolic blood pressure of 1–2 mmHg, and weight loss of about 2 kg have been seen with these agents from glucosuria.

Because of its action, several outcomes trials have been designed to test cardiorenal outcomes. The EMPA-REG OUTCOME,

CANVAS program, and DECLARE-TIMI 58 have shown reductions in major adverse cardiac events with the use of empagliflozin, canagliflozin, and dapagliflozin, respectively. The DAPA-HF (dapagliflozin) and EMPEROR-Reduced (empagliflozin) trials have shown an improvement in heart failure outcomes in patients with or without type 2 diabetes. The CREDENCE (patients with type 2 diabetes) and DAPA-CKD (with and without type 2 diabetes) trials showed improvements in chronic kidney disease outcomes.
- Genitourinary tract infections are one of the often-cited concerns for this class of drugs; the frequency has been reported to be about 5–7% in the first year. In rare cases, Fournier's gangrene has been seen.

Diabetic ketoacidosis (DKA), especially euglycemic DKA, has been reported with SGLT2 inhibitor use. Purported mechanisms include a reduction in either endogenous insulin or exogenous insulin (dose reduction because of improvement in glucose control), and an increase in glucagon production from its action on pancreatic alpha cells. Because of the potential for DKA, it is recommended that these agents be held 3–4 days prior to surgical procedures.

Other oral antidiabetes agents
Colesevelam
- Colesevelam hydrochloride, the bile acid sequestrant used to treat hyperlipidemia, was approved in 2008 in the US for the treatment of type 2 diabetes in conjunction with insulin or other oral agents.
- The average improvement in HbA1c is 0.5–0.6%, though a reduction of 1% has been seen in those with baseline HbA1c >8% (64 mmol/mol).
- The speculated mechanisms include a reduction in gastrointestinal glucose absorption and effects on the incretins.

Side effects
- Gastrointestinal side effects, such as constipation and dyspepsia, are common.

- Its use is contraindicated in patients with a history of bowel obstruction, severe hypertriglyceridemia (>5.65 mmol/L [500 mg/dL]), and hypertriglyceridemia-induced acute pancreatitis.

Bromocriptine
- The quick-release form of bromocriptine (Cycloset®), a dopamine-D2-receptor agonist, has been approved by the US FDA for the management of type 2 diabetes. Though the exact mechanism of its glucose-lowering effect is not known, several observations are noteworthy:
  ◇ In patients with type 2 diabetes, it is believed that there is a decrease in dopaminergic activity, and an increase in sympathetic activity (with concomitant increase in hepatic glucose output), in the early morning.
  ◇ In individuals with obesity, there is also an increase in daytime plasma prolactin levels.
  ◇ With the administration of Cycloset in the morning, the elevated prolactin levels are reduced, possibly reflecting a restoration of dopaminergic tone, and a reduction in postprandial plasma glucose levels is seen.
- Bromocriptine is taken in the morning within two hours of awakening, with food. The initial dose is 0.8 mg per day and can be increased weekly, to a maximum dose of 4.8 mg per day.

Side effects
- Bromocriptine may cause hypotension, exacerbate psychotic disorders, and increase the risk of hypotension in patients with syncopal migraine. There is early evidence that cardiovascular events might be decreased in patients taking Cycloset compared to placebo.

Non-insulin injections

Glucagon-like peptide 1 (GLP-1) analogs
As described above in the section on DPP4 inhibitors, most of the postprandial insulin section in humans is from the incretin effect.

GLP-1 analogs enhance insulin secretion and help reduce postprandial hyperglycemia.

- GLP-1 is the best characterized of the incretins, and in addition to enhancing insulin secretion it suppresses production of the counter-regulatory hormone glucagon, delays gastric emptying, and induces a feeling of greater satiety. The net effect of these actions is to help limit the extent and duration of postprandial hyperglycemia.
- GLP-1 secretion is decreased in type 2 diabetes, making it potentially a target for therapeutic intervention.

To capitalize on the action of GLP-1, agonists to the GLP-1 receptor have been developed; the first one marketed is exenatide.

- Exenatide is a synthetic form of exendin-4, a circulating meal-related peptide isolated originally from the saliva of Heloderma suspectum (the Gila monster). It shares slightly more than 50% homology with human GLP-1 and binds to and stimulates human GLP-1 receptors in vitro. Because of the difference at the site of DPP-4 action, exenatide is not inactivated by the enzyme and therefore has a much longer half-life than native GLP-1 (Figure 14.16) and is given as a subcutaneous injection twice a day. It results in greater reduction in post-meal glucose, but not as much fasting glucose lowering effect, compared to with insulin glargine (Figure 14.17).
- Liraglutide and lixisenatide are GLP-1 agonists injected subcutaneously once daily with comparable glucose-lowering effects to exenatide.

Longer-acting GLP-1 agonists (exenatide extended release, dulaglutide, semaglutide, albiglutide) are injected subcutaneously once weekly.

Oral semaglutide is administered daily. GLP-1 agonists decrease A1c by 1–2% in general.

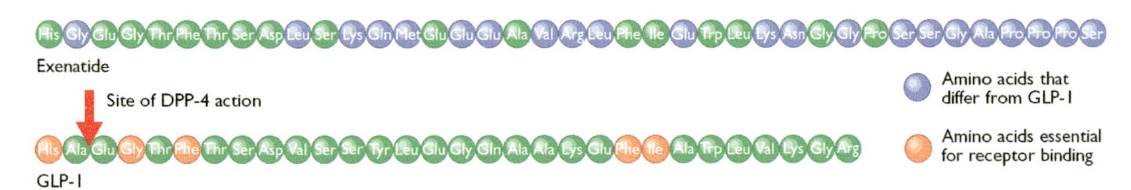

Figure 14.16 GLP-1 analogs. Exenatide is a 39-amino acid peptide, having 50% homology with human GLP-1. Comparative amino acid sequences of exenatide and GLP-1, and the cleavage site of DPP-4 (arrow), are shown.

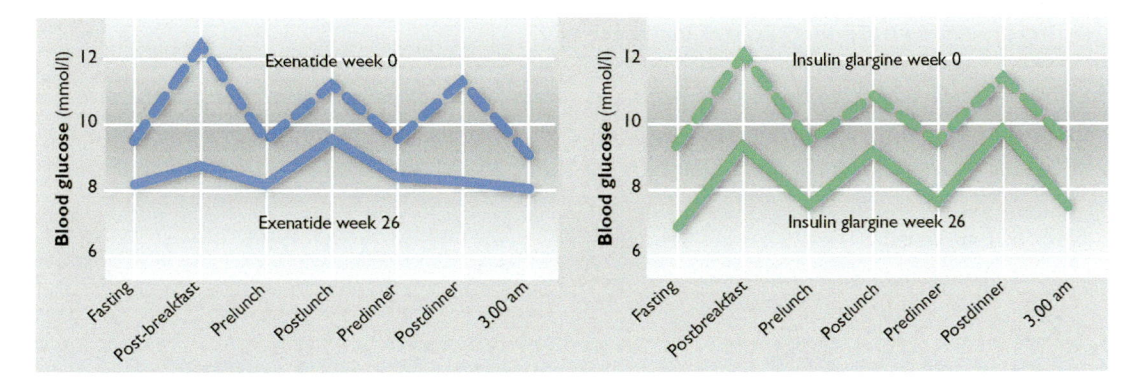

Figure 14.17 Exenatide and glucose levels. In this study, patients treated with exenatide had greater reduction in postprandial glucose than those treated with insulin glargine, but higher fasting glucose.

An average weight loss of 1–3.5 kg can be seen by 26 months of treatment.

Cardiovascular outcomes trials have been conducted on GLP-1 agonists, showing different favorable results. The LEADER (lixisenatide), REWIND (dulaglutide), and SUSTAIN-6 (injectable semaglutide) showed a lower primary composite cardiovascular outcome of death from cardiovascular causes, myocardial infarction, or stroke (3-point major adverse cardiovascular events) from these respectively, compared to placebo. EXSCEL (exenatide extended release) and PIONEER-6 (oral semaglutide) showed a reduction in all-cause mortality compared to placebo.

REWIND, LEADER, and SUSTAIN-6 also showed a reduction in renal outcomes.

Side effects

The risk of hypoglycemia on monotherapy is low.

- The major adverse effects of GLP-I analogs are nausea and vomiting These side effects are usually relatively short lived, settling within 2–4 weeks, but clinical experience shows that at least 10% of patients are unwilling to persist with the drug because of them.
  - A longer-acting form of the medication (Bydureon) is reported to be better tolerated.
- In 2006 the FDA received reports of acute pancreatitis occurring in patients receiving exenatide treatment. Even if many of these patients had other well-recognized pancreatitis risk factor, such as gallstones, heavy alcohol intake, or hypertriglyceridemia, a history of pancreatitis remains as a cautionary condition for the use of many GLP-1 agonists.

Because of its action on slowing down gastric output, caution should be used for patients with gastroparesis.

- Liraglutide was found to causes thyroid C-cell hyperplasia in rodents by activation of GLP-1 receptors. However, thyroid C-cells in humans show much lower expression of GLP-1 receptors than in rodents. Even so, continued vigilance is advised and medullary thyroid carcinoma and multiple endocrine neoplasia type 2 are listed as contraindications to the use of GLP-1 agonists

Combined GLP-1 and GIP agonist

- As of press time, tirzepatide was approved in the US. Studies show A1c improvement of around 2% and weight reduction of up to 9.5 kg.

Pramlintide

- Amylin is a hormone that is co-secreted with insulin by the pancreatic β cells (see Chapter 4); it has been found to reduce glucagon levels after meals, increase satiety, and delay gastric emptying. It is reduced in patients with type 2 diabetes.
- Pramlintide, an amylin analog, is given as a premeal subcutaneous injection in patients on prandial insulin. A reduction in prandial insulin is recommended in patients with relatively good control, to avoid hypoglycemia. Weight loss of about 0.5–1.4 kg has been seen in studies.

Side effects

- Nausea is a common side effect, especially in the first few weeks.
- Pramlintide is contraindicated in patients with confirmed gastroparesis and hypoglycemia unawareness.

CHAPTER 15

Insulin treatment and pancreatic/islet cell transplantation

Overview

- Insulin is found in every vertebrate.
- The active part of the molecule shows few differences between species: in the past, beef and pork insulin were used for treatment. Nowadays, when we talk about insulin, it is largely biosynthetic human insulin.
- The aim of insulin therapy is to mimic insulin action in patients who have a relative or absolute insulin deficiency.

Indications for insulin treatment

- In classical childhood- or adolescent-onset type 1 diabetes the need for insulin treatment is clear and unequivocal.
- When autoimmune diabetes develops later in life the extent of insulin deficiency is initially less severe. Patients are commonly misdiagnosed as having type 2 diabetes, but many progress to insulin treatment.
- In type 2 insulin treatment is generally recommended when the other alternatives have failed to achieve adequate glycemic control, or at least initially and/or temporarily when patients are symptomatic from hyperglycemia.
  - ◇ Many type 2 patients will at some stage benefit from insulin treatment as a part of their routine treatment.
  - ◇ We have traditionally been too slow in confronting the need for insulin in our patients, due to a combination of patient anxiety about insulin treatment and clinical inertia.

Many type 2 diabetes patients will benefit from insulin therapy as a part of their routine treatment.

- Other situations where insulin is accepted as 'the treatment of choice' for the patient with type 2 diabetes, or with hyperglycemia, include:
  - ◇ Pregnancy, when diet therapy alone is not sufficient (though there is literature indicating that some oral agents may be quite safe and effective).
  - ◇ Intercurrent illness, especially infections.
  - ◇ Myocardial infarction.
  - ◇ Surgical (and, with qualification, medical) intensive-care patients.
  - ◇ Hyperosmolar nonketotic coma (HONK).
- Decisions to be made about insulin treatment include:
  - ◇ Type of insulin.
  - ◇ Timing of injections.
  - ◇ Dose of insulin.
  - ◇ Education regarding adjustment of insulin dose.
  - ◇ Need for assistance.
  - ◇ Blood glucose monitoring.
  - ◇ Education regarding hypoglycemia.
  - ◇ Need to carry glucose.
  - ◇ Cost.

Classes of insulin

Insulins are often categorized according to time of onset and duration of action – ultralong-acting, long-acting, intermediate-acting, short-acting, rapid-acting, and ultrarapid-acting. They are also often described as providing basal (regardless of meals) or prandial (mealtime) coverage. Ultralong- and long-acting insulins are used as basal insulins as they lack a relative peak, while short-, rapid- and ultrarapid-acting insulins are used as prandial insulins as they have a peak to coincide with the rise in blood glucose after a meal. Intermediate-acting insulins have both basal and prandial action (Figure 15.1). In patients using continuous subcutaneous insulin infusions (CSII or insulin pumps), only one kind of insulin is used and the pump settings are designed to deliver basal and prandial needs.

Regular insulin

♦ Regular insulin enters the circulation slowly, reaching a peak 2–3 hours after injection, and predisposing to hypoglycemia due to persistent action several hours later.
  ◊ This profile differs from that of natural insulin. Because of this limitation, rapid-acting insulins were developed.

Rapid-acting insulin

♦ Insulin analogs have been manufactured in which the structure of the insulin molecule is modified to change its pharmacokinetics (Figure 15.2). Insulin lispro (for example Humalog, Admelog), insulin aspart (for example Novorapid in the UK or Novolog in the US), and insulin glulisine (for example Apidra) have small modifications of

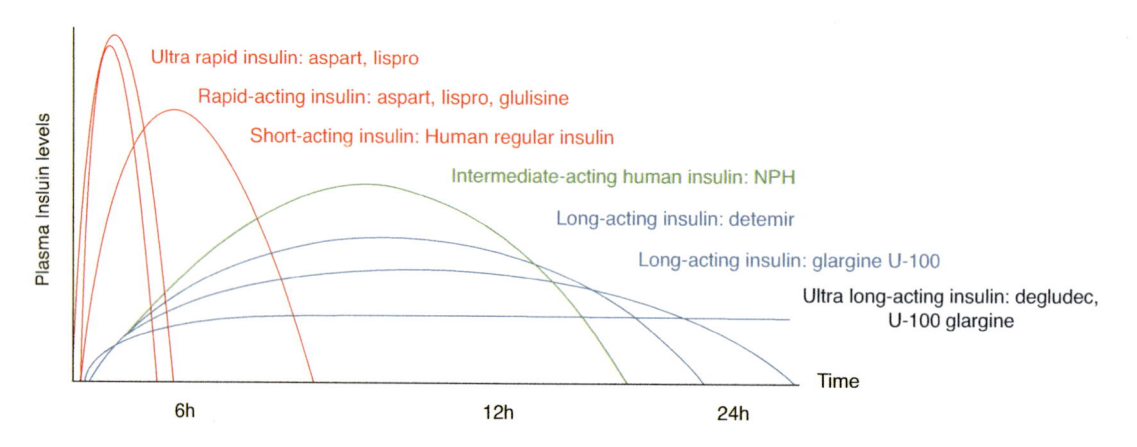

Figure 15.1 **Insulin action profiles.** Conceptual time/action profiles of the different insulin categories.

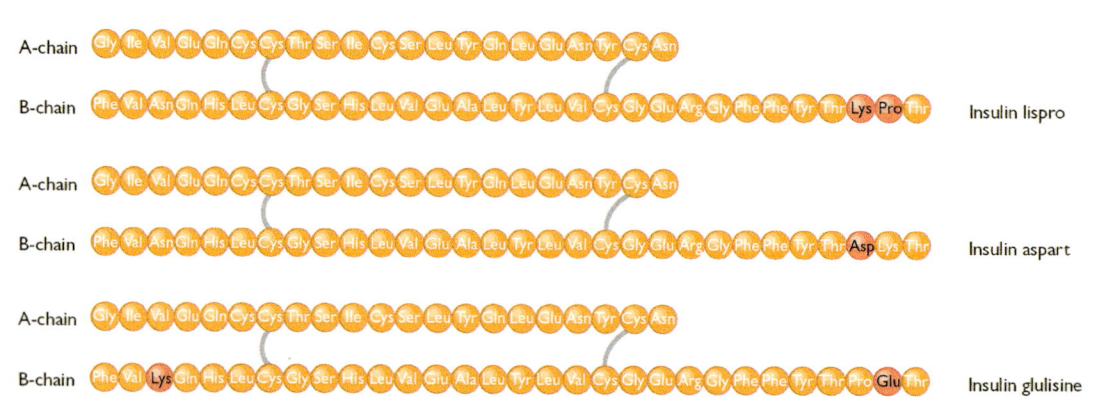

Figure 15.2 **Rapid-acting insulin analogs.** Comparative structures of the available rapid-acting insulin analogs, showing the B-chain amino acid substitutions.

their amino acid residues on the B-chain, enabling them to be absorbed and cleared more rapidly than soluble insulin.

Ultrarapid-acting insulin
These insulins are absorbed faster than their rapid-acting counterparts. For ultrarapid aspart (Fiasp), the molecule is the same as aspart but niacinamide is added to increase the speed of initial absorption (2.5 minutes). Lispro-aabc (Lyumjev) has treprostinil and sodium citrate for rapid absorption (appears in the circulation within 1 minute) (Figure 15.3).

Glargine differs from human insulin in that the A21 amino acid asparagine is replaced by glycine, and two arginines are added to the C-terminus of the B-chain.

Detemir differs from human insulin in that the B30 amino acid threonine is omitted and a 14-carbon fatty acid chain – myristic acid – is attached to lysine at B29.

Degludec likewise has the B30 amino acid threonine removed, and this time a 16-carbon fatty diacid (hexadecanoic diacid) is attached to lysine at B29.

Intermediate-acting insulin
- Protamine can be added to insulins to promote formation of insulin crystals, which dissolve slowly after subcutaneous injection. These insulin preparations are suspensions rather than solutions so they are cloudy in appearance, in contrast to regular and analog insulins (e.g. detemir, glargine), which are clear.
- NPH (neutral protamine Hagedorn) insulin, known as isophane insulin, is an intermediate-acting insulin. To provide basal coverage, it is best given twice a day. When given in the morning, its peak (6 hours later) is taken advantage of as noontime meal coverage. NPH insulin can

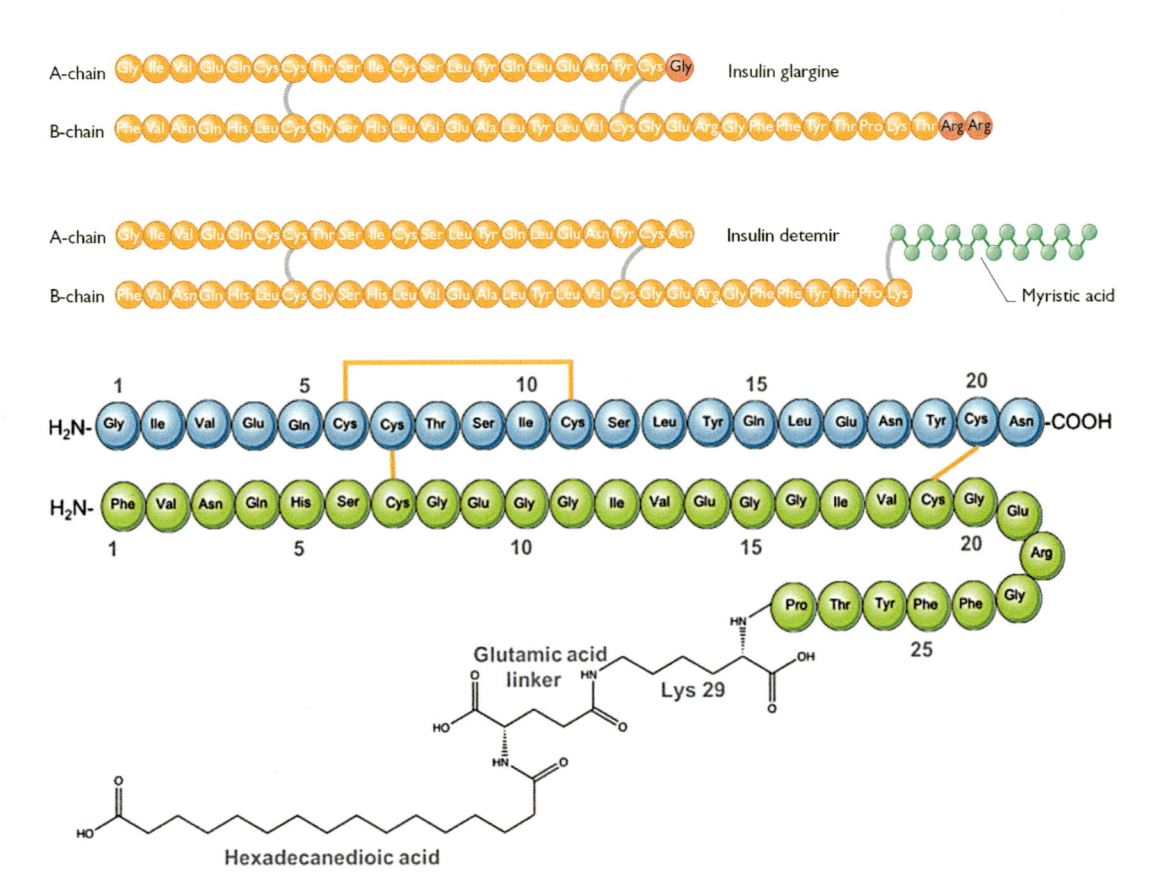

Pancreatic/islet cell transplantation

Figure 15.3 Long-acting insulin analogs. Comparative structures of long-acting insulin analogues showing amino acid substitutions/additions.

Pancreatic/islet cell transplantation

be premixed with soluble insulin to form stable mixtures. A range of these mixtures is available, but the combination of 30% regular insulin with 70% isophane is the most widely used.

Protaminated lispro and protaminated aspart have a similar action as NPH insulin, and are given as part of premixed insulins (see section under Type 2 diabetes later in this chapter).

Regular U500 insulin

Because obesity increases insulin resistance, larger doses of insulin are needed, often exceeding 100 units a day. A smaller volume to be injected is helpful in these situations. Regular insulin is also produced in a formulation that is five times more concentrated than the usual U100 formulation. U100 is the most common concentration of present-day insulins, translating into 100 units in one mL. U500 means there are 500 units in 1 mL. Regular insulin U500 has a time of onset of 30–45 minutes, a peak at 4–6 hours, and duration of action of 10-18 hours, depending on the dose. It is usually given at breakfast and dinner, but a smaller dose at lunchtime might be needed.

Long-acting insulin

- *Insulin glargine* has its structure modified to reduce its solubility at physiological pH, thus prolonging its duration of action (Table 15.1). It is injected as a slightly acidic (pH 4) solution and then precipitates in the tissues, which have a pH of about 7.4. The precipitates then dissolve slowly from the injection site, giving the preparation a relatively peakless action with a duration of approximately 24 hours.
- *Insulin detemir* is another modified insulin with relatively peakless action. Its prolonged action is due to hexamer stabilization, hexamer-hexamer interaction, and binding to albumin.

Ultralong-acting insulin

Glargine U300 is a concentrated form of glargine, with 300 units of insulin in 1 mL.

Table 15.1 Types of insulin. These can be classed according to their pharmacodynamic characteristics: time to onset of action, time of peak action, and duration of action.

Insulin action			
	ONSET (hr)	PEAK (hr)	DURATION (hr)
Rapid- or fast-acting insulin (lispro, aspart, glulisine)	0.25–0.5	1–2	3–4
Short-acting insulin (regular)	0.5	2–3	6–8
Intermediate-acting (NPH)	1–2	4–6	8–16
Long-acting (glargine, detemir)	3–4	Generally no peak	Generally 24 hr for glargine; 9–23 hr for detemir

This higher concentration allows for a smaller amount to be injected, a smaller surface area of the depot and a longer time for it to stay in the subcutaneous tissue, and a slower redissolution rate and more gradual and prolonged absorption compared to glargine U100.

Degludec forms stable and soluble dihexamers, which upon injection further self-associate into multihexamers, forming a depot. The zinc additive then dissociates and the multihexamers disassemble into dimers and monomers.

The need for injections has long been a barrier to insulin treatment in type 2 patients.

Insulin delivery systems

Insulins are still largely delivered via subcutaneous injections

Because of cost, patients in many countries might still prefer the use of insulin in vials, hence need to draw up and inject insulin via syringes. However, insulin pens (either prefilled with insulin and disposable, or with replaceable insulin cartridges) are more convenient (Figure 15.4).

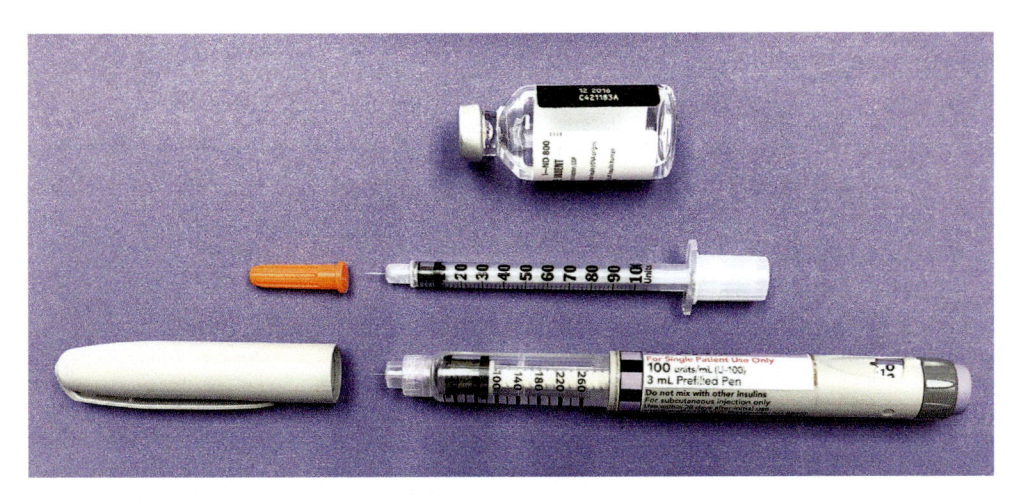

Figure 15.4 Insulin vial, insulin syringe, insulin pen. *Courtesy Susan Suglio, Cleveland Clinic.*

Nowadays, there are smart insulin pens (used with insulin cartridge) with a smart phone app that can calculate mealtime doses based on physician recommendations, and provide helpful reminders and reports. Though not an insulin delivery system per se, there are smart pen caps that fit onto insulin pens, can scan readings from a continuous glucose monitor, and make dose recommendations based on physicians' prescriptions.

- There are alternative insulin delivery systems, although not all of them are widely approved or available:
  - Inhaled insulin.
  - Oral spray. Continuous subcutaneous insulin infusion (CSII or insulin pumps)
  - Implantable insulin pumps.
- *Inhaled insulin.* The first inhaled insulin (Exubera), an inhalation powder of human insulin of recombinant DNA (rDNA) origin, was approved for use in 2006 but withdrawn in 2008 due to lack of commercial success.

  Afrezza is human insulin in powder form also produced by rDNA technology. It is an orally inhaled rapid-acting insulin used for prandial coverage that comes in 4-, 8-, and 12-unit cartridges. It begins working within 12–15 minutes, peaks by 35–55 minutes, and its action lasts 1.5–3 hours. It is contraindicated in patients with chronic lung disease such as asthma and chronic obstructive pulmonary disease because of the risk of bronchospasm. Assessment of lung function by measuring forced expiratory volume in 1 second (FEV1) should be done before initiation, after 6 months of therapy, and yearly.
- *Insulin spray.* An insulin spray (Oral-Lyn, Generex) which delivers human insulin for absorption through the buccal mucous membrane, but not the lungs, has been approved for commercial marketing and prescription since 2005 in various countries (but not Europe or North America).
  - The peak insulin concentration occurs about 25 minutes after administration, with onset of action occurring a little later and peaking at about 45 minutes. There have been no postmarketing reports of this buccal insulin's long-term use.

Implantable insulin pump

This delivers insulin intraperitoneally, and only a few patients are on it. At least two companies (Medtronic and PhysioLogic) are developing this technology further. When insulin pumps are referred to in this chapter, it refers to external insulin pumps rather than implantable pumps.

Continuous subcutaneous insulin infusion or (external) insulin pumps

This method of delivery is discussed below.

Pancreatic/islet cell transplantation

Pancreatic/islet cell transplantation

Insulin regimen: type 1 diabetes

- To establish an insulin regimen, a typical day can be considered to comprise periods of basal insulin production – essentially the fasting and postabsorptive states – interspersed with bursts of prandial and postprandial insulin production.

Table 15.2 Insulin regimens. It is important to match the choice of regimen to the clinical and lifestyle needs of the patient.

Common insulin regimens
A single daily subcutaneous injection of long-acting insulin (in patients with type 2 diabetes)
Two daily injections of premixed fast-acting and intermediate-duration insulins
Four daily injections: three of fast-acting insulin given with each meal and one intermediate or long-acting insulin at bedtime
A subcutaneous infusion of fast-acting insulin given via a pump throughout the day

- In healthy individuals, with normal glucose tolerance and taking three meals a day, basal insulin accounts for about 50% of the total. This will naturally be modified by physical activity and normal diurnal fluctuations in counter-regulatory hormone production. Mealtime or prandial insulin makes up the other 50% of insulin secretion. Secretion of insulin in response to meals is rapid, with a relatively narrow peak, and results in absorption of glucose in tissues, with excess glucose being stored as glycogen in the liver and muscle or converted to lipid.
- While it makes sense to mimic this pattern, there is no rule when it comes to the best regimen, which should be tailored to suit individual needs (Figure 15.5). In patients with type 1 diabetes on insulin pumps, the basal rate seems to be closer to 40% and the prandial doses closer to 60%, but this is again modified depending on the carbohydrate- or meal-related insulin requirements.
- Regimens with multiple subcutaneous injections (Table 15.2) are flexible, and the risk of hypoglycemia can be reduced by using long-acting insulin with minimal peak action for basal needs and rapid-acting insulin analogs for mealtime coverage. This is often called a basal-bolus insulin regimen. Other regimens of combining NPH insulin with regular-or rapid-acting insulins, or premixed insulins

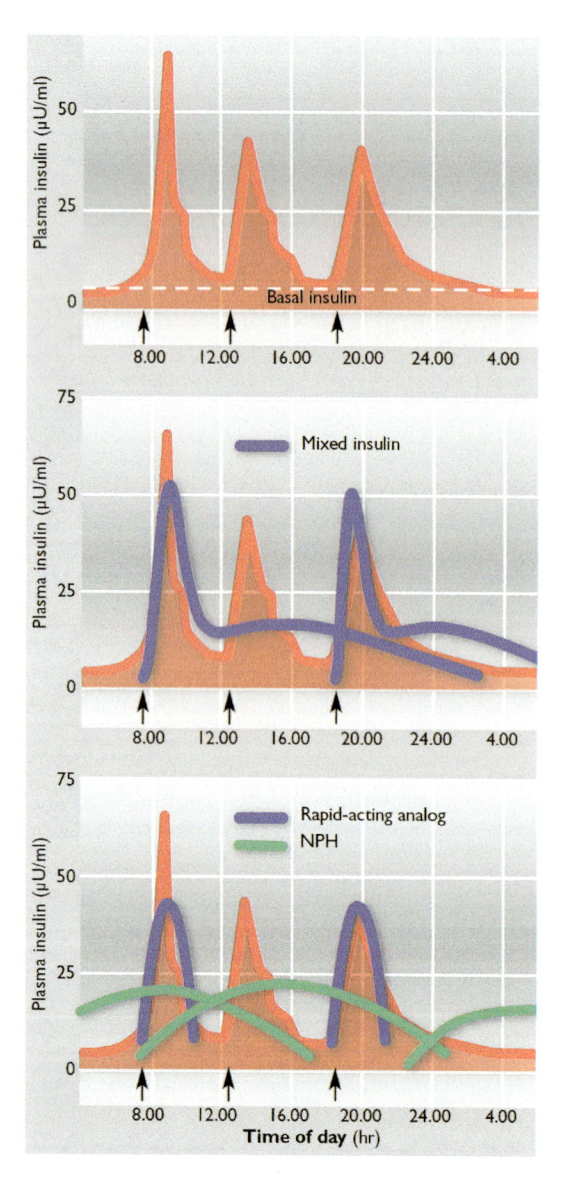

Figure 15.5 Insulin regimens. The pattern of physiological basal-bolus insulin secretion (top), with peak action at mealtimes (arrows), can be mimicked by therapy schedules. These can use both rapid-acting and longer-acting (NPH) insulin or mixed (rapid/longer-acting) insulin or a single injection of long-acting insulin with rapid-acting insulin at mealtimes.

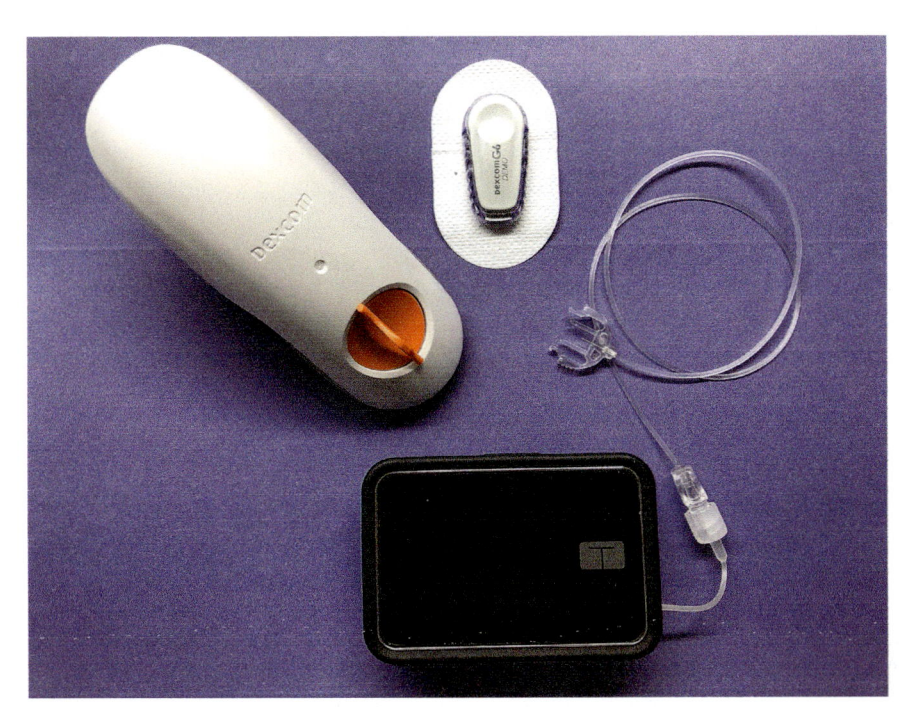

Figure 15.6 CSII. In this sensor-augmented system, clockwise from top left: (a) sensor applicator, (b) sensor, (c) pump with tubing and infusion set. *Photo courtesy of Susan Suglio, Cleveland Clinic.*

- (discussed later in this chapter) may entail fewer injections but are not as flexible with dosing and timing especially in relation to meals.
- The closest we can get to mimicking physiological insulin production (apart from pancreas or islet cell transplantation) is with CSII or insulin pumps (Figure 15.6). CSII could be suggested for most patients with type 1 diabetes, but specific reasons include:
    ◇ Poor metabolic control with hyperglycemia.
    ◇ Poor metabolic control with hypoglycemia.
    ◇ Instability of metabolic control with swings from high to low glucose.
    ◇ Patients who have a significant dawn phenomenon (a rise in blood glucose in the early hours) – since a pump can deliver insulin at different rates or doses at different times of the day.
- For a period (weeks to months) after type 1 diabetes has been diagnosed, there will usually be some residual endogenous insulin secretion and less intensive insulin regimens may achieve excellent glycemic control at that time.
    ◇ Occasionally, insulin treatment can be temporarily withdrawn and blood glucose levels will remain normal. This 'remission' of diabetes is popularly referred to as the 'honeymoon period' and it is important to emphasize to patients that it is, regrettably, a temporary phenomenon.
- Once the honeymoon period is over, patients with type 1 diabetes who have a relatively normal body weight will typically require a daily insulin dose of between 0.5 and 1.0 units/kg.
- The precise distribution of the insulin dosages will depend on a number of factors.

Multiple daily injections

- If the basal coverage is supplied by long-acting insulin that is relatively without peak, then it is reasonable to apportion approximately 50% of the total daily dose to that.
    ◇ For glargine, this can usually be given as a single injection at approximately the same time each day, usually at

bedtime, but chosen to fit in with the individual's lifestyle.
- ◇ In some people – particularly adolescents and young adults – with irregular work and leisure schedules, it may make more sense to split the glargine insulin dose in two to ensure 'round the clock' coverage.
- ◇ In a small percentage of patients, insulin glargine may not last the full 24 hours, making a split-dose regimen more effective.
- ◆ If the basal component is supplied by a long-acting insulin that does have a significant peak – such as isophane/NPH – then that insulin will make a significant contribution to mealtime coverage as well as basal requirements, so that proportionately more basal and less prandial insulin will comprise the total dose.
  - ◇ Insulin detemir probably lies somewhere between glargine and isophane/NPH in this respect, and both detemir and isophane/NPH (plus in selected cases glargine) can be given twice a day when used as basal insulin in type 1 diabetes.

Ultralong-acting insulins are given once a day. Insulin glargine U300 should be given around the same time every day, but insulin degludec can be given in adults any time of day with doses at least 8 hours apart (for children, it should be the same time of day).

Continuous subcutaneous insulin infusion: insulin pump treatment

- ◆ CSII at basal levels in the fasting and postabsorptive states, coupled with mealtime increases, represents an attempt to mimic normal pancreatic β-cell function that can realistically be offered to many, if not most, people with type 1 diabetes.
- ◆ Since the pioneering days in the 1970s of bulky, makeshift pumps, advances in microchip technology have led to the development and availability of quite sophisticated devices that are small enough to be concealed in clothing or 'worn' like a pager or mobile phone (Figure 15.7).

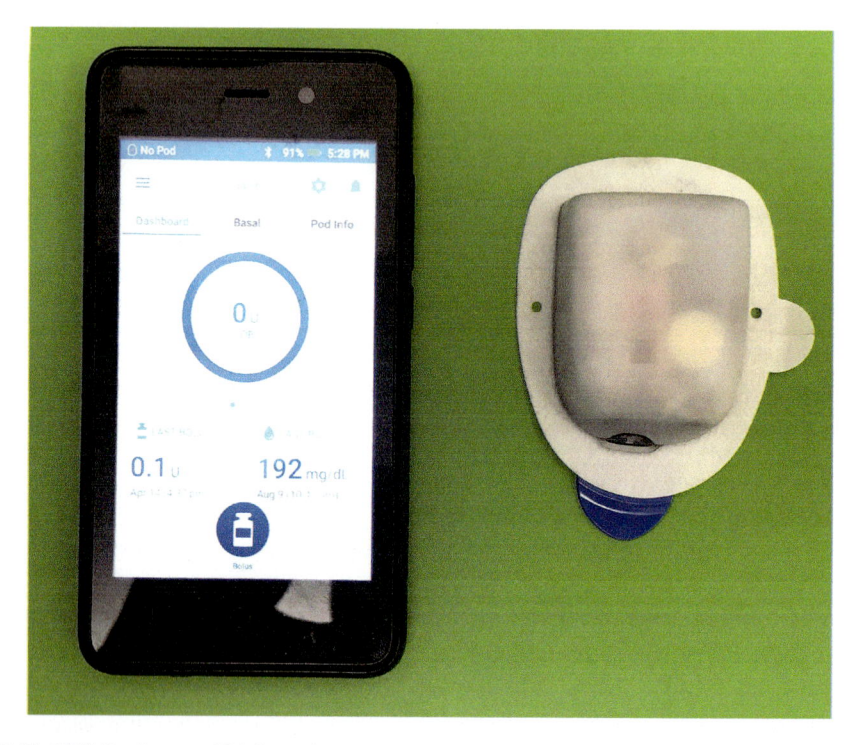

Figure 15.7 CSII. Patch pump. This is a tubeless pump (right) with the personal diabetes manager (left). *Courtesy Nancy Ferritto, Cleveland Clinic.*

- Insulin is fed to the subcutaneous tissue from a reservoir via a fine flexible catheter that is easily inserted by the patient; this catheter is changed every 2 or 3 days.
  - With careful attention to simple hygiene, and relocation of the infusion site each time, there are very few problems with infection or other local adverse effects, such as fibrosis or lipohypertrophy.
- There is general consensus that a rapid-acting insulin analog rather than soluble regular human insulin works best in the pump. Ultrarapid-acting insulins can also be used in insulin pumps.
- Pumps can be programmed to alter the basal rate of infusion many times during a 24-hour period:
  - Some patients find that a single basal rate over 24 hours works well.
  - Many patients do better with different basal rates throughout the day that take account of such things as diurnal changes in counter-regulatory hormones, work patterns, and regular exercise.

Insulin pump technology has advanced from the large unwieldy gadgets to small pager-sized devices, and include the following:

Conventional pumps

These pumps deliver insulin according to settings agreed upon by the prescriber and the patient. In general, these settings include how much insulin is delivered for basal needs (basal rate), how many grams of carbohydrate that 1 unit of insulin is expected to cover for meals (insulin to carbohydrate ratio), and how many mg/dL of blood glucose is expected to be lowered by 1 unit (correction factor or sensitivity factor, similar to a correction scale for subcutaneous insulin injections). Most of these systems comprise the pump, the cannula inserted subcutaneously into the skin, and tubing that conveys insulin from the pump to the cannula.

Sensor-augmented and hybrid closed loop pumps

Some pumps have the ability to receive glucose readings from CGMs, which allows for the basal insulin delivery to be suspended during hypoglycemia, or suspended if hypoglycemia is predicted to occur. There are pumps that can also give a small dose of insulin for hyperglycemia if the basal rate is inadequate. At least two companies have received approval for the pump to determine basal rates according to an algorithm – basal rate settings are entered only as backup.

Patch pumps

Patch pumps deliver insulin via a cannula directly from the device to the skin without tubing. The Omnipod system is an example, but many other systems are smaller and disposable, and can deliver basal and/or bolus doses.

Pumps with both insulin and glucagon are being studied.
- Advice from an experienced diabetes educator and 'pump trainer' can be invaluable.
- Although patients can have the pump effectively deliver basal insulin once the settings are in place, the same is not true of mealtime insulin boluses. Pumps do not yet have sufficient sophistication to anticipate and respond to the increased insulin needs that accompany eating, but this technology is being developed.
  - Modern pumps do offer programs that help calculate the appropriate dose in relation to the composition of the meal, and the choice of delivering the mealtime insulin as a single bolus or a slower delivery over a defined period, or a combination of the two.
  - This aspect of insulin pump therapy still requires as much active input from the patient as any insulin injection regimen, and for this reason it should not be assumed that pump

treatment will necessarily lead to better glucose control.
- ◇ Several studies confirm that forgetting, or neglecting, to deliver a mealtime bolus is one of the commonest problems among (particularly younger) pump-treated patients.
- ◆ It is very important to educate patients that, because this type of insulin delivery does not involve the buildup of a subcutaneous depot of insulin, development of ketoacidosis will occur rapidly in the event of system malfunction, such as blockage of the catheter.
  - ◇ Patients can swing from a state of normoglycemia to severe, and life-threatening, ketoacidosis in as little as 4–6 hours.
  - ◇ 'Before and after' studies generally show that HbA1c can be expected to improve when a patient with inadequate control switches from intensive treatment with injections to CSII, and several such reports emphasize that, particularly for patients who remain on pump therapy for more than 1 year, the improvement in HbA1c can be substantial.

Ketoacidosis will occur rapidly if the pump malfunctions or a catheter is blocked.

- ◆ There are several reasons for thinking that CSII should provide better glycemic control than intensive injection therapy (Table 15.3).
- ◆ Many nonrandomized studies suggest that even if pump therapy does not inevitably lead to a lower HbA1c, it will enable a near-normal HbA1c to be achieved with less risk of hypoglycemia than will intensive-injection regimens, though the use of insulin analogs, especially for basal coverage, has reduced the risk of severe hypoglycemia.

Table 15.3 Advantages of CSII. As well as delivering insulin in a more physiologically precise manner than injections, pump therapy also offers greater flexibility.

Potential advantages of CSII
Decreased variability of insulin absorption
Greater ability to cover snacks as well as main meals
Greater flexibility with meals and snacks
Decreased risk of nocturnal hypoglycemia
Greater ability to counteract 'dawn' phenomenon
Ability to adjust for exercise
Lack of subcutaneous depot of insulin decreases risk of exercise-induced hypoglycemia

- ◆ Theoretically, there is no reason why every patient with type 1 diabetes should not be offered the option of pump treatment. However, the costs (pump plus catheter supplies) are greater than those of injection treatment, and this is a limiting factor.
  - ◇ Self-monitoring of blood glucose (SMBG)

For most people with diabetes, blood glucose is checked with a fingerstick. In general, the higher the risk of hypoglycemia, the more frequent fingerstick check is recommended. For those on basal-bolus insulin, four checks a day is not uncommon. Alternative sites and technology for checking (such as earlobe or wrist) had not quite taken off. However, several continuous glucose monitors (discussed next) have successfully been launched, and stayed in the market (Figure 15.8).

Continuous glucose monitors (CGMs)

- ◆ Frequent and consistent self-monitoring of blood glucose is essential to the success of pump therapy.
- ◆ Concurrent with advances in pump technology there has been development of accurate and reliable sensor devices for glucose levels in interstitial fluid rather than frequent fingerstick testing.

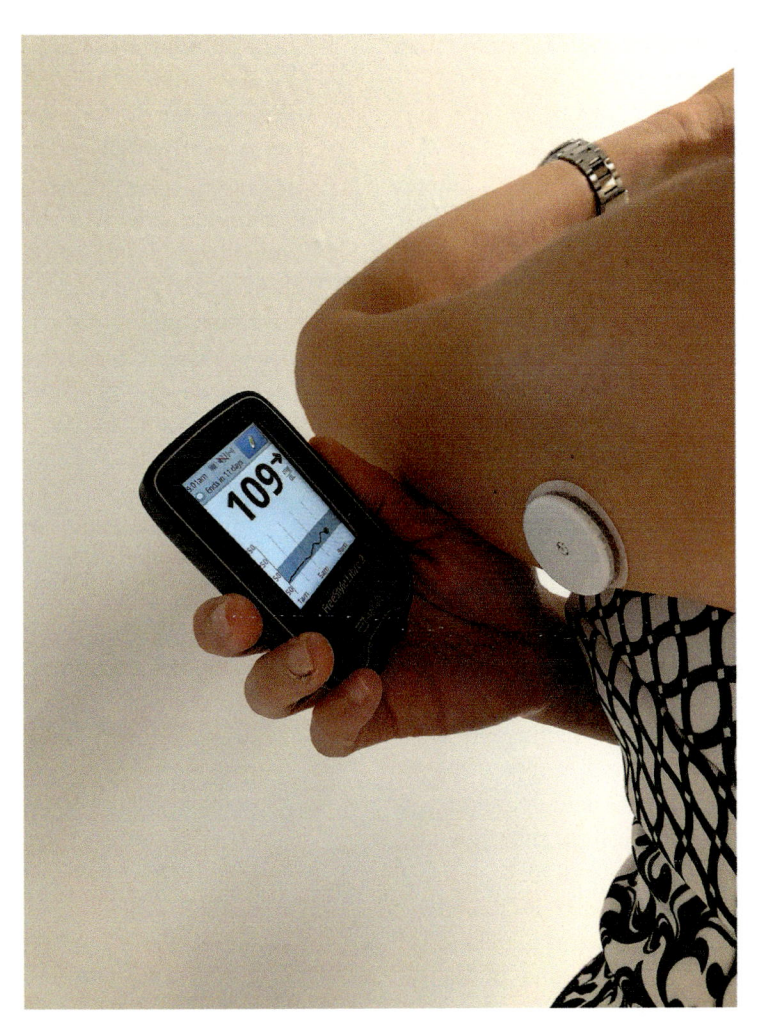

Figure 15.8 Intermittently scanned continuous glucose monitor. *Courtesy M. Cecilia Lansang, Cleveland Clinic.*

- Such devices give results that correlate well with laboratory-measured plasma glucose, but they are expensive and the sensors have to be replaced frequently. Subcutaneously inserted glucose sensors are either real-time or intermittently-scanned. At least one company has developed an implantable sensor that can stay subcutaneously for 6 months. A typical real-time CGM has a sensor (filament that detects glucose in the interstitial fluid), a transmitter (sends information wirelessly from the sensor to the reader), and a reader (receives and displays information every few minutes). An intermittently scanned CGM has a sensor and a reader (a smartphone app can be used instead of a reader in some models) that will display the glucose level when the reader or app is scanned against the sensor.

Insulin regimen: type 2 diabetes

General considerations
- Insulin treatment in type 2 diabetes is most often prescribed when treatment with oral agents or noninsulin injectables has been insufficient.
- Starting patients with type 2 diabetes on insulin has long been hedged around with fears, anxieties, and misunderstanding on the part of patients and physicians. Numerous reasons have been put forward

for failure to get patients on insulin when glycemic control is clearly inadequate despite maximal doses of other diabetes medications.
- ◇ It is understandable that most patients will prefer not to take injections if other satisfactory alternatives are available; the idea that insulin treatment represents any failure on the patient's part should be avoided.
- ◇ Too often the 'threat' of insulin treatment is brandished as a means of achieving better compliance with diet, exercise, and oral agents; this is not just bad psychology – it fails to appreciate that many patients, simply through the nature of the condition, will remain hyperglycemic despite reasonable adherence to prescribed regimens.

♦ A more appropriate approach is to emphasize at the outset that insulin deficiency is an integral part of type 2 diabetes and that, therefore, many patients will require and benefit from insulin treatment at some time.

♦ Because type 2 diabetes so often affects several family members and generations, many patients recount hearing of some relative who seemed to be fine until he or she received insulin late in the stage of the disease, after which there was steady deterioration.

♦ Positive expectations of benefit can outweigh reservations about insulin self-injection (extending to needle phobia, hypoglycemia, and weight gain). This was amply demonstrated by the relative welcome that many patients gave when offered a trial of the noninsulin injectable exenatide because of expectations that it would promote weight loss.

♦ Any insulin treatment brings with it a risk of hypoglycemia, but risk of severe hypoglycemia is considerably less in patients with type 2 diabetes than in those with type 1 diabetes.
- ◇ This may be due partly to increased insulin resistance, and regimens that employ supplementation of basal insulin in the absence of mealtime dosing are also less likely to cause severe hypoglycemia.

♦ Given that hypoglycemia is an unpleasant and potentially serious adverse effect of insulin, it makes sense to start with low doses that will be unlikely to cause hypoglycemia, and gradually increase the dose thereafter; this is true whatever insulin regimen is selected in type 2 diabetes.

♦ There are two components to the insulin-secretory defect in type 2 diabetes: fasting insulin and first-phase insulin response.
- ◇ Loss of first-phase insulin response to ingested food is, perhaps, the earliest abnormality, and this defect is apparent in subjects with fasting glucose levels higher than normal but not yet at the level of 7 mmol/L (126 mg/dL) that defines diabetes.
- ◇ In these individuals, and also those with recently diagnosed type 2 diabetes, the fasting serum insulin level often appears similar to, or even higher than, fasting insulin levels in normal subjects, as insulin deficiency is relative to the higher glucose level and, in effect, at an early stage there is a defect in both mealtime as well as basal insulin secretion.

♦ The choice of insulin treatment could, therefore, lie between augmenting basal and mealtime insulin levels, or a combination of the two. Consideration of the typical 24-hour glucose profile in type 2 diabetes is useful in this respect (Figure 15.9).
- ◇ The major abnormality is that the elevated fasting glucose results in the entire glucose profile shifting upwards; the postprandial glucose excursions are greater in diabetes, and increase as the fasting glucose increases.
- ◇ The entire area under the profile represents the integrated glucose, corresponding to HbA1c level; augmenting basal insulin and reducing the fasting glucose towards normal – effectively

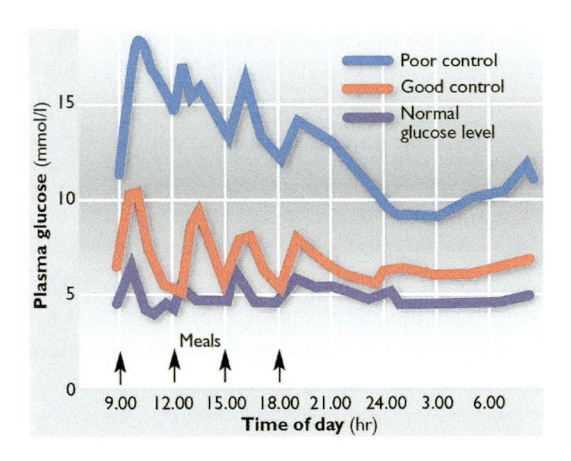

Figure 15.9 24-hour glucose profile. As plasma glucose falls from high towards normal levels, so the basal glucose falls and is an indicator of glucose control. *From Holman RR and Turner RC, 1981.*

shifting the whole line downwards – should lead to a greater overall reduction in glycemia and HbA1c than targeting only the postprandial glucose peaks by giving mealtime insulin.

◇ Fasting and postprandial glucose are not independent variables, however, and action taken to specifically change the one will have a 'knock-on' effect on the other, so either strategy can be expected to have success, and an ideal strategy would be to target both.

◇ At this stage, patient choice, convenience, and economics come into play.

Basal insulin

◆ Isophane or NPH insulin at bedtime has been shown to be an effective means of reducing fasting glucose as its action overnight has the effect of limiting hepatic glucose output.
  ◇ NPH insulin has a significant peak of action some 4–6 hours after subcutaneous injection, so there is a risk of nocturnal hypoglycemia, which might be obviated by a small bedtime snack.
  ◇ A comparison between NPH and glargine as basal insulin treatment in type 2 diabetes found them to be equally effective in reducing fasting glucose and HbA1c (Figure 15.10); nocturnal hypoglycemia occurred approximately twice as frequently with NPH as with glargine, though there was a small increase in daytime hypoglycemia with glargine (Figure 15.11).
  ◇ In one study of patients treated with either metformin or sulfonylurea or both, glargine was also given: at the end of the study the mean HbA1c was just under 7% (53 mmol/mol), from a starting HbA1c of 8.7% (72 mmol/mol).

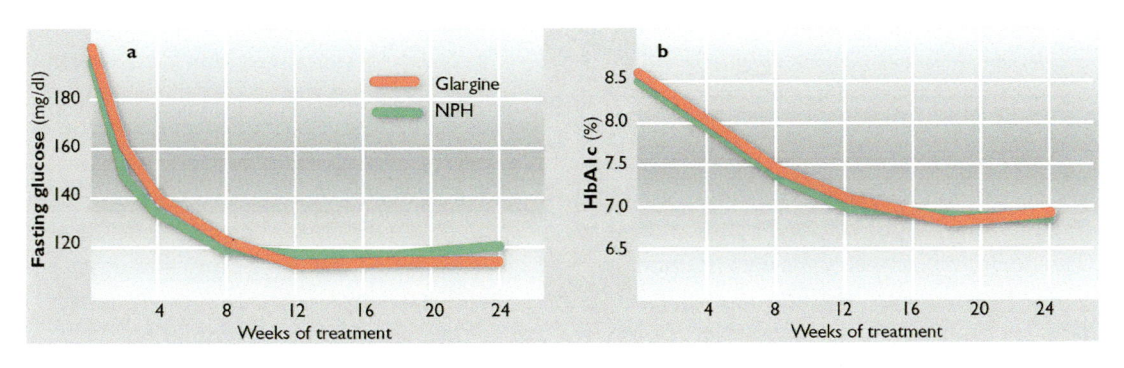

Pancreatic/islet cell transplantation

Figure 15.10 Basal insulin treatment. Insulin glargine and NPH had similar effects on fasting glucose (a) and HbA1c (b) in the Treat-to-Target trial. Insulin dosages were titrated upwards on a weekly basis, depending on the fasting glucose level. *From Riddle MC, Rosenstock J, et al. 2003.*

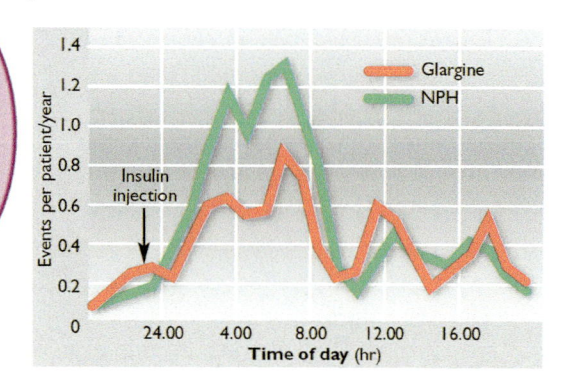

Figure 15.11 Hypoglycemic events. Although both glargine and NPH achieved similar fasting glucose and HbA1c levels in the Treat-to-Target trial, glargine did so with markedly less nocturnal hypoglycemia. *From Riddle MC, Rosenstock J, et al. 2003.*

A truly basal insulin has little or no peak action.

- Basal insulin supplementation of existing diabetes regimens that have failed to achieve a satisfactory HbA1c is now the most common pathway for the introduction of insulin treatment in type 2 diabetes. This typically occurs after the patient has been on a combination of two or three other agents, but it can be applied also when oral monotherapy does not result in a satisfactory HbA1c.
- A single injection each day is easily accepted by most patients when the potential benefits are explained to them. Administering the first injection during the course of a routine clinic visit often convinces even reluctant patients of the ease of the treatment.
    ◇ With long-acting and ultralong-acting insulin, the timing of subsequent injections can be selected by the patient to fit in best with their daily routine and preferences. The important thing is consistency from day to day for long-acting insulin.
    ◇ With NPH insulin, bedtime injection is preferable to lower the fasting glucose.
- Regardless of which particular insulin is selected, it makes sense to start with a relatively low dose that would not be expected to cause hypoglycemia, and then to titrate the dose gradually but steadily, aiming ideally for fasting glucose levels persistently in the range of 4.4–7 mmol/L (about 80–130 mg/dL).
    ◇ This needs to be explained and frequently reinforced to patients, who will often become concerned that the strategy may not be working if, after a few weeks of steadily increasing insulin dosage, the fasting glucose is still not at goal.
- Because of the insulin resistance in type 2 diabetes, the effective dose of basal insulin can seem alarmingly high to patients.
    ◇ It is therefore imperative that patients learn that there is no predetermined 'maximum dose' of insulin, and that some patients require much higher doses, sometimes well over 100 units per day as a single injection, for this regimen to be successful.
- There is no single 'dosage algorithm' that is necessarily better than another to start basal insulin. Some studies have used 10 units daily, or 0.15 to 0.25 unit/kg daily (with the lower dose for patients with chronic kidney disease and the higher doses for those with obesity/insulin resistance), with increases made weekly on the basis of the mean fasting glucose, while others recommend more frequent dose increases, such as an additional single unit every day until the 'target' fasting glucose is achieved fairly consistently. The important thing is for the patient to recognize the need for insulin adjustment and to participate in the process.
- This strategy enables many patients to achieve HbA1c levels of <7% (IFCC 53 mmol/mol), but inevitably some patients will start experiencing hypoglycemia, either nocturnal or daytime, before the target fasting glucose has been achieved.
    ◇ In that case the dose of the basal insulin should be reduced to eliminate the hypoglycemia, and

adjustments to, or addition of, other diabetes medications be made.

Mealtime insulin
- Targeting the postprandial rise in glucose is another potential means of improving all-round glycemia.
- Epidemiological studies suggest that postprandial glucose is a greater determinant of cardiovascular risk than fasting glucose.
- The need for several injections per day makes this option less attractive as an initial insulin treatment for most type 2 patients, though it can be successful in those who try it.

It is important for the patient to recognize the need for insulin and participate actively in the process.

Premixed insulin
- Premixed 'fixed ratio' insulin, consisting of rapid-acting or regular insulin, plus NPH insulin or an intermediate-acting analog (such as protaminated lispro or protaminated aspart), is a convenient way of trying to provide both basal and mealtime insulin supplementation.
    ◇ Common premixed insulins contain either 25% or 30 of regular or rapid-acting insulin, and 75% or 70% of NPH or protaminated lispro or aspart.
- The obvious attraction is the convenience of having both components in one premixed syringe or pen device, and injections are typically given before breakfast and before the evening meal. However, given that these injections are a mix of two insulins combined, there is less flexibility on mealtime dosing compared to the previously described basal-bolus insulin.

Metabolic instability on insulin

- There are several factors surrounding insulin use that might affect glucose control.

- Errors in insulin injection technique:
    ◇ The wrong dose or timing.
    ◇ Air in the syringe.
    ◇ Poor injection technique.
- Alterations in insulin pharmacokinetics:
    ◇ Injection into the wrong place (e.g. into area of lipohypertrophy or intradermal or intramuscular injection) (common) (Figure 15.12).
    ◇ Anti-insulin antibodies bind insulin (rare) (Figure 15.13).
    ◇ Insulin clearance is rapid (rare).
- Alterations in insulin action:
    ◇ Insulin receptor defects.
    ◇ Insulin postreceptor defects (e.g. obesity, type 2 diabetes).
    ◇ Drugs.
    ◇ Counter-regulatory hormone disturbances.

Pancreatic/islet cell transplantation

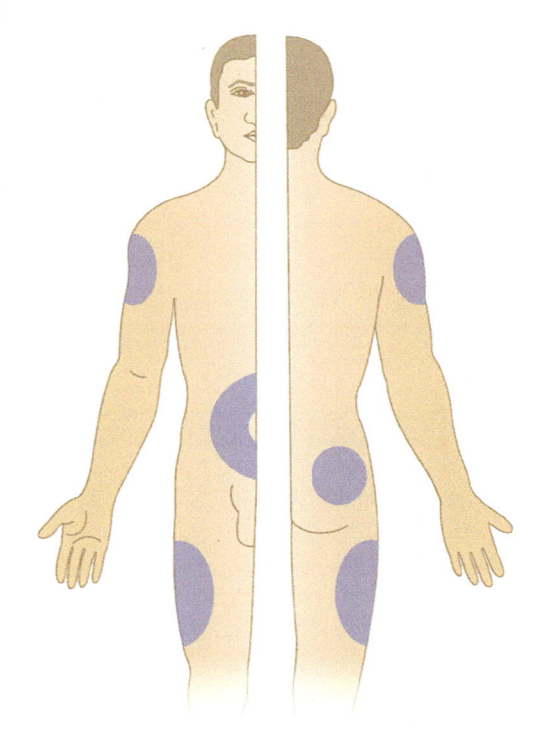

Figure 15.12 Insulin injection sites. Injections should usually be made into the subcutaneous tissue. The abdomen has the fastest rate of absorption, followed by the arms, thighs, and buttocks.

Pancreatic/islet cell transplantation

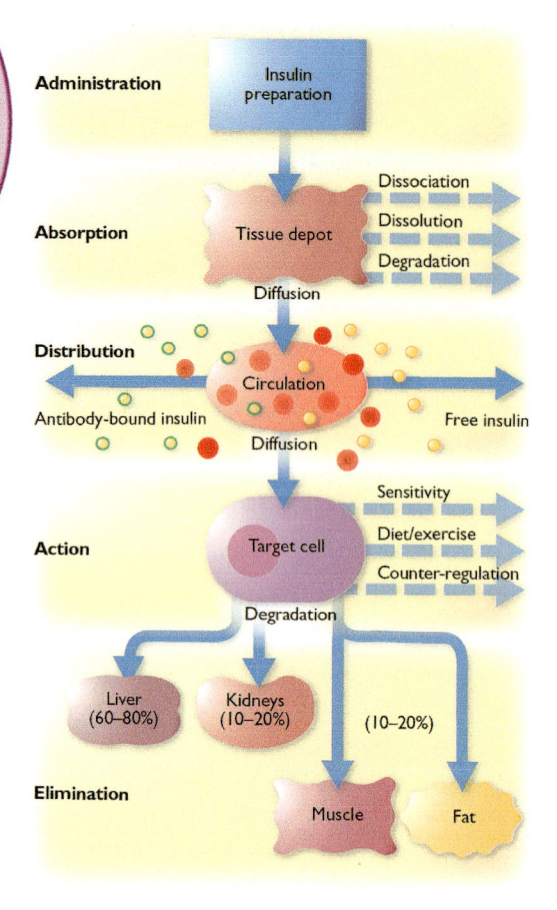

Figure 15.13 Insulin pharmacokinetics. The main steps comprise absorption, distribution – including binding to circulating insulin antibodies, if present, or to insulin receptors – and ultimately degradation and excretion through a variety of processes. Insulin action is determined by the sensitivity of the patient to insulin, amount of exercise, diet, and the various counter-regulatory mechanisms that prevail.

Complications: hypoglycemia

- Hypoglycemia is a common problem in patients on insulin treatment, and to a lesser extent in patients treated with insulin secretagogues.
- Hypoglycemia is potentially the greatest barrier to achieving normoglycemia.
- Virtually all insulin-treated patients experience intermittent symptoms of hypoglycemia, and approximately 10% will have a severe episode requiring assistance each year. A small minority suffer attacks that are so frequent and severe as to be virtually disabling.
- Hypoglycemia results from an imbalance between injected insulin or oral hypoglycemic therapy and a patient's normal diet, activity, and metabolic requirements.
  ◊ For patients on insulin, the times of greatest risk are before meals and during the night.
  ◊ Patients on secretagogues are at greatest risk during the late afternoon.
  ◊ Irregular eating habits, unusual exertion, and alcohol excess may precipitate episodes.
  ◊ Some cases in those on insulin therapy appear to be due simply to variation in insulin absorption.
- Symptoms of hypoglycemia develop when the blood glucose level falls towards 3.5 mmol/L (60–70 mg/dL) and typically develop over a few minutes (Figure 15.14).
- Common symptoms include altered mental alertness, hunger, feeling shaky, and distortion of vision, while physical signs include 'adrenergic' features of pallor, sweating, tremor, and a pounding heartbeat (Table 15.4).
  ◊ Patients progressing to more severe hypoglycemia appear pale, drowsy or detached – signs that their relatives quickly learn to recognize.

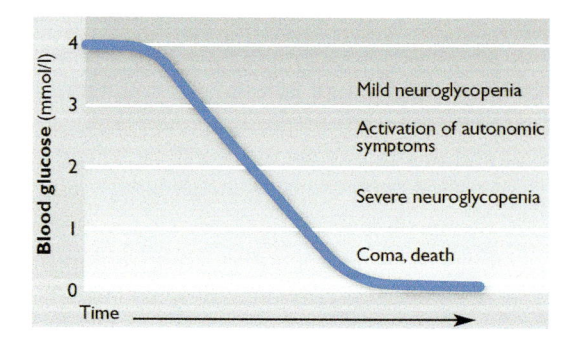

Figure 15.14 Development of hypoglycemia. Glycemic thresholds for release of epinephrine and subsequent activation of autonomic and neuroglycopenic symptoms.

Table 15.4 Hypoglycemia symptoms. Awareness of symptoms and timely intervention can avoid a hypoglycemic event.

Common signs and symptoms of hypoglycemia and actions to be taken by the patient

SYMPTOMS	PHYSIOLOGICAL MECHANISM	BLOOD GLUCOSE AT ONSET (MMOL/L[MG/DL])	INTERVENTION REQUIRED
Hunger, sweating, tremor, palpitations	Autonomic response to subnormal glycemia	Below ≈3.5 [63]	Take glucose-rich sweets, drink or food
Cognitive dysfunction, atypical behavior, speech difficulty, uncoordination, dizziness, drowsiness	Neuroglycopenia (brain deprived of glucose)	Below ≈2.8 [50]	Take glucose-rich sweets, drink or food; seek assistance
Malaise, headache, nausea, reduced consciousness	Severe neuroglycopenia	Below ≈2.0 [36]	Third-party intervention required
Convulsions, coma	Severe neuroglycopenia	Below ≈1.5 [27]	Medical intervention essential

Hypoglycemia is potentially the greatest barrier to achieving normoglycemia.

- Behavior is clumsy or inappropriate, and some patients become irritable or even aggressive.
- Some such patients slip rapidly into hypoglycemic coma.
- Occasionally, patients develop convulsions during hypoglycemic coma, especially at night. It is important not to confuse this with idiopathic epilepsy, especially since patients with frequent hypoglycemia often show EEG abnormalities.
- Another presentation is with a hemiparesis that resolves within a few minutes when glucose is administered.

Hypoglycemic unawareness

- Many patients with long-standing insulin-treated diabetes report loss of these warning symptoms and are at a greater risk of progressing to more severe hypoglycemia.
- This is rarely a problem until diabetes has been present for a number of years. People with diabetes have an impaired ability to counter-regulate glucose levels after hypoglycemia.
- The glucagon response is invariably deficient, even though the α cells are preserved and respond normally to other stimuli.
- The epinephrine response may also fail in patients with a long duration of diabetes, and this is associated with loss of warning symptoms.
- Recurrent hypoglycemia may itself induce a state of hypoglycemia unawareness (Figure 15.15).

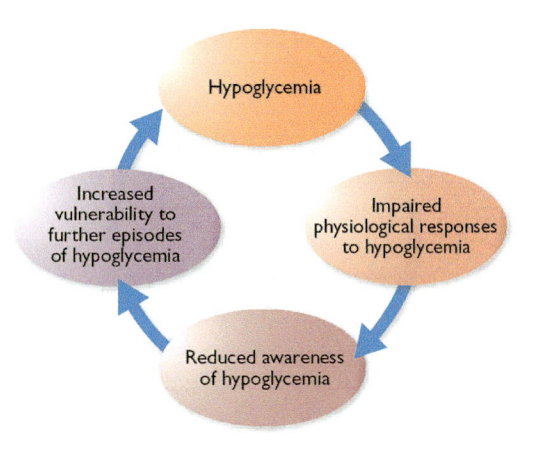

Figure 15.15 Hypoglycemic unawareness. Lack of warning symptoms, or a failure to recognize them, can lead to a vicious circle of repeated hypoglycemia.

The ability to recognize the condition may sometimes be restored by relaxing control for a few weeks.

Nocturnal hypoglycemia
- This is a major cause of anxiety for patients and relatives – particularly parents of children and adolescents with type 1 diabetes. Common experience suggests that nocturnal hypoglycemia, and the thought of falling asleep never to reawaken, hold particular terror for some patients and for many parents.
- Basal insulin requirements fall during the night but increase again from about 4 am onwards, at a time when levels of injected insulin are falling. As a result many patients awake with high blood glucose levels, but find that injecting more insulin at night increases the risk of hypoglycemia in the early hours of the morning.
- Use of longer-acting insulin analogs have been shown to reduce the likelihood of nocturnal hypoglycemia by compared with other intermediate-acting insulins.
- Other strategies that will help to minimize the likelihood of nocturnal hypoglycemia include
    - Checking that a bedtime snack is taken.
    - For patients taking twice-daily mixed insulin to separate their evening dose and take the intermediate insulin at bedtime rather than before supper.
    - Reducing the dose of regular insulin before supper, since the effects of this persist well into the night.
    - Changing patients on a multiple injection regimen with regular insulin to a rapid-acting insulin analog.

Recurrent severe hypoglycemia
- Each year about 10% of patients on insulin will have an episode of severe hypoglycemia requiring intervention by someone else.
    - About 1–3% of patients with type 1 diabetes have recurrent severe hypoglycemia.
    - Most patients with recurrent persistent problems are adults who have had diabetes for more than 10 years with low production of endogenous insulin as estimated by C-peptide.
- Pancreatic α cells are still present in undiminished numbers, but their glucagon response to hypoglycemia is virtually absent and the catecholamine response may be impaired. These patients therefore lack a major component of the hormonal defense against hypoglycemia.
- The following factors predispose to recurrent hypoglycemia:
    - Overtreatment with insulin. Frequent hypoglycemia impairs the response to further hypoglycemia within 2 weeks and lowers the blood glucose level at which symptoms develop.
    - Endocrine causes, including pituitary insufficiency, adrenal insufficiency, hypothyroidism, and premenstrual insulin sensitivity.
    - Gastrointestinal causes, including exocrine pancreatic failure, celiac disease, and diabetic gastroparesis.
    - Renal failure. The kidneys are important for the clearance of insulin and oral hypoglycemics, such as sulfonylureas, and also contribute to gluconeogenesis, which diminishes with declining renal function.
    - Patients may manipulate their therapy or misunderstand it.
    - Alcohol use has been implicated in up to 19% of severe hypoglycemic episodes. Alcohol in excess will suppress hepatic gluconeogenesis and, particularly if taken late in the evening, the effect may coincide with the nocturnal decline in cortisol, predisposing the patient to severe nocturnal hypoglycemia.
    - Other 'recreational' drug use. In a recent report, 10% of diabetic patients under the age of 50 tested positive for illicit drugs at the time of a severe hypoglycemic episode.

Treating hypoglycemia

- Treatment depends on the severity of the hypoglycemia.
- If it is practical to do so, it is useful to confirm the diagnosis with a blood or plasma glucose estimation by fingerstick. However, if hypoglycemia may reasonably be assumed, it is important not to delay treatment simply because of lack of absolute certainty about the diagnosis.
  ◇ Administering treatment for hypoglycemia when in fact hypoglycemia is not present is potentially less harmful than delaying treatment to someone who is truly hypoglycemic, as long as there is adequate assessment and follow-up over several hours.
- All patients and their close relatives and friends should learn about the risks of hypoglycemia and to recognize and treat the symptoms.
- Patients should be warned that taking excessive carbohydrate could be counterproductive, since this may cause rebound hyperglycemia; however, in practice it is notoriously difficult to avoid some degree of overcorrection.
- The dangers of alcohol excess and of hypoglycemia while driving need to be emphasized.

Mild hypoglycemia
- Any form of rapidly absorbed carbohydrate will relieve the early symptoms, and sufferers should always carry a source of glucose.
  Initial treatment with 15 grams of rapidly absorbed carbohydrate such as glucose tablets or liquids (juice, soda) is recommended, with rechecking of glucose levels 15 minutes later.
  ◇ It is also sensible to recommend a small amount of less readily absorbed carbohydrate (30 g) afterwards, particularly when an oral hypoglycemic drug or longer-acting insulin is implicated as a cause of the hypoglycemia, as a proportion of these patients will become hypoglycemic again after treatment.

Severe hypoglycemia
- Patients should carry identification, wear a bracelet or necklace, or employ a phone app identifying themselves as having diabetes, and these should be looked for in unconscious patients. The diagnosis of severe hypoglycemia resulting in confusion or coma is simple and can usually be made on clinical grounds, backed by an 'on the spot' fingerstick blood test.
  ◇ If real doubt exists, blood should be taken for glucose estimation before treatment is given, as long as this does not delay treatment for more than a short period (i.e. 1–2 minutes).
- Unconscious patients should be given either intramuscular, subcutaneous, or inhaled glucagon (1 mg) or intravenous glucose (25–50 ml of 50% dextrose solution) followed by a flush of normal saline to preserve the vein (since 50% dextrose scleroses veins).
  ◇ Glucagon acts by mobilizing hepatic glycogen, and works almost as rapidly as glucose. It is simple to administer and can be given at home by relatives. It does not work after a prolonged fast.
- As with milder hypoglycemia, oral administration of slowly absorbed carbohydrate, once the patient is more alert and able to comply, and continuing careful observation for several hours are important, so that recurrence of hypoglycemia can be prevented or promptly recognized and dealt with.

Preventing hypoglycemia
- If a pattern of hypoglycemic episodes is evident, then hypoglycemic agents such as sulfonylureas and insulin should be adjusted accordingly.
- Patients on insulin, especially basal-bolus insulin, can be taught how to adjust

insulin doses temporarily while waiting to see their treating physician. Ideally, patients would have been taught, and would have understood, that the insulin dose to be lowered is the dose preceding the hypoglycemic events.
  ◇ If a patient frequently has hypoglycemic events mid-morning, it is the rapid-acting insulin at breakfast that has to be decreased.
  ◇ If the patient has hypoglycemic events upon awakening in the morning, then it is the long-acting insulin dose that has to be reduced.
◆ Often, patients who do not recognize that the insulin dose has to be reduced consume extra carbohydrates to prevent low blood glucose.

Other complications or adverse effects from insulin treatment

◆ Hypoglycemia is the most common complication of treatment with insulin or insulin secretagogues, but there are other considerations (Table 15.5).
◆ Weight gain occurs with insulin treatment, since insulin has anabolic effects. Weight gain can also result from hypoglycemic episodes, as patients overcompensate by eating more calories than needed. It is, therefore, especially important to counsel patients on an appropriate diet.
◆ True insulin allergy is rare; allergy is more often due to the additives in the insulin preparations. For true insulin allergy, desensitization can be performed by allergy specialists.
  ◇ Anti-insulin antibodies can develop in response to exogenous insulin, but generally do not affect the therapeutic effect of insulin.
◆ Lipoatrophy and lipohypertrophy may occur at insulin injection sites used repeatedly (Figure 15.16). Management includes avoiding those sites until improvement is seen, and rotating injection sites to avoid these local reactions.
◆ Edema can occur, and may be more frequent when insulin is used in combination with TZDs.

Rotate injection sites to avoid local reactions.

Table 15.5 Complications of treatment. Side-effects of insulin treatment, such as allergic reaction, are rare, but they do occur in some patients.

Complications of insulin treatment
Allergy Local or general
Dose-dependent Hypoglycemia Weight gain (due to the anabolic action of insulin)
Not dose-dependent Lipohypertrophy (due to repeated injections at the same site) Lipoatrophy (rare now with purified insulin) Insulin edema (especially just after the start of treatment)

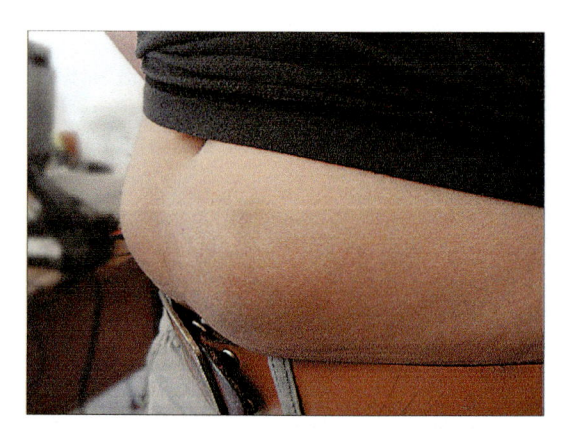

Figure 15.16 Lipohypertrophy at insulin injection sites. Lipohypertrophy may lead to poor glycemic control, as insulin absorption can be significantly delayed.

Pancreas transplantation

Overview and background
- The first successful human pancreas transplant was completed in 1966 in the United States.
- It is the only treatment for patients whom are dependent on exogenous insulin that will restore glycemic control without incurring the risk of hypoglycemia.
- In the setting of improved surgical techniques and also immunosuppression, survival rates for patients and grafts 1-year post-transplant are greater than 95% and 85% respectively.
- Most pancreas transplants occur as simultaneous pancreas-kidney transplants (SPK) or pancreas after kidney transplant (PAK).

Criteria for pancreas transplant
- There are 2 primary criteria for pancreas transplant in those with diabetes as outlined by the American Diabetes Association
  1. The patient has end-stage renal disease and is planned for kidney transplant
  2. Consideration for a pancreas transplant alone in those with complications such as:
     - History of frequent, acute, severe metabolic complications from diabetes (hypoglycemia unawareness, ketoacidosis, severe hyperglycemia)
     - Incapacitating clinical and emotional problems related to exogenous insulin therapy
     - Consistent failure of insulin-based management to prevent acute metabolic problems

Types of pancreas transplant
- The 3 major types of pancreas transplant are:
  - Simultaneous pancreas-kidney transplant (SPK)
  - Pancreas after kidney transplant (PAK)
  - Pancreas alone transplant (PAT)
- The decision of which type of transplant is offered to the patient is dependent on the patient characteristics, availability of organs and, for those in need of the renal transplant, the expected time on dialysis (Figure 15.17).
- SPK is preferred over a kidney transplant alone in a patient with diabetes because of the risk of developing or having worsening diabetic nephropathy in the transplanted kidney.
- The majority (over 75% depending on country and region) are SPK.
- The benefit of a living donor kidney is to avoid dialysis, which carries with it a 33% mortality within the first 5 years, especially when a pancreas cannot be identified at the time.
- While there is some disagreement on this point, pancreas transplant alone (PTA) suffers from higher rates of graft loss and rejection. Additionally, the use of immunosuppression which is nephrotoxic (such as calcineurin inhibitors) can have a deleterious impact on the patient's native kidney function. The 10-year incidence of post-PTA chronic kidney disease when pre-transplant eGFR was >60 mL/minutes is between 10–30%. While PTA is done, it is for these reasons that it is much less commonly performed.
- Pancreas retransplants do occur and account for approximately 6% of all pancreas transplants, typically in those with a failed pancreas graft after simultaneous pancreas-kidney transplants.

Outcomes after pancreas transplant
- In the United States, 5-year patient survival stands at around 93% for SPK, 91% for PAK, and 78% for PTA.
- The 5-year pancreas graft survival is 73% for SPK, 65% for PAK, and 53% for PTA.
- The numbers for other regions such as Europe appear to be similar.
- Overall patient survival is better for SPK than deceased-donor kidney transplant alone with 20–30% lower 10 and 20-year all-cause mortality.

```
                    ┌─────────────────────────────────────┐
                    │ INSULIN DEPENDENT DIABETES MELLITUS │
                    └─────────────────────────────────────┘
                                      │
          ┌───────────────────────────┼───────────────────────────────┐
          │                           │                               │
   ┌──────────────┐                   │                    ┌──────────────────────────────┐
   │ eGFR ≤ 20 mL/1.73m² │            │                    │ ■ Severe metaboloc complications │
   └──────────────┘                   │                    │    -Hypoglycemia              │
          │                           │                    │    -Marked hypoglycemia       │
   ┌──────┴──────┐                    │                    │    -Ketoacidosis              │
   │             │                    │                    │ ■ Incapacitating problems with │
┌─────────┐ ┌─────────┐                │                    │    exogenous insulin therapy  │
│No suitable│ │Suitable  │             │                    │ ■ Failure of insulin based    │
│living donor│ │living donor│           │                    │    management to prevent acute│
│or expected │ │+ expected │             │                    │    complications              │
│time on    │ │time on    │             │                    └──────────────────────────────┘
│dialysis < 1│ │dialysis > 1│
│year       │ │year       │
└─────────┘ └─────────┘
              │
         ┌─────────┐
         │Living donor│
         │  kidney   │
         │ transplant │
         └─────────┘
```

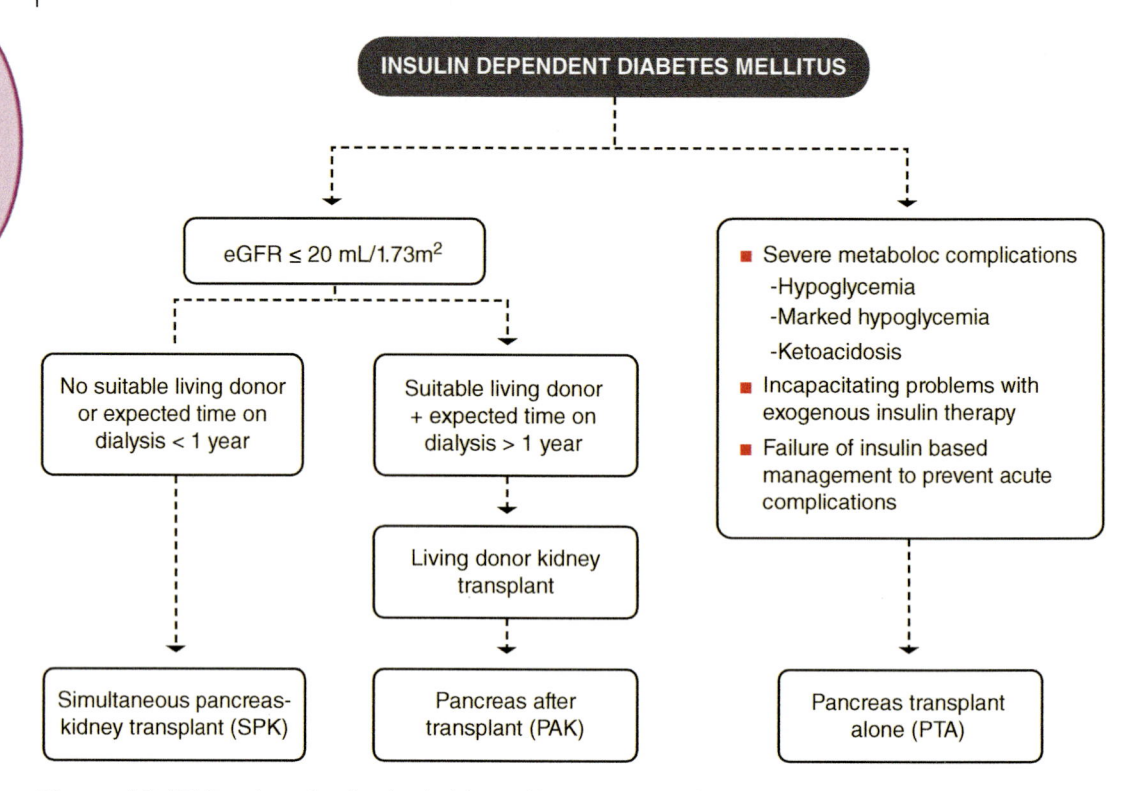

Figure 15.17 Flowchart showing the decision making to the type of pancreas +/− kidney transplant that the patient will receive.

Boxes at bottom: Simultaneous pancreas-kidney transplant (SPK); Pancreas after transplant (PAK); Pancreas transplant alone (PTA).

- After 5 years, over 50% of patients with PTA remain insulin free.
- SPK is clearly associated with improvements in quality of life.
- What is less clear is whether PTA confers a survival benefit over being maintained on medical therapy for patients without significant renal dysfunction.
- Immediate post-transplant complications can include acute rejection in addition to issues directly related to the surgical procedure. Long term, concerns include risk of infection and chronic rejection.

Impact on microvascular and macrovascular complications

- Improvement in pre-existing microvascular complications can be dependent on the premorbid state prior to transplant.
- *Retinopathy* Both SPK and also PTA appear to be able to result in at least stabilization if not improvement of the retinopathy over time.
- *Neuropathy* There is improvement after SPK in somatic neuropathy (i.e. peripheral neuropathy) likely related to an improvement in uremia from the kidney disease.
- *Cardiovascular* There is a reduction in cardiovascular death and also progression of peripheral vascular disease after SPK. There is not enough data to determine if the same holds for PTA.

Islet cell transplant

- There has been increasing interest in the area of islet cell transplantation
- There are two basic divisions:
  ◇ Islet transplantation from donor pancreases
  ◇ Autologous islet cell transplantation done in setting of chronic pancreatitis

Donor islet cell transplantation

- This has been seen as a potential alternative to PTA or even to replace the pancreas transplant portion of PAK.
- The process for extraction of islets is well established (Figure 15.18).

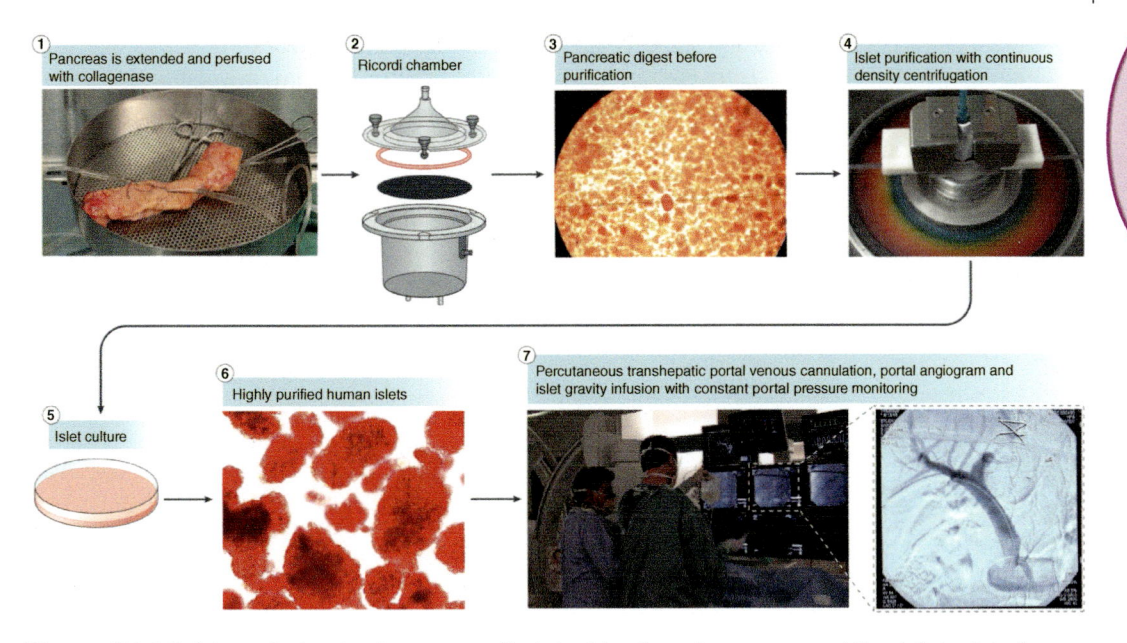

Figure 15.18 Schematic showing the process of isolating islets from the pancreas and then infusing into the portal vein.

- The eligibility criteria include having type 1 diabetes that is complicated by hypoglycemia unawareness, severe hypoglycemia, and/or extreme glycemic variability despite maximal insulin therapy under guidance from an endocrinologist.
- When using donor pancreas, typically 2–4 organs are required to achieve the more than 500,000 islets which are commonly infused as islets represent less than 2% of the pancreas.
- This has been a major barrier to more widespread uptake as it can be challenging to procure the sufficient donor pancreases for the transplant.
- Typically mortality is very low at less than 3% and typically not a direct consequence of the procedure. Most common side effect is simply some discomfort at the site of infusion.
- Immediately after the procedure, up to 80% of patients can achieve insulin independence under favorable conditions, which includes infusion with >5,000 IEQ/kg.
- In the presence of appropriate induction immunosuppressive therapy and anti-inflammatory therapy, about 50% of patients can be maintained insulin free at 5 years out from transplant.
- Even those in whom there is insulin-dependence continue to be relatively protected from hypoglycemia.

Autologous islet cell transplantation

- The eligibility for Total Pancreatectomy with Islet Autologous Transplant (TP-IAT) includes having chronic pancreatitis without type 1 diabetes or c-peptide negative diabetes. The purpose is to treat the chronic pain and reduced quality of life in those with chronic pancreatitis.
- There is still no way to prognosticate post-transplant islet function but there is a definitive correlation with the number of islets that can be successfully transplanted. When >5,000 IEQ/kg can eb transplanted, 72% of those patients were insulin-independent still after 3 years.
- Outcomes after transplant follow the rule of thirds, meaning that a third of patients will be insulin free, a third will have partial islet function requiring some support from insulin, and the final third will be

- fully insulin dependent in the setting of graft failure.
- ◆ Adjuvant therapies such as GLP-1 analogs and IL-8 inhibitors have been under study to see if they can support continued islet cell function and reduce islet loss acutely after islet infusion.

CHAPTER 16

Special management considerations

Inpatient diabetes considerations

- Diabetes is a chronic illness, mostly managed in the outpatient setting. When a patient with diabetes is admitted to the hospital for reasons other than diabetes, the focus of treatment is the illness triggering the admission.
- Patients with diabetes who have poor control before admission may continue to have poor control in the hospital. Patients who lack dietary discipline may experience unexpected hypoglycemia and a decrease in insulin requirements with imposed dietary compliance caused by hospitalization.
- Patients who were in good control before admission now find themselves with elevated blood glucoses since they are sick, and the dosing of their insulin is left to physicians who may not pay careful attention to their glycemic control.
- The risk of mortality and complications increases as the level of hyperglycemia increases (Figure 16.1).
  ◇ Mortality is higher in hyperglycemic versus nonhyperglycemic patients.
  ◇ Mortality in those without a previous diagnosis of diabetes (i.e. patients who have new hyperglycemia) has been shown to be even greater in a few studies – either because hyperglycemia is a marker for worse prognosis or because newly diagnosed diabetes was frequently left untreated (Figure 16.2). In support of the latter, patients known to have diabetes have

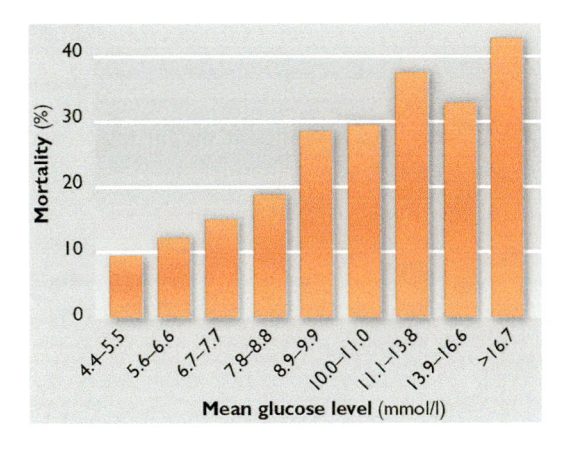

Figure 16.1 Hyperglycemia in critically ill patients. Hyperglycemia is associated with a significantly increased risk of mortality. *From Krinsley JS, 2003.*

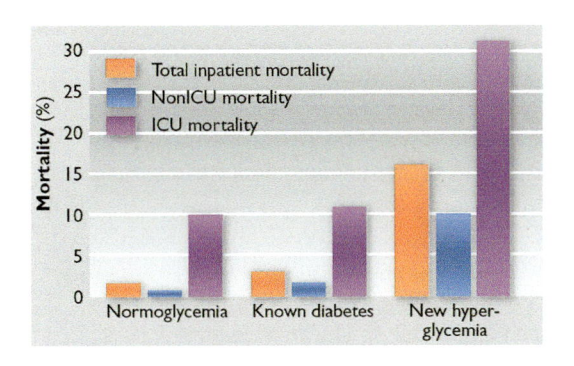

Figure 16.2 Inpatient mortality. Patients with new hyperglycemia admitted to both critical care areas and general wards had a significantly higher mortality rate than patients with a known history of diabetes or normoglycemia. *From Umpierrez GE, et al, 2002.*

Special management considerations

improved outcomes when aggressively managed with insulin.
- In the critically ill, the use of insulin infusion protocols in the intensive care unit has facilitated the control of hyperglycemia.
- Morbidity and mortality are lower in intensively treated patients achieving excellent glucose control.
  ◇ In one study of hyperglycemic patients admitted to the surgical intensive care unit, the use of an insulin infusion protocol to achieve blood glucose levels of <6.0 mmol/L (108 mg/dL) was associated with significantly less mortality and less incidence of complications (such as acute renal failure, critical care neuropathy, septicemia, and the need for blood transfusions) compared to conventional treatment. Of note, only 13% of these patients had a known history of diabetes.
  ◇ The same study was performed in the medical intensive care unit; in this group, intensive insulin infusion reduced morbidity but not mortality.
  ◇ In cardiothoracic surgery, the use of insulin infusion protocols in patients immediately following coronary artery bypass graft resulted in a reduced incidence of deep sternal wound infection, and thus a decreased length of hospital stay.
- However, subsequent studies in critically ill patients suggest that a tight glucose target of 4.4–6.1 mmol/L (80–110 mg/dL) may have to be reevaluated. Studies such as the VISEP and the largest study, NICE-SUGAR, show either no benefit or a greater risk of hypoglycemia and mortality with tighter control.
- Insulin infusions are broadly recommended for perioperative care, and details of such management are to be found in more specialized sources.
- In the noncritically ill patient on the regular hospital ward, the ongoing use of retroactive sliding scale insulin therapy, despite recommendations to the contrary, is one of the reasons why hyperglycemia is perpetuated.
- In general, the use of basal insulin (in the form of NPH [isophane] insulin, detemir insulin or glargine U100 and U300) and, if necessary, prandial insulin, can prevent hyperglycemia, whereas sliding scales are reactive and only treat patients when the blood glucoses are high.
- Detemir or glargine 10 IU daily for insulin-naïve patients, or 0.15 IU/kg daily for patients with features of insulin resistance, is a typical starting dose to provide patients with basal insulin in the hospital. However, many acutely ill patients will require doses of 0.3 IU/kg or higher.
- Insulin pumps present a unique problem: patients with these are usually independent and attuned to their insulin needs. However, if they are too ill to manipulate their pumps and calculate insulin doses, it may be better to put these patients on basal and prandial subcutaneous insulin if the hospital staff cannot operate the pump. This decision can be arrived at based on the patient's clinical state and the individual hospital's policy, if any exists, regarding allowing the patient to self-administer insulin.
- Since the beginning of the COVID-19 pandemic, there has been increased used of outpatient continuous glucose monitoring devices on the inpatient side and studies that have demonstrated sufficient accuracy of these devices compared with point-of-care glucometers approved for inpatient use.

Diabetes and surgery

- It is accepted, and supported by clinical trial results, that efforts to achieve near-normal glycemia during and after major surgery, particularly cardiothoracic surgery, and in surgical intensive care patients, will significantly decrease mortality and postoperative infection, and may also decrease the need for

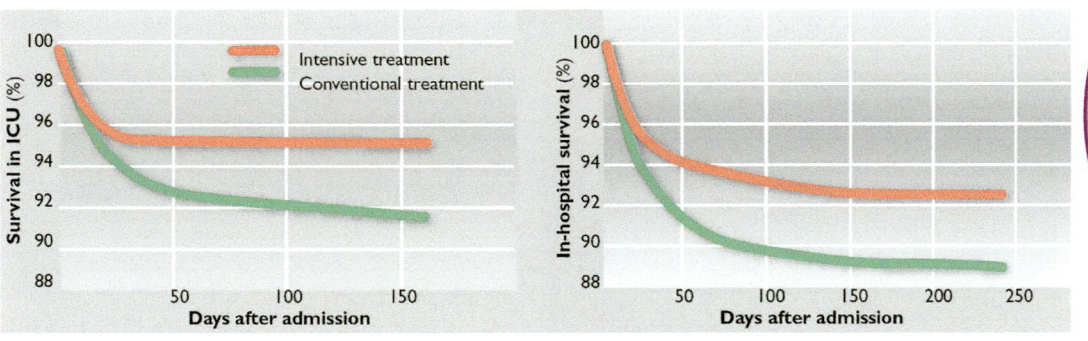

Figure 16.3 Intensive insulin therapy in critically ill patients. In a study of 1548 patients, intensive therapy reduced both ICU and general in-hospital mortality. *From van den Berghe G, et al, 2001.*

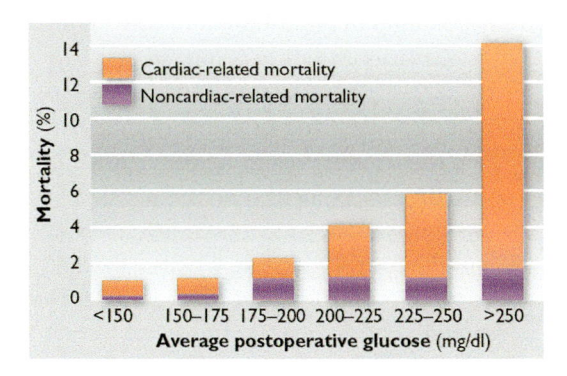

Figure 16.4 Coronary artery bypass graft surgery and hyperglycemia. There is a clear relationship between high glucose levels and high in-hospital cardiac-related mortality. *From Furnary AP, Gao G, et al, 2003.*

transfusion, need for dialysis, and critical care neuropathy (Figure 16.3).

- When an emergency major surgical procedure is required in a patient with diabetes it is therefore mandatory to institute immediately an insulin infusion regimen that aims to achieve and sustain near normal glucose levels (4–8 mmol/L [72–144 mg/dL]) (Figure 16.4).
  - Relevant medical, nursing, and intensive care staff should be trained in the use of an algorithm-based insulin infusion regimen (Table 16.1).
- Experienced medical and nursing staff may assume that hypoglycemia is the major risk to the severely ill postoperative patient, but the adverse consequences of hyperglycemia probably outweigh the minor risks posed by hypoglycemia in such patients.

Table 16.1 Insulin therapy for hospitalized patients. Staff should be trained in administration of an insulin infusion.

Insulin-treated diabetes regimen
Stop long-acting and/or intermediate insulin the day before surgery, substitute short-acting insulin, and start insulin infusion
Use intravenous 10% dextrose (500 ml infused at 100 ml/h) and soluble (regular in US) insulin (1–3 IU/h) perioperatively with potassium chloride (10 mmol [10 mEq] in 500 ml)
Postoperatively, the infusion is maintained until the patient is able to eat. Other fluids must be given through a separate intravenous line
Monitor glucose and potassium levels and adjust amounts in infusion while keeping the rate constant
When transitioning patient from infusion to subcutaneous insulin, the first injection of basal insulin should be administered at least 2 h before the infusion is discontinued

Major surgery

- For major surgery that is elective, rather than emergency, efforts should be made to optimize glycemic control and electrolytes before admission to hospital (Table 16.2).
  - If that seems unlikely to be achieved on an outpatient basis, consider admitting the patient a day early for intensive insulin management preoperatively.
  - An alternative is to significantly reduce the long-acting and/or intermediate acting insulin the day

Special management considerations

Table 16.2 Elective surgery. Plan to optimize glycemic control.

Diabetes management for surgery
Management is by a team; liaison between the diabetes team and the anesthetist is ideal
Metabolic control should be optimized before the operation. For emergency surgery, metabolic disturbances should be carefully managed
Use insulin therapy when in doubt
Put the patient at the beginning of the list at the start of the day, if practicable
Electrolyte disturbances should be corrected before surgery, when feasible

Table 16.3 Hospitalized patients and oral therapy. Oral anti-hyperglycemic therapy should be discontinued and insulin therapy initiated if needed.

Diet- or tablet-treated diabetes
Omit short-acting agents (e.g. sulfonylureas) on the morning of the operation
Omit long-acting sulfonylureas (e.g. glibenclamide/glyburide) at least 24 h before nonemergency surgery, and manage glycemia with insulin
Avoid glucose- and lactate-containing fluids in minor operations when possible
Avoid metformin perioperatively and if radiological contrast is required
For all major operations consider need for insulin treatment. For relatively minor procedures it may be sufficient simply to omit oral agents on the morning of surgery, and resume when the patient starts eating again

before and day of the surgery and hold all scheduled short-acting insulin while the patient is being maintained without nutrition. In this situation an insulin infusion would not be needed.
- Tight glycemic control postoperatively should be just as outlined for emergency surgery.
- These principles should apply equally to type 1 and type 2 diabetes.
- Where the patient's usual treatment is with oral agents, these should be discontinued at least 24 hours before surgery, and insulin instituted (Table 16.3).
- In particular, SGLT2 inhibitors should be discontinued about 2–3 days prior to surgery due to the risk of diabetic ketoacidosis.
- Ideally, the operation should be scheduled at the start of the operating list, if practicable.

Minor surgery
- For minor surgery there can be a more individualized approach, with some basic ground rules:
  ◇ Insulin secretagogues, especially the longer acting, should be discontinued at least 24 hours before surgery.
  ◇ If use of contrast material in imaging peri- or postoperatively is anticipated, metformin should be discontinued the day before.
- Insulin glargine or detemir, given the evening before surgery, may be an alternative to insulin infusion, but published data are lacking.
- Once weekly GLP1 receptor agonists should be held if due to be given the morning of surgery.
- For short and very simple procedures it may be sufficient to omit oral agents or short-acting insulin on the morning of surgery.

Surgery and blood pressure
- As a general medical consideration it is accepted that control of blood pressure should be achieved before elective surgery.

Conception, contraception, and pregnancy

- Diabetes, both type 1 and type 2, confers a greater maternal and fetal risk than in women without diabetes. Diabetes management extends to all periods of pregnancy and includes the prepregnancy planning period and the postnatal phase (Tables 16.4 and 16.5).
- Modern management of pregnancy in women with diabetes means that

Table 16.4 Management points. Optimization of blood glucose is key to successful management.

Management points for diabetes in pregnancy
Prepregnancy counseling to optimize blood glucose control and thereby limit risk of congenital malformations
Optimize blood glucose control with 1 h postprandial blood glucose between 4 and 8 mmol/L (72–144 mg/dL) and HbA1c (or fructosamine) in the normal range
Monitor blood glucose control. Ketoacidosis in pregnancy carries a 50% fetal mortality, but maternal hypoglycemia is relatively well tolerated by the fetus
Limit calorie intake in obesity (30% decrease) and avoid refined carbohydrate
Insulin therapy if blood glucose does not achieve targets. Use multiple injections or insulin subcutaneous pump, as insulin requirement rises progressively during the 2nd trimester, levelling off thereafter
Avoid oral hypoglycemic agents unless strong indication
Review in joint diabetes/antenatal clinic at intervals of ≤2 weeks. The aim should be outpatient management with a spontaneous vaginal delivery at term. Retinopathy and nephropathy may deteriorate Expert fundoscopy and urine testing for protein undertaken at booking, at 28 weeks, and before delivery
Delivery should be in hospital. Obstetric problems include stillbirth, fetopelvic disproportion, hydramnios and pre-eclampsia. Assess pregnancy staging using ultrasound. Cesarean section is often required

Table 16.5 Management plan. Management of early pregnancy is important to reduce the risk of congenital anomalies.

Management plan for diabetes in the three trimesters	
FIRST TRIMESTER	
Mother	Folate supplements (to reduce congenital malformation risk)
	Stop smoking; avoid alcohol, ACEIs, statins
	Optimize glycemic control
	Screen for diabetes complications
Baby	Ultrasound scan (for congenital anomalies)
SECOND TRIMESTER	
Mother	Stop smoking, avoid alcohol
	Optimize glycemic control (insulin dose increases)
	Screen and treat diabetes complications
	Monitor and treat blood pressure
Baby	Ultrasound scan (for congenital anomalies, growth)
THIRD TRIMESTER	
Mother	Stop smoking, avoid alcohol, check drugs
	Optimize glycemic control (insulin dose increases to 34–36 weeks)
	Screen and treat diabetes complications
	Monitor and treat blood pressure
	Check for pre-eclampsia (twice as common as normal)
Baby	Ultrasound scan (for congenital anomalies, growth)
	Plan delivery

outcomes in specialized centers approach those in pregnancy without diabetes.

◇ Before the discovery of insulin in 1921, most women with type 1 diabetes did not survive to reproductive age; the few pregnancies reported suffered a 50% perinatal and maternal mortality rate. Even 50 years ago both the maternal and neonatal morbidity and mortality were substantial.

◇ The subsequent transformation was due to meticulous metabolic control throughout the three trimesters of pregnancy and general improvements in medical and obstetric management (Figure 16.5).

◆ Glycemic control at the time of conception and in the early weeks of pregnancy is particularly important, as maternal hyperglycemia and/or accompanying metabolic disturbance during organogenesis increase the risk of congenital malformation in the fetus.

◆ However, even with good glycemic control and improved obstetric services, rates of congenital malformation and perinatal death associated with pregnancy in type

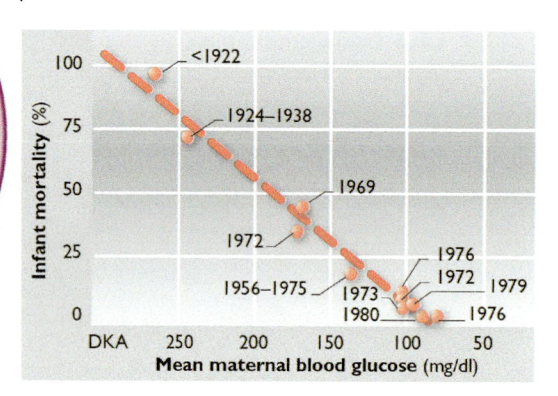

Figure 16.5 Infant mortality. A review of the major studies over the last century revealed that as maternal blood glucose concentrations decreased, infant mortality also decreased. *From Jovanovic and Peterson.*

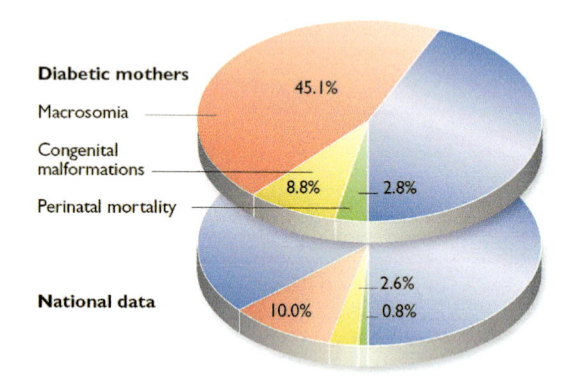

Figure 16.6 Perinatal outcomes. Women with type 1 diabetes in the Netherlands in 1999–2000 showed a 3–4-fold greater risk of obstetric complications compared to national data. *From Evers IM, de Valk HW, et al, 2004.*

1 diabetes continue to exceed those in women without diabetes (Figure 16.6).
◇ Whether this is because not all women with diabetes receive obstetric care in specialized centers is a matter of conjecture, and while a case can be made for such a policy, its implementation would be difficult to enforce in most healthcare systems.

Diabetes management should cover the prepregnancy planning period.

Contraception and diabetes

◆ Because the issue of periconceptual glycemic control is so important, pregnancy in diabetes should preferably be planned; therefore, contraception is an important part of management.
◆ There may sometimes be situations related to diabetes in which it is better to advise against pregnancy altogether, though that decision is ultimately for the patient to make (see p. 182).
◆ The options for contraception are as for individuals without diabetes, and an individual approach should be taken to deciding which is appropriate for the particular patient. Methods other than the contraceptive pill, tubal ligation, and vasectomy have significant 'failure' rates – perhaps as high as 4–5% for IUCD and condom, rising to at least 20% for the rhythm method.
◆ Regarding the contraceptive pill, the only specific point of relevance in diabetes relates to the metabolic effects associated with estrogen.
   ◇ High-dose estrogen combined pills may cause an increase in glycemia, necessitating an increase in insulin dosage; this is not the case with low-dose estrogen pills, which are prescribed much more.
   ◇ Lipid levels are less likely to be perturbed by low-dose than high-dose combined pills.
   ◇ In women with clinical macrovascular disease or with other significant risk factors such as strong family history, smoking, hypertension, or hyperlipidemia, the use of combined estrogen-progesterone contraception needs to be carefully considered, as would be the case in women without diabetes. An increased risk of thromboembolic disease accompanies use of a combined oral contraceptive pill, though it is less with low-dose formulations.

High-dose estrogen combined contraceptive pills may cause an increase in glycemia.

- Progestogen-only pills are not associated with metabolic or lipid disturbance, and therefore may be considered particularly suitable for women with diabetes. They can lead to menstrual irregularity such as intermenstrual bleeding, or sometimes amenorrhea.
  - Intermenstrual bleeding may be resolved by increasing the dose temporarily for a few cycles.
  - Once it has been established that the onset of amenorrhea is associated with a negative pregnancy test the patient can be reassured that the amenorrhea is a natural effect of the progestogen inhibiting ovulation.

Glucose monitoring and glycemic goals in pregnancy

- The optimal method of glucose monitoring in pregnancy has been reasonably well, indeed uniquely, studied.
  - Most studies of the utility of glucose monitoring in insulin-treated diabetes apart from pregnancy have concentrated on preprandial and fasting glucose.
  - However, a study of preprandial glucose monitoring in women with insulin-treated gestational diabetes suggested that this strategy did not adequately reflect strict glycemic control or decrease the risk of macrosomia.
  - A subsequent randomized study in a similar cohort showed that, in comparison to preprandial monitoring, postprandial testing led to a greater decrease in HbA1c, lower mean infant birth weight with fewer 'weight-related' complications such as cephalopelvic disproportion, and less likelihood of cesarean section and neonatal hypoglycemia. However, this study has been criticized on the grounds that the preprandial glucose target was set at a relatively high level (3.3–5.9 mmol/L [60–106 mg/dL]) whereas the postprandial target was relatively low (7.8 mmol/L [140 mg/dL]).
  - A randomized study with glucose targets identical to those in the preceding study, but carried out in women with type 1 diabetes from 16 weeks' gestation, showed that postprandial monitoring, as compared with preprandial, was associated with greater success in achieving glycemic targets in the second and third trimesters and significantly less likelihood of pre-eclampsia (Table 16.6).
- There is now a consensus that in pregnancy the aim should be to achieve glucose levels of less than 7.8 mmol/L (140 mg/dL) 1 hour after meals. There is more debate about appropriate preprandial targets, with some investigators suggesting a target of 3.3–4.4 mmol/L (60–80 mg/dL) rather than the more conservative one of <5.9 mmol/L (106 mg/dL).
- With the rise in use of continuous glucose monitoring, recent recommendations have been released from the Advanced Technologies and Treatments for Diabetes in 2019 on the targets for individuals in pregnancy. Every 5% increase in time in range is associated with benefit for pregnancy in individuals with type 1 diabetes (Table 16.7).

In pregnancy, the aim should be to achieve postprandial glucose levels of less than 7.8 mmol/L.

Type 1 diabetes patients
- Prepregnancy counseling, with efforts to achieve near normal glycemia, and the planned introduction of folate 5 mg, should ideally be the rule at an early stage in adult life.

Table 16.6 Glucose monitoring. In this study, 61 women with type 1 diabetes were randomly assigned at 16 weeks' gestation to preprandial or postprandial blood glucose monitoring throughout pregnancy. Maternal age, parity, age of onset of diabetes, number of previous miscarriages, smoking status, social class, weight gain in pregnancy, and compliance with therapy were similar in both groups. The postprandial monitoring group had a significantly reduced incidence of preeclampsia and greater success in achieving glycemic targets.

Obstetric outcome in relation to pre- and postprandial blood glucose monitoring

VARIABLE	PREPRANDIAL (n = 31)	POSTPRANDIAL (n = 30)
Delivery gestational age (wks)	36.9 (1.5)	36.7 (2.5)
Weight gain (kg)	15.0 (5.2)	15.9 (6.5)
Insulin dose		
Prepregnancy	50.0 (23.2)	51.3 (25.1)
Units/day	105.0 (51.3)	120.4 (32.3)
Units/kg	1.2 (0.5)	1.4 (0.5)
Change	50.2 (35.7)	65 (49.0)
Cesarean section		
Total	21/31 (68%)	14/30 (47%)
For suspected disproportion	8/31 (26%)	7/30 (23%)
Pre-eclampsia	6/28 (21%)	1/30 (3%)
Mean glycated hemoglobin (%) [mmol/mol]		
Initial	7.6 [59]	7.4 [56]
Final	6.3 [46]	6.0 [42]
Mean capillary glucose (mmol/L) [mg/dL]		
Trimester 2 (before breakfast)	7.7 [138.6] (1.8)	7.0 [126.0] (2.0)
Trimester 3 (before breakfast)	7.0 [126.0] (1.3)	7.0 [126.0] (2.0)
Fructosamine (μmol/L)		
Trimester 2	250.4 (37.6)	240.3 (33.2)
Trimester 3	214.4 (27.2)	213.4 (32.8)
Success in glycemic control (%)		
Trimester 2	29.4 (11)	51.6 (19)
Trimester 3	30.3 (11)	55.5 (20)

Data presented as mean (SD) or number (%) where appropriate.
Source: Adapted, with permission, from Manderson JG, Patterson CC, Hadden DR, et al, 2003.

Table 16.7 Targets for continuous glucose monitoring in pregnancy. TIR Time in range TBR Time below range TAR Time above range.

	Percent Time
TIR (3.5–7.8 mmol/L)	>70%
TAR (>7.8 mmol/L)	<25%
TBR (<3.5 mmol/L)	<5%

- Inevitably, many women become pregnant when HbA1c is still elevated.
- An appreciation of the effect of pregnancy on insulin needs is crucial.
- During the first trimester insulin requirements are fairly stable, though the actual diagnosis of pregnancy will often lead to a change in the level of self-care, and if dietary habits alter (i.e. calorie intake decreases) there may be a need for adjusting the insulin dosage downwards. On the other hand, in those women

with elevated HbA1c an alteration in the insulin dose (usually an increase) will be required to optimize glycemic control rapidly.
- ◇ Patients not already on an intensive insulin regimen of multiple injections or a subcutaneous insulin infusion pump should be strongly advised to adopt one or the other.
- ◆ In the second trimester, insulin needs rise steadily, often to more than double the prepregnancy dose, and then tend to level off or occasionally even fall slightly in the final few weeks (Figure 16.7).
  - ◇ The precise cause of the increasing insulin need is not known, but is probably related to the rise in hormones like cortisol, progesterone, and human placental lactogen.
- ◆ Management of glycemia during labor is best achieved by intravenous infusion of insulin and glucose, the aim being to maintain normal glucose levels.
- ◆ Immediately postpartum the insulin resistance of pregnancy decreases, so the insulin dose may decrease to low levels, even zero, for a few days; thereafter, insulin should be resumed at a dosage appropriate for prepregnancy needs.

An appreciation of the effect of pregnancy on insulin needs is crucial.

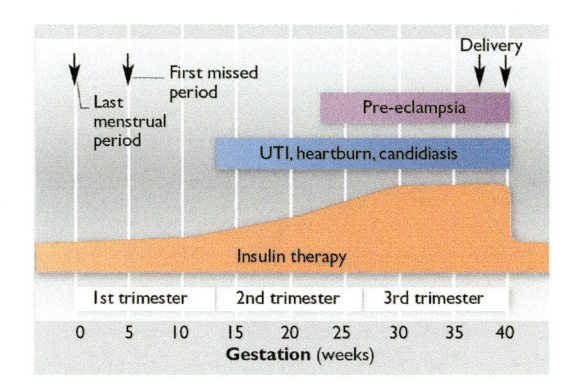

Figure 16.7 Impact of diabetes on the mother. Insulin needs rise rapidly in the second trimester.

- ◆ In the sense that insulin therapy is a necessity for women with type 1 diabetes, its 'safety' in pregnancy has been established through common usage; the outcome for both the mother and the fetus would be clearly disastrous in the absence of insulin therapy.
- ◆ Insulin analogs, prescribed increasingly along with or in preference to human insulin in nonpregnant patients with diabetes, have not been specifically tested for safety in human pregnancy. Inevitably, therefore, the package inserts of analog insulins caution against the lack of safety data as to their use in pregnancy.
  - ◇ With each new analog, concerns are raised about potential for harm, for example through affinity for placental receptors of insulin-like growth factors. However, to date, the lack of evidence for adverse effects supports the emerging view that insulin analogs are probably just as safe as human and animal insulin.
  - ◇ It is unlikely that the safety issue will ever be strictly tested in randomized controlled trials in pregnancy, and probably true that the majority of diabetologists with wide experience in pregnancy treatment would regard current insulin analogs as safe for use.
  - ◇ Each woman and her partner need to make an informed choice between the lack of evidence of an adverse effect of insulin analogs, the known risk of diabetic pregnancy, and the risk of poor diabetes control versus the potential benefit of good glucose control using insulin analogs.

Type 2 diabetes patients
- ◆ The rising prevalence of type 2 diabetes in women of childbearing age has resulted in increasing numbers of pregnant women with preexisting diabetes.
- ◆ Unless stringent glycemic control is readily achieved through dietary management the consensus is that insulin treatment is appropriate.

Table 16.8 Oral glucose-lowering agents in pregnancy. In an analysis of 379 women with type 2 diabetes using oral hypoglycemic agents (metformin and glibenclamide) subdivided into three groups according to therapy, increased perinatal mortality was associated with the use of sulfonylureas or sulfonylureas plus metformin. Conversion from oral agents to insulin was protective for perinatal mortality compared with oral agents alone.

Comparison of insulin and oral glucose-lowering agents in pregnancy

	ORAL AGENTS ALONE	ORAL AGENTS → INSULIN	DIET/INSULIN
Birth weight (g)	3185.2 ± 103.3 (n = 90)	3259.0 ± 52.3 (n = 244)	3238.8 ± 140.5 (n = 29)
No. of outcomes/no of pregnancies			
Perinatal mortality	11/88 (12.5%)	7/248 (2.8%)	1/30 (3.3%)
Stillbirth rate	8/88 (9.1%)	5/248 (2.0%)	1/30 (3.3%)
Neonatal death rate	3/87 (3.4%)	2/248 (0.8%)	0/30 (0.0%)
No. of outcomes/no of pregnancies			
Fetal anomaly	5/88 (5.7%)	5/248 (2.0%)	0/30 (0.0%)
Cesarean section	55/88 (62.5%)	146/244 (59.8%)	18/31 (58.1%)
Neonatal hypoglycemia	18/75 (24%)	37/196 (18.9%)	5/22 (22.7%)
Macrosomia	21/90 (23.3%)	44/245 (18%)	5/29 (17.2%)
Pre-eclampsia	3/87 (3.4%)	5/239 (2.1%)	0/33 (0.0%)
Neonatal jaundice	14/75 (18.7%)	21/199 (10.6%)	2/22 (9.1%)

Source: Adapted, with permission, from Ekpebegh CO, Coetzee EJ, van der Merwe L, et al, 2007.

- ◇ Initial insulin needs are likely to be greater than in type 1 diabetes because of the preexisting insulin resistance associated with type 2 diabetes, but the principles of treatment are essentially the same.
- ◆ Many women with diabetes, on learning that they are pregnant, make a renewed effort with dietary care and their general well-being. So, in theory at least, since glycemia in type 2 diabetes is potentially more responsive to lifestyle change than in type 1 diabetes, insulin requirements may be individually more variable.
- ◆ It is likely that some women with type 2 diabetes could maintain satisfactory control with oral agents, but studies of this are limited.
  - ◇ At present the use of oral agents is not acknowledged as the 'standard of care', though many patients with diabetes and polycystic ovary syndrome are becoming pregnant whilst on metformin, and results to date suggest that the drug has no adverse effect on the fetus.
- ◆ A retrospective survey in South Africa found that, despite the achievement of comparable glycemic control when glibenclamide and metformin were used rather than insulin, there were higher perinatal mortality and stillbirth rates (Table 16.8), but such adverse effects from these oral agents have not been confimed in other studies.

Risks to the mother with diabetes

- ◆ Theoretically the risk of maternal mortality is higher in the diabetic than non-diabetic pregnancy (Figure 16.8 and Table 16.9). This relates to:
  - ◇ Risk of ketoacidosis if appropriate attention is not paid to glycemic control.
  - ◇ Increased labor risks if there is fetal macrosomia.
  - ◇ Increased risk of cardiac or renal failure in the presence of established advanced microvascular or macrovascular disease.
  - ◇ Increased risk of pre-eclampsia.

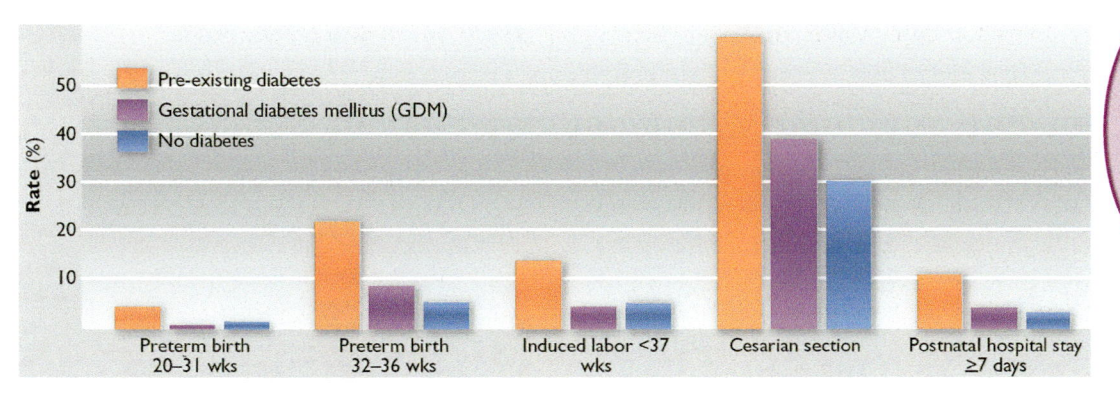

Figure 16.8 Pregnancy outcomes. The Australian Institute of Health and Welfare analysis of National Perinatal Data Collection data found that mothers with pre-existing diabetes have higher rates of adverse pregnancy outcomes than mothers without diabetes or with GDM.

Table 16.9 Pregnancy risks. Diabetes during pregnancy significantly increases the risks to both mother and child.

Risks of diabetic pregnancy
MATERNAL RISKS
Metabolic deterioration
Microvascular complications progress
Macrovascular complications
Risk of urinary tract infection increased
Risk of pre-eclampsia increased
Rates of cesarean section increased
FETAL RISKS
Risk of congenital malformations increased (cardiac, sacral agenesis, spina bifida)
Rates of stillbirth increased
Perinatal morbidity and mortality increased
Neonatal complications increased (fetal distress, jaundice, hypoglycemia)
Risk of diabetes in later life increased

- It is important to screen all pregnant women with diabetes for the presence of microvascular complications as soon as pregnancy is diagnosed.
- The pre-existence of complications is not necessarily a reason to advise against pregnancy, but women with diabetes should be made aware that microvascular complications can worsen suddenly and considerably during pregnancy despite improving glycemic control. Reasons for strongly advising against pregnancy include:
  ◇ Clinical ischemic heart disease holds greatly increased maternal risk of mortality, and with the increasing prevalence of type 2 diabetes in younger patients, we may expect to see more patients in that situation.
  ◇ Advanced nephropathy, particularly with severe hypertension or proteinuria, is associated with greatly increased risk to both mother and fetus.
  ◇ Active proliferative retinopathy.
  ◇ Severe symptomatic autonomic neuropathy.

Microvascular complications can worsen considerably during pregnancy, despite improving glycemic control.

Gestational diabetes mellitus (GDM)
- GDM occurs when abnormal glucose tolerance develops during pregnancy in a woman not known to have diabetes before pregnancy, unless she has had GDM in a previous pregnancy.
- Usually the abnormal glucose tolerance resolves after delivery, but women with GDM are quite likely to develop it again

in a subsequent pregnancy, and are at considerably increased risk of developing type 2 diabetes in the future.
- ◇ Progression to diabetes is around 30% over 7–10 years, or in some particularly susceptible populations as high as 50% in 5 years, suggesting that GDM is a 'prediabetes' state.
- ◇ Women who are obese, older, have first-degree relatives with diabetes, have a previous history of poor pregnancy outcome, have a history of large-for-gestational-age babies, or belong to an ethnic/racial group with a known high prevalence of type 2 diabetes are particularly at risk for GDM.
- ◆ About 2% of pregnant white Europeans develop gestational diabetes. A small percentage of cases have diabetes-associated antibodies and progress to type 1 diabetes mellitus.
- ◆ Screening. All women over age 25 and with a BMI above normal should be assessed for diabetes early in pregnancy, unless they have absolutely none of the risk factors mentioned above. If they are found not to have GDM they should be tested again between 24 and 28 weeks and more frequently if at particularly high risk.
- ◆ GDM is usually asymptomatic.
- ◆ Diagnostic criteria have been established for GDM (Table 16.10). The definition is based on either a 3-hour/100-g (ADA, 2001) or a 2-hour/75-g (WHO, 1999) oral glucose tolerance test (OGTT). These criteria are still a matter for debate, though there is a general move towards standardization.
  - ◇ The International Association of the Diabetes and Pregnancy Study Groups (IADPSG) fetal outcome-based definition, using 2-hour 75 g OGTT data from the worldwide Hyperglycemia and Adverse Pregnancy Outcome (HAPO) study, is being adopted in many countries.
- ◆ IADPSG has also published a strategy to detect unrecognized type 2 diabetes at

Table 16.10 Diagnostic criteria. The definition of GDM is based on an oral glucose tolerance test (OGTT). The IADPSG threshold values of venous plasma glucose (one or more to be equalled or exceeded) are listed, as well as previous systems from the WHO and ADA, which are still used in some centers.

Diagnostic criteria for GDM			
Plasma glucose (mmol/L [mg/dL])	IADPSG	WHO	ADA
Fasting	5.1 [92]	7.0 [126]	5.3 [95]
1 hour	10.0 [180]	–	10.0 [180]
2 hour	8.5 [153]	7.8 [140]	8.6 [155]
3 hour*	–	–	7.8 [140]

* 100-g load only

the first prenatal visit, so that therapy can be started immediately.
- ◆ Initial treatment for GDM is with diet, though there is no consensus as to which one is best. There have been no randomized trials addressing this issue and there are no data, other than a possible reduction in the risk of macrosomia, to support any particular intervention.
- ◆ Insulin treatment, required in about 30% of cases, is initiated if postprandial glucose cannot be maintained at less than 7.8 mmol/L (140 mg/dL) with diet.
  - ◇ Insulin does not cross the placenta.
- ◆ Oral agents such as metformin and second-generation sulfonylureas may be of value when the hyperglycemia is just above target levels, though caution should be exercised, and these agents remain the second line of treatment.
- ◆ GDM is associated with the obstetric and neonatal problems described for pre-existing diabetes, except that there is no increase in the rate of congenital abnormalities. The later onset of glucose intolerance in gestational diabetes means that such abnormalities – a result of glucose intolerance in the first trimester – do not occur.

- Hospital admission may be required if the patient is symptomatic, has ketonuria or a marked hyperglycemia (>15 mmol/L, 270 mg/dL).
- Fetal macrosomia is the major risk, affecting up to 40%. This in turn increases the risk of birth injuries due to the large size of the fetus, but earlier delivery to avoid birth injuries inevitably increases the risks associated with prematurity.
    ◇ Keeping the postprandial glucose below 7.8 mmol/L (140 mg/dL) has been shown to reduce the likelihood of macrosomia and its attendant risks, though it does not completely normalize the risk.
- The occurrence of GDM must be regarded as an indication for preventive measures postpartum against the development of type 2 diabetes in the future.
    ◇ All such women should be encouraged to continue lifestyle measures (diet and exercise) after pregnancy even if glucose levels have returned to normal.
    ◇ Interest in the possible role of TZD treatment in the prevention of type 2 diabetes in this population (see p. 147) is now limited due to safety concerns.

Labor and delivery
- Labor and delivery are potentially hazardous for the mother with diabetes and her baby. The need for cesarean section – used more commonly in diabetes – should be frequently reviewed; the aim should be for natural childbirth as near to term as possible.
- Indications for elective delivery by the abdomen include:
    ◇ Malpresentation.
    ◇ Disproportion between child and birth canal.
    ◇ Intrauterine growth retardation.
    ◇ Fetal distress.
    ◇ Pre-eclampsia.
- Insulin requirements are low during labor and insulin can be given by continuous intravenous insulin infusion (typically 2–4 IU/hour of fast-acting soluble insulin) plus 10% glucose infusion at 125 ml/hour (i.e. 1 l every 8 h) with regular blood glucose (usually capillary sample) monitoring.
- After delivery the insulin requirements fall to prepregnancy levels and the insulin infusion rate should be reduced by half initially.

Neonatal problems

- Neonatal hypoglycemia may occur in infants born to a mother with diabetes.
- The mechanism of neonatal hypoglycemia is as follows:
    ◇ Maternal glucose crosses the placenta, but insulin does not.
    ◇ The fetal islets hypersecrete to combat maternal hyperglycemia.
    ◇ The neonatal glucose falls to hypoglycemic levels when the umbilical cord is severed.
- Other problems in neonates include
    ◇ Respiratory distress syndrome or hyaline membrane disease (a disease of the lung membrane that causes respiratory difficulty; uncommon now).
    ◇ Transient hypertrophic cardiomyopathy (30% affected on ultrasound).
    ◇ Hypocalcemia (50%) and hypomagnesemia (80%).
    ◇ Polycythemia (12%) and jaundice (60%).
- Maternal diabetes, especially when poorly controlled, is associated with fetal macrosomia (defined as large-for-gestational dates) (Figure 16.9) and accelerated fetal growth (Figure 16.10).
- The infant of a mother with diabetes is more susceptible to congenital malformations and also to hyaline membrane disease than infants of similar maturity of mothers without diabetes (Table 16.11 and Figure 16.11).
    ◇ These abnormalities are principally related to hyperglycemia, congenital malformations being

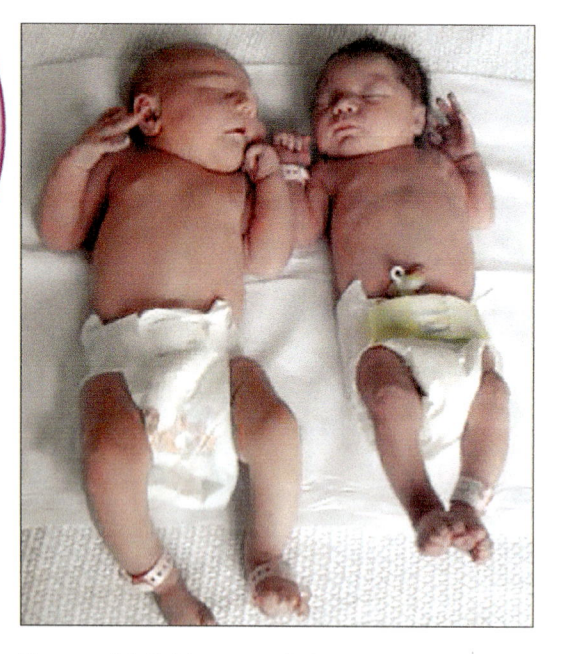

Figure 16.9 Macrosomia. Macrosomia in an infant of a mother with diabetes (left), compared with a normal-sized infant of a mother without diabetes (right). *Photo courtesy Dr Anne Dornhorst.*

Table 16.11 Congenital malformations. Diabetes is associated with an increased risk of major and minor fetal abnormality.

Common major congenital malformations	
Cardiac	Great vessel anomalies Septal defects
Central nervous system	Anencephaly Spina bifida
Skeletal and facial	Caudal regression syndrome Cleft palate or lip Arthrogryposis
Genitourinary tract	Renal agenesis Ureteric duplication

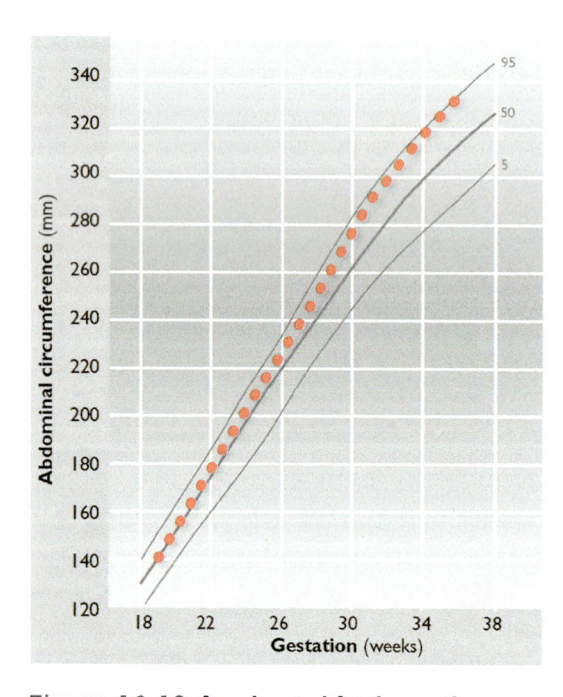

Figure 16.10 Accelerated fetal growth. Abdominal circumference in the fetus of a mother with type 2 diabetes.

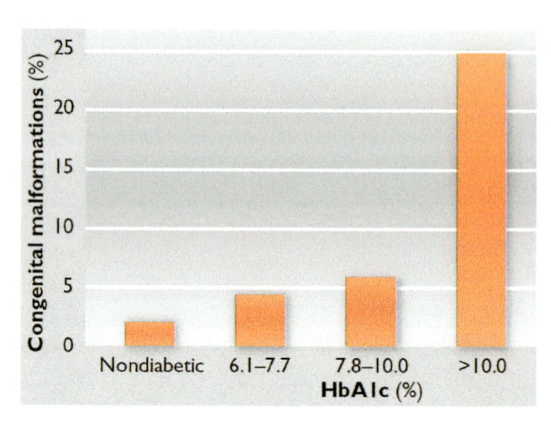

Figure 16.11 Malformation risk. The risk of congenital malformations in newborns of women with type 1 diabetes is about twice as high as in the general population, even when HbA1c is normal. The risk increases sharply with poor blood glucose control. *From Taylor and Davison, 2007.*

largely determined by hyperglycemia in the first trimester – the critical period with regard to organogenesis (Figure 16.12).
◇ As such, when a pregnancy is planned, optimal metabolic control should be sought before conception.

Glucose control in the first trimester is critical.

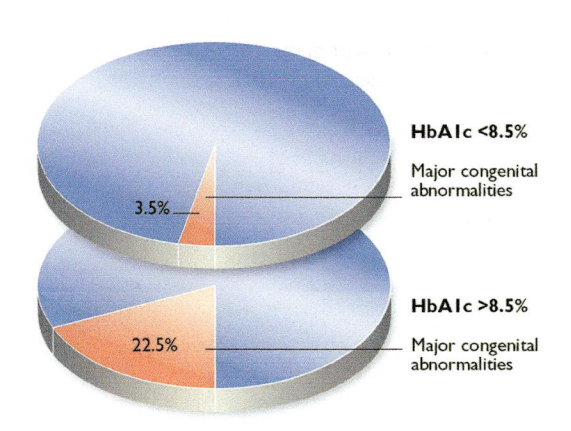

Figure 16.12 First-trimester hyperglycemia. HbA1c above 8.5% in early pregnancy is associated with an almost 7-fold increase in major congenital abnormalities.

HbA1c <8.5% — Major congenital abnormalities 3.5%

HbA1c >8.5% — Major congenital abnormalities 22.5%

Special management considerations

References

Achenbach P, Hawa MI, Krause S, Lampasona V, Jerram ST, Williams AJK, Bonifacio E, Ziegler AG, Leslie RD; Action LADA Consortium. Autoantibodies to N-terminally truncated GAD improve clinical phenotyping of individuals with adult-onset diabetes: Action LADA 12. *Diabetologia*. 2018 Jul;61(7):1644–1649.

Agarwal S, Mathew J, Davis GM, Shephardson A, Levine A, Louard R, Urrutia A, Perez-Guzman C, Umpierrez GE, Peng L, Pasquel FJ. Continuous Glucose Monitoring in the Intensive Care Unit During the COVID-19 Pandemic. *Diabetes Care*. 2021 Mar;44(3):847–849.

Agarwal S et al. Montefiore subcutaneous insulin DKA protocol n.d.

American Diabetes Association. Economic Costs of Diabetes in the U.S. in 2017. *Diabetes Care* 2018;41:917–928.

Aref A, Zayan T, Pararajasingam R, Sharma A, Halawa A. Pancreatic transplantation: Brief review of the current evidence. *World J Transplant*. 2019 Aug 26;9(4):81–93.

Bagdade JD, Nielson KL, Bulger RJ. Reversible abnormalities in phagocytic function in poorly controlled diabetic patients. *Am J Med Sci*. 1972;263(6):451–6.

Battelino T, Danne T, Bergenstal RM, Amiel SA, Beck R, Biester T, Bosi E, Buckingham BA, Cefalu WT, Close KL, Cobelli C, Dassau E, DeVries JH, Donaghue KC, Dovc K, Doyle FJ 3rd, Garg S, Grunberger G, Heller S, Heinemann L, Hirsch IB, Hovorka R, Jia W, Kordonouri O, Kovatchev B, Kowalski A, Laffel L, Levine B, Mayorov A, Mathieu C, Murphy HR, Nimri R, Nørgaard K, Parkin CG, Renard E, Rodbard D, Saboo B, Schatz D, Stoner K, Urakami T, Weinzimer SA, Phillip M. Clinical targets for continuous glucose monitoring data interpretation: Recommendations from the international consensus on time in range. *Diabetes Care*. 2019 Aug;42(8):1593–1603.

Belgam Syed SY, Lipoff JB, Chatterjee K. Acrochordon. [Updated 2021 Aug 11]. In: *StatPearls* [Internet]. Treasure Island (FL): StatPearls Publishing; 2021 Jan. Available from: https://www.ncbi.nlm.nih.gov/books/NBK448169/

Bersoff-Matcha SJ, Chamberlain C, Cao C, Kortepeter C, Chong WH. Fournier gangrene associated with sodium-glucose cotransporter-2 inhibitors: A review of spontaneous postmarketing cases. *Ann Intern Med*. 2019 Jun 4;170(11):764–769.

Bhatt DL, Marso SP, Lincoff AM, Wolski KE, Ellis SG, Topol EJ. Abciximab reduces mortality in diabetics following percutaneous coronary intervention. *J Am Coll Cardiol*. 2000 Mar 15; 35(4): 922–8. doi: 10.1016/s0735-1097(99)00650-6. PMID: 10732889.

Boggi U, Vistoli F, Andres A, Arbogast HP, Badet L, Baronti W, Bartlett STB et al. First World Consensus Conference on pancreas transplantation: Part II - recommendations. *Am J Transplant*. 2021 Sep;21 Suppl 3(Suppl 3):17–59.

Buchanan TA, Xiang AH, Peters RK Preservation of pancreatic beta-cell function and prevention of type 2 diabetes by pharmacological treatment of insulin resistance in high-risk hispanic women. *Diabetes* 2002; 51(9): 2796–803.

Buse JB, Wexler DJ, Tsapas A, Rossing P, Mingrone G, Mathieu C, D'Alessio DA, Davies MJ. 2019 Update to: Management of Hyperglycemia in Type 2 Diabetes, 2018. A Consensus Report by the American Diabetes Association (ADA) and the

European Association for the Study of Diabetes (EASD). *Diabetes Care*. 2020 Feb;**43**(2):487–493.

Carey IM, Critchley JA, DeWilde S, Harris T, Hosking FJ, Cook DG. Risk of infection in Type 1 and Type 2 diabetes compared with the general population: A matched cohort study. *Diabetes Care*. 2018;**41**(3):513–521.

Cathcart S, Cantrell W, Elewski B. Onychomycosis and diabetes. *J Eur Acad Dermatol Venereol*. 2009;**23**(10):1119–22.

Chen J, Li S, Li C. Mechanisms of melanocyte death in vitiligo. *Med Res Rev*. 2021 Mar;**41**(2):1138–1166. doi: 10.1002/med.21754

Cheng NC, Tai HC, Chang SC, Chang CH, Lai HS. Necrotizing fasciitis in patients with diabetes mellitus: clinical characteristics and risk factors for mortality. *BMC Infect Dis*. 2015 Oct 13;**15**:417.

Chernyadyev SA, Ufimtseva MA, Vishnevskaya IF, Bochkarev YM, Ushakov AA, Beresneva TA, Galimzyanov FV, Khodakov VV. Fournier's Gangrene: Literature Review and Clinical Cases. *Urol Int*. 2018;**101**(1):91–97.

Chiasson, J.L., Josse, R.G., Gomis, R., Hanefeld, M., Karasik, A. and Laakso, M. Acarbose for Prevention of Type 2 Diabetes Mellitus: The STOP-NIDDM Randomised Trial. *The Lancet* 2002; **359**, 2072–2077. doi: 10.1016/S0140-6736(02)08905-5

Colhoun HM, Betteridge DJ, Durrington PN, Hitman GA, Neil HA, Livingstone SJ, Thomason MJ, Mackness MI, Charlton-Menys V, Fuller JH CARDS investigators. Primary prevention of cardiovascular disease with atorvastatin in type 2 diabetes in the Collaborative Atorvastatin Diabetes Study (CARDS): multicentre randomised placebo-controlled trial. *Lancet* 2004 Aug 21–27; **364**(9435): 685–96. doi: 10.1016/S0140-6736(04)16895-5. PMID: 15325833

Collison KS, Parhar RS, Saleh SS, Meyer BF, Kwaasi AA, Hammami MM, Schmidt AM, Stern DM, Al-Mohanna FA. RAGE-mediated neutrophil dysfunction is evoked by advanced glycation end products (AGEs). *J Leukoc Biol*. 2002;**71**(3):433–44.

Cost of diabetes report. v2Jan 2014 V2. Diabetes.org.uk. Accessed Dec 2021.

Czupryniak L, Dicker D, Lehmann R, Prázný M, Schernthaner G. The management of type 2 diabetes before, during and after Covid-19 infection: what is the evidence? *Cardiovasc Diabetol*. 2021 Oct 1;**20**(1):198.

Davies MJ, D'Alessio DA, Fradkin J, Kernan WN, Mathieu C, Mingrone G, Rossing P, Tsapas A, Wexler DJ, Buse JB. Management of Hyperglycemia in Type 2 Diabetes, 2018. A Consensus Report by the American Diabetes Association (ADA) and the European Association for the Study of Diabetes (EASD). *Diabetes Care*. 2018 Dec;**41**(12):2669–2701.

de Macedo GM, Nunes S, Barreto T. Skin disorders in diabetes mellitus: an epidemiology and physiopathology review. *Diabetol Metab Syndr*. 2016 Aug 30;**8**(1):63.

Dean PG, Kukla A, Stegall MD, Kudva YC. Pancreas transplantation. *BMJ*. 2017 Apr 3;**357**:j1321.

Defronzo, Ralph. From the Triumvirate to the Ominous Octet: A New Paradigm for the Treatment of Type 2 Diabetes Mellitus. *Diabetes* 2009; **58**:773–95. doi: 10.2337/db09-9028

Delamaire M, Maugendre D, Moreno M, Le Goff MC, Allannic H, Genetet B. Impaired leucocyte functions in diabetic patients. *Diabet Med*. 1997;**14**(1):29–34.

Diepersloot RJ, Bouter KP, Beyer WE, Hoekstra JB, Masurel N. Humoral immune response and delayed type hypersensitivity to influenza vaccine in patients with diabetes mellitus. *Diabetologia*. 1987;**30**(6):397–401.

Dryden M, Baguneid M, Eckmann C, Corman S, Stephens J, Solem C, Li J, Charbonneau C, Baillon-Plot N, Haider S. Pathophysiology and burden of infection in patients with diabetes mellitus and peripheral vascular disease: focus on skin and soft-tissue infections. *Clin Microbiol Infect*. 2015 Sep;**21** Suppl 2:S27–S32.

Duff M, Demidova O, Blackburn S, Shubrook J. Cutaneous manifestations of diabetes mellitus. *Clin Diabetes*. 2015 Jan;**33**(1):40–8.

Eikawa S, Nishida M, Mizukami S, Yamazaki C, Nakayama E, Udono H. Immune-mediated antitumor effect by type 2 diabetes drug, metformin. *Proc Natl Acad Sci USA*. 2015;**112**(6):1809–14.

Erener S. Diabetes, infection risk and COVID-19. *Mol Metab*. 2020 Sep;**39**:101044.

Esmeijer K, Hoogeveen EK, van den Boog PJM, Konijn C, Mallat MJK, Baranski AG, Dekkers OM, de Fijter JW; Dutch Transplant Centers; Dutch Kidney Transplant Centres. Superior Long-term Survival for Simultaneous Pancreas-Kidney Transplantation as Renal Replacement Therapy: 30-Year Follow-up of a Nationwide Cohort. *Diabetes Care*. 2020 Feb;**43**(2):321–328.

Esper AM, Moss M, Martin GS. The effect of diabetes mellitus on organ dysfunction with sepsis: an epidemiological study. *Crit Care*. 2009;**13**:R18.

Evers IM, de Valk HW, Visser GH. Risk of complications of pregnancy in women with type 1 diabetes: nationwide prospective study in the Netherlands. *BMJ*. 2004 Apr 17; **328**(7445): 915. doi: 10.1136/bmj.38043.583160.EE. Epub 2004 Apr 5. PMID: 15066886; PMCID: PMC390158

Falcone M, Meier JJ, Marini MG, Caccialanza R, Aguado JM, Del Prato S, Menichetti F. Diabetes and acute bacterial skin and skin structure infections. *Diabetes Res Clin Pract*. 2021 Apr;**174**:108732.

Faulds ER, Boutsicaris A, Sumner L, Jones L, McNett M, Smetana KS, May CC, Buschur E, Exline MC, Ringel MD, Dungan K. Use of continuous glucose monitor in critically Ill COVID-19 patients requiring insulin infusion: An observational study. *J Clin Endocrinol Metab*. 2021 Sep 27;**106**(10):e4007–e4016.

Feig DS, Donovan LE, Corcoy R, Murphy KE, Amiel SA, Hunt KF, Asztalos E, Barrett JFR, Sanchez JJ, de Leiva A, Hod M, Jovanovic L, Keely E, McManus R, Hutton EK, Meek CL, Stewart ZA, Wysocki T, O'Brien R, Ruedy K, Kollman C, Tomlinson G, Murphy HR; CONCEPTT Collaborative Group. Continuous glucose monitoring in pregnant women with type 1 diabetes (CONCEPTT): a multicentre international randomised controlled trial. *Lancet*. 2017 Nov 25;**390**(10110):2347–2359.

Feldman, EL. et al. A practical two-step quantitative clinical and electrophysiological assessment for the diagnosis and staging of diabetic neuropathy. *Diabetes Care* Nov 1994 **17** 11.

Forbes J.M., Cooper M.E. Mechanisms of diabetic complications. *Physiological Reviews*. 2013;**93**(1):137–188.

Furnary AP, Gao G, Grunkemeier GL, Wu Y, Zerr KJ, Bookin SO, Floten HS, Starr A. Continuous insulin infusion reduces mortality in patients with diabetes undergoing coronary artery bypass grafting. *J Thorac Cardiovasc Surg*. 2003 May; **125**(5): 1007–21. doi: 10.1067/mtc.2003.181. PMID: 12771873

Furnary AP, Zerr KJ, Grunkemeier GL, Starr A. Continuous intravenous insulin infusion reduces the incidence of deep sternal wound infection in diabetic patients after cardiac surgical procedures. *Ann Thorac Surg*. 1999;**67**:352–360.

Geerlings S, Fonseca V, Castro-Diaz D, List J, Parikh S. Genital and urinary tract infections in diabetes: impact of pharmacologically-induced glucosuria. *Diabetes Res Clin Pract*. 2014 Mar;**103**(3):373–81.

George SM, Walton S. Diabetic dermopathy. *Br J Diabetes Vasc Dis*. 2014;**14**:95–7.

Ghosh SK, Bandyopadhyay D, Chatterjee G. Bullosis diabeticorum: A distinctive blistering eruption in diabetes mellitus. *Int J Diabetes Dev Ctries*. 2009 Jan;**29**(1):41–2.

Gianani R, Eisenbarth GS. The stages of type 1A diabetes: 2005. *Immunol Rev*. 2005 Apr;**204**:232–49.

Gill JM, Malkova D. Physical activity, fitness and cardiovascular disease risk in adults: interactions with insulin resistance and obesity. *Clin Sci (Lond)*. 2006 Apr; **110**(4): 409–25. doi: 10.1042/CS20050207. PMID: 16526946

Goldstein BJ, Feinglos MN, Lunceford JK, Johnson J, Williams-Herman DE. Sitagliptin 036 Study Group. Effect of initial combination therapy with sitagliptin, a dipeptidyl peptidase-4 inhibitor, and metformin on glycemic control in patients with type 2 diabetes. *Diabetes Care*, 2007; **30**:1979–87.

Goodpaster BH, Katsiaras A, Kelley DE. Enhanced fat oxidation through physical activity is associated with improvements in insulin sensitivity in obesity. *Diabetes*. 2003 Sep; **52**(9):2191–7. doi: 10.2337/diabetes.52.9.2191. PMID: 12941756

Gregg EW, Sophiea MK, Weldegiorgis M. Diabetes and COVID-19: Population Impact 18 Months Into the Pandemic. *Diabetes Care*. 2021 Sep;**44**(9):1916–1923.

Gruessner RW, Gruessner AC. The current state of pancreas transplantation. *Nat Rev Endocrinol*. 2013 Sep;**9**(9):555–62.

Gürlek A, Firat C, Oztürk AE, Alaybeyoğlu N, Fariz A, Aslan S. Management of necrotizing fasciitis in diabetic patients. *J Diabetes Complications*. 2007 Jul-Aug;**21**(4):265–71.

Hammerstad SS, Grock SF, Lee HJ, Hasham A, Sundaram N, Tomer Y. Diabetes and Hepatitis C: A Two-Way Association. *Front Endocrinol (Lausanne)*. 2015 Sep 14;**6**:134.

He C, Yang Z, Lu NH. Helicobacter pylori infection and diabetes: is it a myth or fact? *World J Gastroenterol*. 2014 Apr 28;**20**(16):4607–17.

Holman RR, Turner RC. The basal plasma glucose: a simple relevant index of maturity-onset diabetes. *Clin Endocrinol (Oxf)*. 1981 Mar; **14**(3):279–86. doi: 10.1111/j.1365-2265.1981.tb00196.x. PMID: 7021010

Hong YS, Chang Y, Ryu S, Cainzos-Achirica M, Kwon MJ, Zhang Y, Choi Y, Ahn J, Rampal S, Zhao D, Pastor-Barriuso R, Lazo M, Shin H, Cho J, Guallar E. Hepatitis B and C virus infection and diabetes mellitus: A cohort study. *Sci Rep*. 2017 Jul 4;**7**(1):4606.

Horton WB, Taylor JS, Ragland TJ, Subauste AR. Diabetic muscle infarction: a systematic review. *BMJ Open Diabetes Res Care*. 2015 Apr 24;**3**(1):e000082.

Hruska LA, Smith JM, Hendy MP, Fritz VL, McAdams S. Continuous insulin infusion reduces infectious complications in diabetics following coronary surgery. *J Card Surg*. 2005;**20**(5):403–7.

Hulme KD, Gallo LA, Short KR. Influenza Virus and Glycemic Variability in Diabetes: A Killer Combination? *Front Microbiol*. 2017 May 22;**8**:861.

International Diabetes Federation Clinical Guidelines Task Force. Global guideline for type 2 diabetes. IDF-Guideline-for-Type-2-Diabetes.pdf accessed December 2021.

Jafar N, Edriss H, Nugent K. The Effect of Short-Term Hyperglycemia on the Innate Immune System. *Am J Med Sci*. 2016;**351**(2):201–11.

Jovanovic L, Peterson CM. Optimal insulin delivery for the pregnant diabetic patient. *Diabetes Care*. 1982 May–Jun; **5**(**Suppl 1**):24–37. PMID: 6765120.

Kahn, S., Hull, R. & Utzschneider, K. Mechanisms linking obesity to insulin resistance and type 2 diabetes. *Nature* 2006; 444, 840–846. doi: 10.1038/nature05482

Kaya İ, Sezgin B, Eraslan S, Öztürk K, Göde S, Bilgen C, Kirazlı T. Malignant otitis externa: A retrospective analysis and treatment outcomes. *Turk Arch Otorhinolaryngol*. 2018 Jun; 56(2):106–110.

Kayar Y, Pamukçu Ö, Eroğlu H, Kalkan Erol K, Ilhan A, Kocaman O. Relationship between Helicobacter pylori Infections in Diabetic Patients and Inflammations, Metabolic Syndrome, and Complications. *Int J Chronic Dis*. 2015;**2015**:290128.

Kesseli SJ, Smith KA, Gardner TB. Total pancreatectomy with islet autologous transplantation: the cure for chronic pancreatitis? *Clin Transl Gastroenterol*. 2015 Jan 29;6(1):e73.

Khanna M, Challa S, Kabeil AS, Inyang B, Gondal FJ, Abah GA, Minnal Dhandapani M, Manne M, Mohammed L. Risk of Mucormycosis in Diabetes Mellitus: A Systematic Review. *Cureus*. 2021 Oct 16;**13**(10):e18827.

Khunti K, Knighton P, Zaccardi F, Bakhai C, Barron E, Holman N, Kar P, Meace C, Sattar N, Sharp S, Wareham NJ, Weaver A, Woch E, Young B, Valabhji J. Prescription of glucose-lowering therapies and risk of COVID-19 mortality in people with type 2 diabetes: a nationwide observational study in England. *Lancet Diabetes Endocrinol*. 2021 May;9(5):293–303.

Kim JH, Park K, Lee SB, Kang S, Park JS, Ahn CW, Nam JS. Relationship between natural killer cell activity and glucose control in patients with type 2 diabetes and prediabetes. *J Diabetes Investig*. 2019;**10**(5):1223–1228.

Knapp S Diabetes and infection: is there a link?—A mini-review. *Gerontology*. 2013;**59**(2):99–104.

Knowler WC, Barrett-Connor E, Fowler SE, Hamman RF, Lachin JM, Walker EA, Nathan DM Diabetes prevention program research group. Reduction in the incidence of type 2 diabetes with lifestyle intervention or metformin. *N Engl J Med*. 2002 Feb 7; 346(6): 393–403. doi: 10.1056/NEJMoa012512. PMID: 11832527; PMCID: PMC1370926

Korbel L, Spencer JD. Diabetes mellitus and infection: an evaluation of hospital utilization and management costs in the United States. *J Diabetes Complications*. 2015;29(2):192–5.

Kornum JB, Thomsen RW, Riis A, Lervang HH, Schønheyder HC, Sørensen HT. Type 2 diabetes and pneumonia outcomes: a population-based cohort study. *Diabetes Care*. 2007 Sep;30(9):2251–7.

Krinsley JS. Association between hyperglycemia and increased hospital mortality in a heterogeneous population of critically ill patients. *Mayo Clin Proc*. 2003 Dec; **78**(12): 1471–8. doi: 10.4065/78.12.1471. PMID: 14661676

Kristensen K, Ögge LE, Sengpiel V, Kjölhede K, Dotevall A, Elfvin A, Knop FK, Wiberg N, Katsarou A, Shaat N, Kristensen L, Berntorp K. Continuous glucose monitoring in pregnant women with type 1 diabetes: an observational cohort study of 186 pregnancies. *Diabetologia*. 2019 Jul;62(7):1143–1153.

Landstra CP, de Koning EJP. COVID-19 and Diabetes: Understanding the Interrelationship and Risks for a Severe Course. *Front Endocrinol (Lausanne)*. 2021 Jun 17;**12**:649525.

Lean MEJ, Leslie WS, Barnes AC, Brosnahan N, Thom G, McCombie L, Peters C, Zhyzhneuskaya S, Al-Mrabeh A, Hollingsworth KG, Rodrigues AM, Rehackova L, Adamson AJ, Sniehotta FF, Mathers JC, Ross HM, McIlvenna Y, Welsh P, Kean S, Ford I, McConnachie A, Messow CM, Sattar N, Taylor R. Durability of a primary care-led weight-management intervention for remission of type 2 diabetes: 2-year results of the DiRECT open-label, cluster-randomised trial. *Lancet Diabetes Endocrinol.* 2019 May;7(5):344–355.

Lepe K, Riley CA, Salazar FJ. Necrobiosis Lipoidica. [Updated 2021 Aug 26]. In: *StatPearls* [Internet]. Treasure Island (FL): StatPearls Publishing; 2021 Jan. Available from: https://www.ncbi.nlm.nih.gov/books/NBK459318/

Leslie, RD. Predicting Adult-Onset Autoimmune Diabetes: Clarity from Complexity. *Diabetes*, 2010 **59**(2), 330–331. doi: 10.2337/db09-1620

Leslie, RD, et al. Adult-Onset Type 1 Diabetes: Current Understanding and Challenges. *Diabetes Care.* 2021 Nov;**44**(11):2449–2456. doi: 10.2337/dc21-0770

Llewelyn D, Llewelyn JG. Diabetic amyotrophy: a painful radiculoplexus neuropathy. *Pract Neurol.* 2019 Apr;**19**(2):164–167.

Mader R, Verlaan JJ, Eshed I, Bruges-Armas J, Puttini PS, Atzeni F, Buskila D, Reinshtein E, Novofastovski I, Fawaz A, Kurt V, Baraliakos X. Diffuse idiopathic skeletal hyperostosis (DISH): where we are now and where to go next. *RMD Open.* 2017 Jun 21;**3**(1):e000472.

Martín C, Requena L, Manrique K, Manzarbeitia FD, Rovira A. Scleredema diabeticorum in a patient with type 2 diabetes mellitus. *Case Rep Endocrinol.* 2011;**2011**:560273.

Martins M, Boavida JM, Raposo JF, Froes F, Nunes B, Ribeiro RT, Macedo MP, Penha-Gonçalves C. Diabetes hinders community-acquired pneumonia outcomes in hospitalized patients. *BMJ Open Diabetes Res Care.* 2016;**4**(1):e000181.

Meirelles Júnior RF, Salvalaggio P, Pacheco-Silva A. Pancreas transplantation: review. *Einstein* (Sao Paulo). 2015 Apr-Jun;**13**(2):305–9.

Merashli M, Chowdhury TA, Jawad AS. Musculoskeletal manifestations of diabetes mellitus. *QJM.* 2015 Nov;**108**(11):853–7.

Metlay JP, Waterer GW, Long AC, Anzueto A, Brozek J, Crothers K, Cooley LA, Dean NC, Fine MJ, Flanders SA, Griffin MR, Metersky ML, Musher DM, Restrepo MI, Whitney CG. Diagnosis and treatment of adults with community-acquired pneumonia: An official clinical practice guideline of the american thoracic society and infectious diseases society of America. *Am J Respir Crit Care Med.* 2019;**200**(7):e45–e67.

Mnif MF, Kamoun M, Kacem FH, Bouaziz Z, Charfi N, Mnif F, Naceur BB, Rekik N, Abid M. Complicated urinary tract infections associated with diabetes mellitus: Pathogenesis, diagnosis and management. *Indian J Endocrinol Metab.* 2013 May;**17**(3):442–5.

Mokta JK, Mokta KK, Panda P. Insulin lipodystrophy and lipohypertrophy. *Indian J Endocrinol Metab.* 2013 Jul;**17**(4):773–4.

Mooradian AD, Reed RL, Meredith KE, Scuderi P. Serum levels of tumor necrosis factor and IL-1 alpha and IL-1 beta in diabetic patients. *Diabetes Care.* 1991;**14**(1):63–5. doi: 10.2337/diacare.14.1.63. PMID: 1991438

Moutschen MP, Scheen AJ, Lefebvre PJ. Impaired immune responses in diabetes mellitus: analysis of the factors and mechanisms involved. Relevance to the increased susceptibility of diabetic patients to specific infections. *Diabete Metab.* 1992 May-Jun;**18**(3):187–201.

Mowat A, Baum J. Chemotaxis of polymorphonuclear leukocytes from patients with diabetes mellitus. *N Engl J Med.* 1971;**284**(12):621–7.

Nitzan O, Elias M, Chazan B, Saliba W. Urinary tract infections in patients with type 2 diabetes mellitus: review of prevalence, diagnosis, and management. *Diabetes Metab Syndr Obes.* 2015 Feb 26;**8**:129–36.

Nyirjesy P, Sobel JD. Genital mycotic infections in patients with diabetes. *Postgrad Med*. 2013 May;**125**(3):33–46.

Ogawa A, Shikata K, Uchida HA, Shinoura S, Yokomichi N, Ogawa D, Sato-Horiguchi C, Yagi T, Wada J, Makino H. Case of emphysematous cholecystitis in a patient with type 2 diabetes mellitus associated with schizophrenia. *J Diabetes Investig*. 2012 Dec 20;**3**(6):534–5.

Ohno Y, Aoki N, Nishimura A. In vitro production of interleukin-1, interleukin-6, and tumor necrosis factor-alpha in insulin-dependent diabetes mellitus. *J Clin Endocrinol Metab*. 1993;**77**(4):1072–7.

Oomichi, T, Emoto, M, Tabata, T, Morioka, T, Tsujimoto, Y, Tahara, H, Shoji, T, Nishizawa, Y. Impact of glycemic control on survival of diabetic patients on chronic regular hemodialysis a 7-year observational study. *Diabetes care*. 2006. **29**:1496–500. doi: 10.2337/dc05-1887

Paschou SA, Dede AD, Anagnostis PG, Vryonidou A, Morganstein D, Goulis DG. Type 2 Diabetes and Osteoporosis: A Guide to Optimal Management. *J Clin Endocrinol Metab*. 2017 Oct 1;**102**(10):3621–3634.

Piette EW, Rosenbach M. Granuloma Annulare. *JAMA Dermatol*. 2015;**151**(6):692.

Priyambada L, Wolfsdorf JI, Brink SJ, Fritsch M, Codner E, Donaghue KC, Craig ME. ISPAD Clinical Practice Consensus Guideline: Diabetic ketoacidosis in the time of COVID-19 and resource-limited settings-role of subcutaneous insulin. *Pediatr Diabetes*. 2020 Dec;**21**(8):1394–1402. doi: 10.1111/pedi.13118. Epub 2020 Oct 12. PMID: 32935435

Rajamani, K. et al, Effect of fenofibrate on amputation events in people with type 2 diabetes mellitus (FIELD study): a prespecified analysis of a randomised controlled trial. *Lancet* 2009 May 23; **373**(9677). doi: 10.1016/S0140-6736(09)60698-X

Reaven GM, Reaven EP. Age, glucose intolerance, and non-insulin-dependent diabetes mellitus. *J Am Geriatr Soc*. 1985 Apr; **33**(4):286–90. doi: 10.1111/j.1532-5415.1985.tb07118.x. PMID: 3886767

Reid G, Lynch JP 3rd, Fishbein MC, Clark NM. Mucormycosis. *Semin Respir Crit Care Med*. 2020 Feb;**41**(1):99–114.

Rendon A, Schäkel K. Psoriasis Pathogenesis and Treatment. *Int J Mol Sci*. 2019 Mar 23;**20**(6):1475.

Repine JE, Clawson CC, Goetz FC. Bactericidal function of neutrophils from patients with acute bacterial infections and from diabetics. *J Infect Dis*. 1980;**142**(6):869–75.

Restrepo BI. Diabetes and tuberculosis. *Microbiol Spectr*. 2016 Dec;**4**(6):doi: 10.1128/microbiolspec.TNMI7-0023-2016

Riddle MC, Rosenstock J, Gerich J. Insulin Glargine 4002 Study Investigators. The treat-to-target trial: randomized addition of glargine or human NPH insulin to oral therapy of type 2 diabetic patients. *Diabetes Care*. 2003 Nov; **26**(11): 3080–6. doi: 10.2337/diacare.26.11.3080. PMID: 14578243

Rosen J, Yosipovitch G. Skin manifestations of diabetes mellitus. [Updated 2018 Jan 4]. In: Feingold KR, Anawalt B, Boyce A, et al., editors. *Endotext* [Internet]. South Dartmouth (MA): MDText.com, Inc.; 2000. Available from https://www.ncbi.nlm.nih.gov/books/NBK481900/

Rosenbloom AL, Silverstein JH, Lezotte DC, Richardson K, McCallum M. Limited joint mobility in childhood diabetes mellitus indicates increased risk for microvascular disease. *N Engl J Med*. 1981 Jul 23;**305**(4):191–4.

Saibal MA, Rahman SH, Nishat L, Sikder NH, Begum SA, Islam MJ, Uddin KN. Community acquired pneumonia in diabetic and non-diabetic hospitalized patients: presentation, causative pathogens and outcome. *Bangladesh Med Res Counc Bull*. 2012 Dec;**38**(3):98–103.

Schauer PR, Bhatt DL, Kirwan JP, Wolski K, Aminian A, Brethauer SA, Navaneethan SD, Singh RP, Pothier CE, Nissen SE, Kashyap SR; STAMPEDE Investigators. Bariatric Surgery versus Intensive Medical Therapy for Diabetes—5-Year Outcomes. *N Engl J Med*. 2017 Feb 16;**376**(7):641–651.

Shah BR, Hux JE. Quantifying the risk of infectious diseases for people with diabetes. *Diabetes Care*. 2003;**26**(2):510–3.

Shapiro AM, Pokrywczynska M, Ricordi C. Clinical pancreatic islet transplantation. *Nat Rev Endocrinol*. 2017 May;**13**(5):268–277.

Smith LL, Burnet SP, McNeil JD Musculoskeletal manifestations of diabetes mellitus, *British Journal of Sports Medicine*. 2003;**37**:30–35.

Sözen T, Başaran NÇ, Tınazlı M, Özışık L. Musculoskeletal problems in diabetes mellitus. *Eur J Rheumatol*. 2018 Dec;**5**(4):258–265.

Starup-Linde J, Vestergaard P. Management of endocrine disease: Diabetes and osteoporosis: cause for concern? *Eur J Endocrinol*. 2015 Sep;**173**(3):R93–9.

Swerdlow AJ, Laing SP, Qiao Z, Slater SD, Burden AC, Botha JL, Waugh NR, Morris AD, Gatling W, Gale EA, Patterson CC, Keen H. Cancer incidence and mortality in patients with insulin-treated diabetes: a UK cohort study. *Br J Cancer*. 2005 Jun 6;**92**(11):2070–5. doi: 10.1038/sj.bjc.6602611

Taylor R, Davison JM. Type 1 diabetes and pregnancy. *BMJ*. 2007; **334**(7596): 742–745. doi:10.1136/bmj.39154.700417.BE

Todd JA. Etiology of type 1 diabetes. *Immunity*. 2010 Apr 23;**32**(4):457–67.

Umpierrez GE, Isaacs SD, Bazargan N, You X, Thaler LM, Kitabchi AE. Hyperglycemia: An independent marker of in-hospital mortality in patients with undiagnosed diabetes. *The Journal of Clinical Endocrinology & Metabolism*. March 1 2002; **87**(3):978–982. doi:10.1210/jcem.87.3.8341

Van den Berghe, G. et al, Intensive insulin therapy in critically ill patients. *N Engl J Med* 2001; **345**: 1359–1367. doi: 10.1056/NEJMoa011300

Walthall J, Anand P, Rehman UH. Dupuytren Contracture. [Updated 2021 Sep 14]. In: *StatPearls* [Internet]. Treasure Island (FL): StatPearls Publishing; 2021 Jan. Available from: https://www.ncbi.nlm.nih.gov/books/NBK526074/

Weng J. et al. Effect of intensive insulin therapy on beta-cell function and glycaemic control in patients with newly diagnosed type 2 diabetes: a multicentre randomised parallel-group trial. *Lancet*, 2008 May 24; **371**(9626): 1753–60. doi: 10.1016/S0140-6736(08)60762-X. PMID: 18502299

Wysocki, T. et al, Absence of adverse effects of severe hypoglycemia of cognitive function in school-aged children with diabetes over 18 months. *Diabetes Care*, Apr 2003; 26, 4.

Zacay G, Hershkowitz Sikron F, Heymann AD. Glycemic Control and Risk of Cellulitis. *Diabetes Care*. 2021 Feb;**44**(2):367–372.

Zerr KJ, Furnary AP, Grunkemeier GL, Bookin S, Kanhere V, Starr A. Glucose control lowers the risk of wound infection in diabetics after open heart operations. *Ann Thorac Surg*. 1997;**63**(2):356–61.

Resources: Research and support organizations

American Diabetes Association
Center for Information
2451 Crystal Drive, Suite 900 Arlington, VA 22202
USA
Website: www.diabetes.org

European Association for the Study of Diabetes (EASD)
Rheindorfer Weg 3
40591 Düsseldorf
Germany
Website: www.easd.org
Email: secretariat@easd.org

European Foundation for the Study of Diabetes (EFSD)
Rheindorfer Weg 3
40591 Düsseldorf
Germany
Website: www.europeandiabetesfoundation.org
Email: foundation@easd.org

Foundation of European Nurses in Diabetes (FEND)
37 Earls Drive
Newcastle on Tyne
NE15 7AL
UK
Website: www.fend.org

International Diabetes Federation (IDF)
Avenue Hermann-Debroux 54
B-1160 Brussels
Belgium
Website: www.idf.org
Email: info@idf.org

International Society for Paediatric and Adolescent Diabetes (ISPAD)
c/o KIT, Kurfürstendamm 71
10709 Berlin
Germany
Website: www.ispad.org
Email: secretariat@ispad.org

JDRF (formerly Juvenile Diabetes Research Foundation) International office
200 Vesey Street, 285h Floor
New York
NY 10281
USA
Website: www.jdrf.org
E-mail: info@jdrf.org

JDRF London
17/18 Angel Gate
City Road
London
EC1V 2PT
UK
Website: www.jdrf.org.uk
Email: info@jdrf.org.uk

National Institute for Health and Clinical Excellence (NICE)
2nd Floor, 2 Redman Place
London
E20 1JQ
UK
Website: www.nice.org.uk
Email: nice@nice.org.uk

World Diabetes Foundation (WDF)
Krogshojvej 30A
Building 8Y
DK-2880 Bagsvaerd
Denmark
Website: www.worlddiabetesfoundation.org

World Health Organization (WHO)
Avenue Appia 2
1211 Geneva 27
Switzerland
Website: www.who.int
Email: info@who.int

Glossary

A

Accelerator hypothesis This proposes that the onset of type 1 diabetes occurs earlier in those with insulin resistance or heavier weight (i.e. with predisposition to type 2 diabetes).

Adenosine triphosphate (ATP) A coenzyme used in the intracellular metabolism of energy.

Adiponectin A cytokine derived from adipocytes that is associated with improved glycemic control and lipid profiles in patients with diabetes.

Advanced glycation end-product (AGE) Formed when excess glucose combines nonenzymatically with tissue or circulating proteins. AGEs are increased in diabetes, and contribute to microvascular complications.

Aldose reductase Some of the glucose that enters the cell is metabolized by this enzyme into sorbitol, which in turn is implicated as a factor for some microvascular complications.

Allele One of a pair of genes found in a specific location on a chromosome.

Alpha-glucosidase inhibitors A class of diabetes drugs that decrease intestinal absorption of glucose by inhibiting the breakdown of carbohydrates into monosaccharides in the small bowel.

Amylin An amino acid stored in the beta cells of the pancreas and co-secreted with insulin, that can decrease postprandial glucagon, increase satiety and slow down gastric emptying.

Angiotensin-converting enzyme inhibitors (ACEIs) A class of drugs that inhibit the conversion of angiotensin I into angiotensin II – a vasoconstrictor. ACEIs also inhibit kininases – enzymes that inactivate kinins (plasma proteins important in vasodilation).

Angiotensin receptor blockers (ARBs) A class of drugs that block the action of angiotensin II on the type 1 angiotensin II receptor, resulting in vasodilation and decreased blood pressure.

Atherosclerosis Thickening of the arterial wall as a result of fat deposition. Patients with diabetes have accelerated atherosclerotic vascular disease.

Autoantibody An antibody that reacts to the patient's own cells or tissues. Islet cell autoantibodies are strongly associated with the development of type 1 diabetes.

Autoantigen An antigen that is present in the endogenous tissue, and stimulates the production of antibodies (autoantibodies).

Autonomic neuropathy Damage of the nerves that are not in the patient's conscious control (such as nerves of the cardiovascular, gastrointestinal, and genitourinary systems).

B

Bariatric surgery Surgery to promote weight loss by altering the gastrointestinal anatomy.

Basal-bolus insulin secretion The physiological pattern of insulin secretion whereby a relatively constant amount of insulin is secreted in the fasting state, and a rise in insulin secretion is seen in response to meals.

Beta cell A type of cell located in the pancreatic islet of Langerhans that produces insulin and amylin. Type 1 diabetes is caused by the autoimmune destruction or dysfunction of most of the β cells, while in type 2 diabetes they fail gradually over time.

Body mass index (BMI)   A measurement to estimate body fat, calculated by dividing a person's weight in kilograms by their height in square meters (kg/m^2). A BMI of less than 18 is considered underweight, 18 to 24.9 is normal, 25 to 29.9 is overweight, and 30 and above is obese.

Brittle diabetes   Diabetes with labile blood glucoses and episodes of hypoglycemia and/or ketoacidosis.

C

Calcium channel   A voltage-gated ion channel on the cell membrane, the opening of which allows calcium to enter the cell, with resultant release of insulin.

Charcot's arthropathy   Deformity of the foot resulting from sensory neuropathy, the most common cause of which is diabetes.

C-peptide   In humans, proinsulin is cleaved into C-peptide and insulin. C-peptide can be used as an indicator of beta-cell function or insulin secretion.

Creatinine   A metabolic by-product of creatine, an amino acid found in muscle. The creatinine blood level is used to measure kidney function.

D

Dawn phenomenon   An increase in blood glucoses in the early morning, thought to be a result of a rise in counterregulatory hormones (cortisol, catecholamines, and growth hormone).

Diabetes insipidus   A disorder of the posterior pituitary gland that leads to decreased levels of antidiuretic hormone, resulting in polyuria and polydipsia.

Diabetic ketoacidosis (DKA)   Severe metabolic disturbance seen in diabetes, consisting of a triad of hyperglycemia, ketonemia, and anion gap acidosis.

Dipeptidyl peptidase-4 (DPP-4) inhibitors   A class of diabetes drugs that inhibit dipeptidyl peptidase-4, the enzyme that degrades glucagon-like peptide-1 (GLP-1). This results in lowering of glucose levels, especially during the mealtime excursions.

Double diabetes   Diabetes with features of both type 1 and type 2 diabetes.

Dyslipidemia   Derangement in lipid (cholesterol and triglyceride) levels and composition. Dyslipidemia contributes to atherosclerosis.

E

Enteroinsular axis   The physiologic pathway involving the intestinal hormones (incretins) and pancreatic hormones (insulin, glucagon) that leads to glucose homeostasis.

Epithelium   A layer of cells that line the cavities and surfaces of structures throughout the body.

F

Fasting plasma glucose (FPG)   A measurement of plasma glucose in the morning (typically around 8 am) after fasting for at least 8 hours overnight.

Free fatty acids (FFA)   Also known as non-esterified fatty acids (NEFA), these are long-chain (typically 14–18 carbon atoms) carboxylic acids, which are one of the main forms of lipid in the circulation, used by the body as fuel. NEFA molecules may be of different chain lengths and be saturated or unsaturated. Elevated plasma levels of FFA are a major cause of insulin resistance in the liver and skeletal muscle.

G

Gestational diabetes mellitus (GDM)   Elevation of plasma glucose to diabetic levels, occurring during the course of a pregnancy and typically remitting after the pregnancy.

Glomerular filtration rate (GFR)   The volume of blood flow per minute through the renal glomeruli.

Glucagon   A hormone produced by the alpha cells of the islets of Langerhans; it has generally anti-insulin effects and forms part of the feedback loop that stabilizes glucose levels.

Glucagon-like peptide-1 (GLP-1)   A hormone released from the L cells of the distal end of the small bowel and the proximal end of the large bowel, usually in response to eating.

Glucokinase   An enzyme that facilitates phosphorylation of glucose to glucose-6-phosphate.

Gluconeogenesis   The synthesis of glucose from non-carbohydrate substrates, such as amino acids and fatty acids.

Glucose   A simple carbohydrate (monosaccharide), $C_6H_{12}O_6$, used by cells as the primary source of energy.

Glucose intolerance   Abnormally high levels of plasma glucose, defined after oral ingestion of (75 g) glucose; typically refers to levels above normal but less than would define diabetes.

Glucose transporter (GLUT)   One of a group of membrane proteins that facilitate the transport of glucose across tissue membranes.

Glucotoxicity/glycotoxicity   Adverse effects ascribed to persistent elevation of plasma glucose.

Glycemic index (GI)   An estimation of the extent to which a specific foodstuff will elevate plasma glucose; sometimes taken to refer specifically to the carbohydrate content of the foodstuff.

Glycogen   A polysaccharide; the principal storage form of glucose in humans, found mainly in the liver and muscles.

Glycogenesis   The process of glycogen synthesis from glucose.

Glycogenolysis   The process of breakdown of glycogen to glucose.

Glycolysis   The intracellular metabolic pathway that converts glucose into high-energy compounds, principally ATP.

Glycosuria   The presence of glucose in the urine. This is usually indicative of impaired glucose tolerance or diabetes.

H

Hemoglobin A1c (HbA1c/glycated hemoglobin)   A form of hemoglobin to which glucose is bound; now universally accepted as a useful clinical measure of long-term glycemic control in diabetes.

High-density lipoproteins (HDL)   Circulating lipoproteins of density >1.063 g/ml, that collect cholesterol from the tissues and return it to the liver, where it is metabolized and excreted, and to the adrenal glands and gonads for synthesis of steroid hormones. HDL are sometimes referred to as the 'good cholesterol' lipoproteins.

Histocompatibility leukocyte antigen (HLA)   The major histocompatibility complex (MHC) in human chromosomes, it comprises a number of genes related to immune function, such as rejection of foreign tissue and expression of autoimmune disease.

Hyperglycemia   Excessive levels of glucose in the blood plasma.

Hyperinsulinemia   Excessive levels of insulin in the blood relative to the level of glucose.

Hyperosmolality   Increased concentration of solutes in a body fluid, e.g. blood, expressed as osmoles of solute per kilogram of serum.

Hyperosmolar nonketotic hyperglycemia (HONK)   Also known as hyperosmolar hyperglycemic state (HHS), this condition is seen more often in type 2 than in type 1 diabetes. It is associated with extremely high plasma glucose, raised urea, electrolyte disturbance, and severe dehydration.

Hypoglycemia   An abnormally low level of plasma glucose and a common complication of insulin treatment. Hypoglycemia results from an imbalance between injected insulin or oral therapy and a patient's diet, activity, and metabolic requirements.

I

Impaired glucose tolerance (IGT)   An abnormal glycemic state, defined as a plasma glucose level of 140 to 199 mg/dL (7–8 to 11.1 mmol/1) 2 hours after the oral ingestion of 75 g of glucose; frequently a precursor to the development of type 2 diabetes.

Incidence   A measurement of the number of new individuals who contract a disease during a particular period of time. Usually expressed as the number of cases per year per population. *See also* prevalence.

Incretin effect   The greater increase in plasma insulin occurring after oral ingestion of glucose compared to the rise seen after the same amount given intravenously. It is caused by the release of gut hormones known as incretins, and accounts for probably 50–70% of the insulin rise.

Insulin   A hormone produced by the β cells of the islets of Langerhans that is the principal hormone regulating glucose, but is also important in regulating fat and carbohydrate metabolism.

Insulin analog   An altered, synthetic form of insulin, in which certain amino acids are modified to affect the time course of the insulin action.

Insulin deficiency   Inability to produce sufficient insulin; the state of having insufficient insulin relative to the prevailing glucose level.

Insulin-like growth factor (IGF)   A protein with a structure similar to insulin, which may interact with insulin receptors and share some actions with insulin.

Insulin receptor   A cell membrane receptor activated by insulin to initiate a signaling cascade that stimulates glucose uptake.

Insulin resistance   A condition in which cells and tissues respond suboptimally to insulin stimulation. Untreated insulin resistance can lead to type 2 diabetes.

Insulin secretagogue   A substance that stimulates the secretion of insulin from the pancreas. Sulfonylureas, repaglinide, and nateglinide are all in this category of drugs.

Insulin sensitivity   A measure of how well an individual responds to insulin.

Intraretinal microvascular abnormality (IRMA)   A very small abnormality of the retinal blood vessels, representing or serving as a precursor to new vessel formation.

Islets of Langerhans   The endocrine tissue of the pancreas, containing alpha, beta, and delta cells; they are discrete microscopic 'islands' of tissue scattered throughout the pancreas, and the source of insulin, glucagon, and other hormones.

K

Ketoacidosis   A metabolic acidosis with the organic acid forms of ketone bodies as the major anions involved. *See also* diabetic ketoacidosis.

Ketone/ketone body   One of a family of organic ketones or their organic acid forms, namely acetoacetate, β-hydroxybutyrate, or acetate.

L

Lactic acidosis A metabolic acidosis with lactic acid as the major anion involved.

Latent autoimmune diabetes of adults (LADA) A slow-onset form of diabetes occurring in adults, closely related to type 1 diabetes.

Leptin A hormone released almost entirely from white adipose tissue; its absence causes insatiable hunger, reduction in metabolic rate, and infertility, among other effects.

Lipoatrophy Atrophy of adipose tissue, which can have a variety of causes, including subcutaneous insulin injection.

Lipohypertrophy Hypertrophy of adipose tissue, usually as a consequence of chronic local insulin injection.

Lipolysis Breakdown of fat, usually triglyceride, which can be either circulating or intracellular.

Lipoprotein A spherical structure composed of lipids and proteins surrounding a core of cholesterol and triglycerides, used to transport these fats through the bloodstream. They can be classified according to density, of which there are five types: chylomicrons; very-low-density lipoproteins (VLDL); intermediate-density lipoproteins (IDL); low-density lipoproteins (LDL); high-density lipoproteins (HDL). *See also* individual types.

Lipotoxicity The concept that excess availability of lipid (which may be of several forms) inhibits normal function of glucoregulatory mechanisms.

Low-density lipoproteins (LDL) Circulating lipoproteins of density 1.019–1.063 g/ml that transport cholesterol from the liver to the tissues. Cholesterol carried in LDL particles is especially atherogenic and hence these are colloquially called 'bad cholesterol' lipoproteins.

M

Macroalbuminuria Albuminuria of sufficient degree to be detectable with routine urine testing strips (>300 mg/24 hr or >300 mg/1 on a spot sample).

Macrosomia Also known as 'big baby syndrome' or 'large for gestational age', macrosomia describes excessive intra-uterine growth. In neonates, it is usually defined as a weight of more than 4000–4500 g.

Maculopathy A pathological condition of the macula (the area of the retina specialized for high acuity vision), particularly that caused by diabetic retinopathy.

Major histocompatibility complex (MHC) A group of cell-surface molecules that mediate cell interactions with the immune system.

Maturity onset diabetes of the young (MODY) A group of forms of diabetes that are strongly hereditable – usually as autosomal dominant traits – that occur typically before mid-life, but not requiring insulin.

Metabolic syndrome A group of co-segregating medical disorders that independently or together increase the risk of developing cardiovascular disease and diabetes. Defining criteria include central obesity, dyslipidemia, raised BP, raised FPG, microalbuminuria, and hypertension.

Metformin A biguanide drug, now the first-line therapy for type 2 diabetes.

Michaelis constant (abbreviated K_m) The substrate concentration at which a reaction obeying Michaelis–Menton kinetics (a model which describes the rate of enzymatic reactions) is at half-maximum rate. Different

K_m values of different glucose transporters (GLUTs) enable specific functions.

Microalbuminuria Albuminuria of modest degree, not detectable with routine urine testing strips (<300 mg/L on a spot sample).

Mononeuritis multiplex Damage to one or more peripheral nerves occurring within a relatively short time.

Mononeuropathy Damage to a single nerve or nerve group, which results in loss of movement, sensation, or other function of that nerve.

N

Nephropathy Kidney damage, caused in diabetes by glomerular and vascular changes.

Neuroglycopenia The consequences of a shortage of glucose supply to the brain, usually caused by severe hypoglycemia.

Neuropathy Nerve damage, possibly caused in diabetes by microvascular injury. Diabetic neuropathy can affect peripheral nerves, autonomic nerves, and cranial nerves.

Nonesterified fatty acids (NEFA) *See* free fatty acids (FFA).

Nonproliferative diabetic retinopathy (NPDR) The earliest stage of diabetic retinopathy, in which damaged blood vessels in the retina begin to leak fluid and small amounts of blood into the back of the eye.

O

Osmolal gap The difference between measured serum osmolality and calculated serum osmolarity, usually <10 mOsm/kg, but may be increased by large amounts of alcohols, proteins or unmeasured sugar (e.g. mannose).

Osmolality, serum A measure of electrolyte-water balance, estimated as the amount of dissoved chemicals (notably sodium, potassium, glucose, and urea) in a given volume of blood serum; it is measured in osmoles (Osm) of solute per kilogram of solvent (Osm/kg).

Osmolarity Very similar in clinical relevance to osmolality, it is a measure of the osmoles of solute per liter of solution (osmol/L or Osm/L).

Osteomyelitis Acute or chronic bone infection; one of a range of foot complications affecting diabetic patients.

Oxidative stress An imbalance between reactive oxygen species and a biological system's ability to detoxify the reactive intermediates or to repair the resulting damage. The term has no close, or agreed, definition.

P

Peripheral arterial disease (PAD) A disease associated with atherosclerosis in those peripheral arteries that carry blood to the body and especially – in disease terms – to the head and limbs.

Peroxisome proliferative-activated receptor (PPAR) One of a group of receptor proteins, found in the cell nucleus, which activate the transcription of the genes that regulate cell differentiation, function, and metabolism – notably the response to insulin stimulus.

Polydipsia Excessive thirst; a clinical hallmark of hyperglycemia.

Polyphagia Excessive hunger/appetite due to poor glucose metabolism.

Polyuria Excessive production or passage of urine (at least 2.5 or 3.0l over 24 hours in adults). Polyuria is a typical clinical feature of high blood glucose due to diabetes.

Potassium channel An ion channel on the cell membrane that allows potassium to pass into and out of the cell. ATP-gated potassium channels are important in the secretion of insulin and the action of sulfonylureas.

Pre-eclampsia A condition associated with both hypertension that arises in pregnancy (pregnancy-induced hypertension) and with significant amounts of protein in the urine; it is a dangerous complication with risk to both mother and baby.

Prevalence A measurement of the total (as distinct from new) number of cases in a population at a given time. It can be used to estimate how common a condition is. Sometimes given as 'lifetime prevalence', if referring to individuals who have had a diagnosis at some point in their lives, or 'current prevalence' to describe the percentage of people who currently have a diagnosis. *See also* incidence.

Proinsulin The prohormone precursor to insulin, which is converted inside the insulin-secreting cells to insulin and C-peptide.

Proliferative diabetic retinopathy (PDR) A serious complication of diabetes. Ischemic damage to the retinal blood vessels leads to the secretion of growth factors which cause abnormal blood vessels to grow on the surface of the retina (neovascularization). These new vessels are fragile and prone to hemorrhage; blindness can result.

Protein kinase C-beta (PKC-β) One of a family of protein kinase enzymes that modify other proteins through the addition of a phosphate group to one of the amino acids. This phosphorylation usually effects a functional change in the target protein. Activation of PKC-β by high intracellular glucose affects vasoconstriction, for instance.

Proteinuria The presence of serum proteins in the urine; this is a hallmark of diabetic kidney disease, especially when there is no blood in the urine.

Pyelonephritis An ascending urinary tract infection that has reached the renal pelvis or pyelum to cause inflammation of the kidney; also referred to as pyelitis.

R

Reactive oxygen species (ROS) Chemically reactive molecules containing oxygen, generated as by-products of cellular metabolism. High intracellular glucose causes increased ROS production, leading to oxidative stress and cell damage.

S

Second messenger system Molecules that relay signals from intercellular (primary) messengers – such as hormones or neurotransmitters – from receptors on the cell surface to target molecules in the cytoplasm or nucleus.

Secondary diabetes A form of diabetes that develops as a result of another disease or condition. For example, endocrine diseases such as Cushing's disease, pancreatitis, and steroid therapy can each cause secondary diabetes.

Sensorimotor neuropathy A process that damages nerve cells, nerve fibers (axons), and nerve coverings (myelin sheath) so that nerve signals are less rapid. Nerves that supply sensation to the feet are often damaged in diabetes.

Sodium-glucose co-transporter (SGLT) One of a family of glucose transporters found in the mucosa of the small intestine (SGLT1) and the proximal tubule of the nephron (SGLT2). SGLT2 plays an important role in renal glucose reabsorption and SGLT2 inhibitors represent a new strategy in antihyperglycemic therapy.

Sorbitol A polyol or sugar alcohol, occurring naturally in fruit and used as a sweetener in many foods. Sorbitol is converted to fructose in the liver, which is not dependent on insulin for metabolism. However, the process of oxidizing accumulated sorbitol in the cells, particularly those of the retina, can lead to intracellular damage.

Sudomotor dysfunction An abnormality of the sweat glands leading to inappropriate sweating. It is a feature of nerve damage in diabetes.

Sulfonylurea (SU)   One of a class of glucose-lowering drugs that are used in the management of type 2 diabetes. They act by increasing insulin release from the pancreatic β cells through the activation of potassium channel receptors.

T

Thiazolidinedione (TZD)   One of a class of drugs, also known as glitazones, used in the treatment of type 2 diabetes. They work by activating nuclear receptors (PPARs) to increase insulin sensitivity.

Triglyceride   A single molecule of glycerol combined with three fatty acids, triglycerides are the principal type of fat stored in the body. High triglyceride levels in the blood tend to coexist with low levels of HDL, contributing to diabetic dyslipidemia, and are associated with an increased risk of atherosclerosis.

Type 1 diabetes   A form of diabetes mellitus that results from autoimmune destruction of the insulin-producing β cells of the pancreas. The subsequent lack of insulin leads to increased blood and urine glucose and often, but not always, requires insulin treatment.

Type 1B diabetes   Also referred to as idiopathic diabetes, or diabetes of unknown origin, this form of type 1 diabetes is not autoimmune in nature and may be due to a viral infection. People with type 1b have an acute onset of insulin deficiency and even ketoacidosis (due to very high blood glucose).

Type 2 diabetes   A metabolic disorder that is characterized by high blood glucose in the context of decreased insulin sensitivity and relatively decreased insulin secretion. This is the most prevalent form of diabetes and largely accounts for the current global 'epidemic'.

U

Ulcer (ischemic/neuropathic foot)   A break in the skin leading to wounds or open sores. The result of peripheral neuropathy, peripheral arterial disease, and other factors, foot ulcers are an important complication of diabetes, as they may lead to infection and amputation.

V

Vagal neuropathy   A condition in which the vagal nerve is damaged. The vagal nerve is involved in the function of several organs, notably the stomach and its acid production, so vagal neuropathy is associated with abnormal clearance of food from the gut.

Vascular endothelial growth factor (VEGF)   A signal protein that is produced by cells and stimulates the production of new blood vessels. It is part of the system that restores the oxygen supply to tissues when blood circulation is inadequate, but can lead to inappropriate new vessel formation in the eyes. *See also* retinopathy, proliferative diabetic.

Very-low-density lipoproteins (VLDL)   Circulating lipoproteins of density 0.95–1.006 g/ml that can newly synthesized triglycerides from the liver to the adipose tissues. They break down in the bloodstream to become IDL and LDL.

Vitreous hemorrhage   The leakage of blood into the vitreous humor of the eye – in diabetes, particularly from weak, new vessels – which can cause acute loss of vision. *See also* retinopathy, proliferative diabetic.

Index

Pages in *italics* refer figures and **bold** refer tables.

A

abciximab therapy, and PTCA, *73*
acanthosis nigricans, 118, *119*
accelerated fetal growth, *218*
accelerator hypothesis, 230
ACEIs, *see* angiotensin-converting enzyme inhibitor
acid-base balance, in ketoacidosis management, 151
acrochordons, 119–120, *120*
acute motor neuropathy, 90
    treatment and management, 92–93
acute sensory neuropathy, 89
    treatment and management, 92
ADA/EASD guidelines, for management of type 2 diabetes, *71*, *158*, *167*
adaptive immunity, change in, 137
adenosine triphosphate (ATP), 12, *14*, *20*, 230
adiponectin, 46, 173, 230
advanced glycation end products (AGEs), 76, 230
    reactions, *76*
albuminuria, *103*; *see also* microalbuminuria
alcohol, 162
aldose reductase, 76–77, 230
alpha-glucosidase inhibitors, 174–175, *175*, 230
    side effects, 175
altered sensorium, in ketoacidosis management, 151
amputation, 134
amylin, 44–45, 180, 230
angina, symptoms, *72*
angiography, fluorescein, *98*
angiotensin-converting enzyme inhibitors (ACEIs), 58, 66, 79, *107*, 112, 114–115, 230
angiotensin receptor blockers (ARBs), 79–80, *107*, 112, 114, 230
antithrombotic agents, and cardiovascular disease, 83–84
ARBs, *see* angiotensin receptor blockers
aspirin, *see* antithrombotic agents
atherosclerosis, *65*, 230
ATP, *see* adenosine triphosphate
autoantibodies, **26**, 28, **28**, *31*, 32–33, 230
autoantigens, 28, 230
autonomic neuropathy, 90–92, 230
    in feet, 129
    symptoms, **90**
    treatment and management, 93–94

B

bariatric surgery, 164–165, 230
    types, *165*
basal-bolus insulin secretion, *186*, 230
basal insulin, 193–195
    treatment, *193*
beta cells, *1*, 230–231
    decline in function, *167*
bladder involvement, and autonomic neuropathy, 91, 93
blood pressure
    monitoring, *159*
    and nephropathy, 112, 114
body mass index (BMI), 35, 160, 231
brittle diabetes mellitus, 155, 231
bromocriptine, 178

C

calcium channel, 231
    blockers, 79–80, 114
calorie intake, 160–161
capillary changes, *97*
carbohydrates, 161
cardiovascular disease
    and glucose-lowering drugs, 67, 71
    impact of pancreas transplant, 202
    and lipid-lowering drugs, 71–72
    and physical activity, *163*
    and thiazolidinediones (TZDs), 174
cardiovascular outcome studies
    with antidiabetes medications in type 2 diabetes, **68–70**
    with SGLT-2i, **109–111**
cardiovascular risk, *64*, 78
cardiovascular system, and autonomic neuropathy, 90–91, 93
carpal tunnel syndrome, 124
cataracts, 95, 99
    treatment and management, 101
cellular dysfunction, 136
cellular recruitment, 136
cellulitis, 141
cerebral edema, and ketoacidosis, 151
CGMs, *see* continuous glucose monitors
Charcot's arthropathy, 129, *129*, 134–135, *135*, 231
childhood diabetes, **53**
    treating, 52–56
    type 1, 25–26
    types, 52–53
chronic sensory polyneuropathy, 87, 89
classification
    AABCs of, **26**
    categories, **5–6**
clinical presentations, 9
colesevelam, 178
coma and impaired consciousness, **150**
community care, 59–60
complement system, 136
complications, 9–10, *32*
    hyperosmolar hyperglycemic state (HHS), 155
    insulin treatment, 196–200, **200**
    macrovascular, 65–66
    microvascular, 73–77
    screening for, 50–52
congenital malformations, **218**
continuous glucose monitors (CGMs), 190–191
    intermittently scanned, *191*
continuous subcutaneous insulin infusion, *see* CSII
contraception, and diabetes, 210–211

238

cost of diabetes, 10–11, *11*
COVID-19, and diabetes, 144, *145*
C-peptide, 19, *25*, 33, 231
creatinine, 51, 104–106, 112, 115, 231
CSII
   advantages, **190**
   insulin pump treatment, 188–190
   patch pump, *188*
   sensor-augmented system, *187*
cytokine signaling dysfunction, 136–137

D

DAN, *see* autonomic neuropathy
dawn phenomenon, 187, 231
deep venous thrombosis, in ketoacidosis management, 152
diabetes insipidus, 1, 231
diabetes mellitus, 1–2
diabetes self-management education (DSME), 59
diabetic amyotrophy, 127–128
diabetic autonomic neuropathy (DAN), *see* autonomic neuropathy
diabetic bullae, 121, *121*
diabetic cheiroarthropathy, 126, *126*
diabetic dermopathy, 118–119, *119*
diabetic foot, 128–134
   treatment and management, 131–134
diabetic ketoacidosis (DKA), *see* ketoacidosis
diabetic kidney disease (DKD), *see* nephropathy
diabetic microangiopathy, pathogenesis, 74
diabetic muscle infarction, 127
diabetic nephropathy, *see* nephropathy
diabetic neuropathy, *see* neuropathy
diabetic retinopathy, *see* retinopathy
diagnosis
   differential, **8**, **106**
   glucose values, **4**
   of nephropathy, 106
   of neuropathy, 86–87
   of UTIs, *143*
   WHO criteria for, 2–4, **3**
dietary management, 159–160, 164
   prescribing a diet, 162

diffuse idiopathic skeletal hyperostosis (DISH), 128
   Resnick criteria, **128**
dipeptidyl peptidase-4 (DPP-4) inhibitors, 175–176, 231
   action, *176*
   effectiveness, *177*
   side effects, 177
DISH, *see* diffuse idiopathic skeletal hyperostosis
DKA, *see* ketoacidosis
DKD, *see* nephropathy
double diabetes, 26, 231
DPP-4 inhibitors, *see* dipeptidyl peptidase-4 inhibitors
driving, 61–63
DSME, *see* diabetes self-management education
Dupuytren's contracture, 124, *125*
dyslipidemia, 80–82, 231
   therapies, **81**

E

elderly people
   with diabetes, 56–58
   therapy key points, **58**
electrolytes, in ketoacidosis management, 151
emphysematous cholecystitis, 140–141
emphysematous cystitis, 142
emphysematous pyelonephritis, 142–143
employment, 60
   restrictions, **60**
end-stage renal disease (ESRD), 105–106
enteroinsular axis, *175*
environmental risk factors, for type 2 diabetes, 35–36
epidemiology, 2
   type 1 diabetes, 25–26
   type 2 diabetes, 34–35
erectile dysfunction
   and autonomic neuropathy, 91–94
   oral therapy, *93*
   penile implant surgery, *94*
   screening, 52
ESRD, *see* end-stage renal disease
ethnic minorities, and diabetes, *37*, 58
exenatide, and glucose levels, *179*
exercise, 162–164
   glycemic response, **163**
   guidelines, **162–163**
   and insulin sensitivity, *163*

eye disease, 95
   examinations, **96**
   screening, 50, *51*; *see also* cataracts; glaucoma; maculopathy; ocular nerve palsies; retinopathy

F

fasting plasma glucose (FPG), *173*, 231
fats, 161
feet
   screening, 52, *52* ; *see also* Charcot's arthropathy; diabetic foot; foot care; foot infections; ulcers
FFA, *see* free fatty acids
fibrates, effect of, *82*
finance, 60
flexor tenosynovitis, 124–125, *125*
fluid replacement, in ketoacidosis management, 150
focal sensory mononeuropathies, treatment and management, 92
foot care, **132**
foot infections, 130
   treatment and management, 132–133
Fournier gangrene, 142
FPG, *see* fasting plasma glucose
free fatty acids (FFA), 12, *22*, **42**, 149, 231
frozen shoulder, 126–127, *126*

G

gastrointestinal tract, and autonomic neuropathy, 91, 93
GCK, *see* glucokinase
genetic factors
   type 1 diabetes, 28–31, *29*
   type 2 diabetes, 36–37
gestational diabetes mellitus (GDM), 7–8, 215–217, 231–232
   diagnostic criteria, **216**
   labor and delivery, 217
GI, *see* glycemic index
glaucoma, 95, 100
   treatment and management, 102
glinides, 171–172
   side effects, 172
glitazones, *see* thiazolidinediones
glomerular filtration rate (GFR), 232

glomerular particle filtration, *104*
glomerulosclerosis, late changes of, *105*
GLP-1, *see* glucagon-like peptide-1, oral glucagon-like peptide 1
GLP-IRAs, and nephropathy, **113**
glucagon, 12, *12*, 14–15, 44, 147, 199, 232
glucagon-like peptide-1 (GLP-1), 18, 232
    analogs, 178–180, *179*
glucokinase (GCK), 7, 18, 232
gluconeogenesis, 14–15, *14*, 232
glucoregulatory defects, in type 2 diabetes, 42
glucose, 232
    homeostasis, 12, 15
    intolerance, 232
    monitoring, in pregnancy, 211, **212**
    resistance, 16
    role and regulation of, 12–18
glucose control
    and macrovascular disease, 66–67
    and nephropathy, 108, *108*
glucose levels
    commonly used goals, **160**
    and diabetes, 13–14
glucose-lowering drugs
    and cardiovascular disease, 67, 71
    in nephropathy, 108–112
    in pregnancy, **214**
glucose metabolism
    in the elderly, 56
    normal, 14–16
glucose profile, 24-hour, *193*
glucose transporters (GLUTs), 16–18, **17**, 232
glucose values, for diagnosis, **4**
glucotoxicity, 232
    and type 2 diabetes, 45–46, *45*
GLUTs, *see* glucose transporters
glycemic control
    and infection outcomes, 145
    and survival, 57, 67
glycemic goals, in pregnancy, 211
glycemic index (GI), 161, *161*, 232
glycogen, *12*, 15, 232
glycogenesis, 15, 232
glycogenolysis, *14*, 15, 232
glycolysis, **4**, 15, *20*, 75, 232
glycosuria, 9, 148, 232
glycotoxicity, *see* glucotoxicity
gout, 127, *127*
granuloma annulare, 121–122, *122*

H

hand conditions, associated with diabetes, 124–126
HbA1c, *see* hemoglobin A1c
HDL, *see* high-density lipoproteins
helicobacter pylori (H. pylori), 140, *141*
hemodialysis, 116
hemodynamic changes, 77
hemoglobin A1c (HbA1c), 4, 232
    and diabetes risk, *5*
hepatitis, 139–140
HHS, *see* hyperosmolar hyperglycemic state
high-density lipoproteins (HDL), 40, 232
high intracellular glucose, and microvascular disease, 75
high plantar pressure, 130
    treatment and management, 133–134
histocompatibility leukocyte antigen (HLA), 26, 29–30, 232
holidays, 61
HONK, *see* hyperosmolar hyperglycemic state
H. pylori, *see* helicobacter pylori
hyperglycemia, 1, 232
    calorie intake, 160–161
    carbohydrates, 161
    and cardiovascular disease, 83
    and coronary artery bypass graft surgery, *207*
    in critically ill patients, *205*
    dietary management, 159–160, 162
    in early pregnancy, *219*
    exercise, 162–164
    fats, 161
    long-term management, 157
    and microvascular disease, 75
    protein, 161–162
    symptoms, 14
    therapeutic targets, **159**
    treatment algorithm, *158*
    treatment targets, 158–159
    and type 2 diabetes, 38–39
hyperinsulinemia, 232
    and type 2 diabetes, 38–39
hyperosmolality, 153–154, 233
hyperosmolar hyperglycemic state (HHS), 146, 153–154
    clinical features, 154
    compared with DKA, *146*, **146**, *154*
    complications, 155
    investigations, 154–155
    precipitating factors, *154*
    prognosis, 155
    treatment, 155
    treatment algorithm, *152*
hyperosmolar nonketotic coma (HONK), 233; *see also* hyperosmolar hyperglycemic state
hypertension
    and cardiovascular disease, 79–80
    drug therapy, **81**
    and type 2 diabetes, 39
hypoglycemia, 233
    in children, 54
    development, *196*
    in the elderly, 57–58
    on insulin treatment, 196–198
    mild, 199
    nocturnal, 198
    preventing, 199–200
    recurrent severe, 198–199
    symptoms, **197**
    treating, 199–200
hypoglycemic events, *194*
hypoglycemic unawareness, 197–198, *197*
hypotension, in ketoacidosis management, 151
hypothermia, and ketoacidosis, 151

I

idiopathic diabetes, *see* type 1B diabetes
IFG, *see* impaired fasting glycemia
IGFs, *see* insulin-like growth factors (IGFs)
IGT, *see* impaired glucose tolerance (IGT)
immune system, changes in, **137**
impaired fasting glycemia (IFG), 4
impaired glucose tolerance (IGT), 4, 233
    in childhood and adolescence, 53
incretin effect, 233
    of orally administered glucose, *176*
incretins, 18, 44
infant mortality, and maternal blood glucose, *210*
infections, 136, *137*
    of foot, 130, 132–133
    gastrointestinal and liver, 139–141
    genitourinary, 142–144
    and glycemic control, 145

head and neck, 137–138
pathophysiology, 136–137
respiratory, 138–139
skin and soft tissue, 141–142
influenza, 139
inhaled insulin, 185
injections
    insulin, 184–185, *195*
    multiple daily, 187–188
    non-insulin, 178–180
innate immunity, change in, 136–137
inpatient management, 205–206
insulin, 181, 233
    action profiles, *182*
    actions of, 22–24, *22*, **23**
    analogs, 182, *182–183*, 198, 213, 233
    classes, 182–184
    delivery systems, 184–185, *185*
    and metabolic instability, 195–196
    pharmacokinetics, *196*
    response to glucose, and type 2 diabetes, 45
    role and regulation of, 18–24
    spray, 185
    structure of, 18–19, *19*
    testing kit, *62*
    types, **184**
insulin deficiency, 1, 233
    in ketoacidosis management, 150–151
insulin-dependent glucose uptake, *17*
insulin injections, 184–185
    sites, *195*
insulin-like growth factors (IGFs), 24, 233
insulin pumps
    continuous infusion, *see* CSII, insulin pump treatment
    conventional, 189
    implantable, 185
    patch pumps, *188*
    sensor-augmented, *187*, 189
insulin receptor, 21–22, 233
    action, *21*
insulin regimens, **186**, *186*
    type 1 diabetes, 186–190
    type 2 diabetes, 191–195
insulin resistance, 1, 31, 233
    and skin disorders, 118–120
    and type 2 diabetes, 43–44
insulin secretagogues, 170–171, 200, 208, 233

insulin secretion and kinetics, *20*
    abnormalities, 24
    normal, 19–21
insulin sensitivity, 5, 31, 233
    and exercise, *163*
insulin treatment
    complications, 196–200, **200**
    for hospitalized patients, **207–208**
    hypoglycemia, 196–198
    indications for, 181
insulitis, 28
intensive insulin therapy, *158*
    in critically ill patients, 207
intermediate-acting insulin, 183–184
intraretinal microvascular abnormality (IRMA), 96, *98*, 233
irbesartan, and nephropathy, *114*
ischemic foot, *see* ulcers
islet autoimmunity, 28
islet cell implantation, 117
islet cell transplantation, 202
    autologous, 203–204
    donor, 202–203, *203*
islets of Langerhans, *1*, 18, 233

J

joint conditions, associated with diabetes, 126–127
joints of the hand
    limited mobility, *see* diabetic cheiroarthropathy

K

ketoacidosis, 146–147, 231, 233
    acute management, 150–152
    clinical features, 149, *149*
    compared with HHS, **146**, *154*
    investigations, 149–150, **150**
    monitoring, **151**
    pathogenesis, 147–149, *149*
    physiological disturbances, *148*
    recurrent, 156
    and SGLT2 inhibitor use, 178
    subsequent management, 152–153
    treatment algorithm, *152*
ketone bodies, 12, 15, 44, 148–149, 233–234
ketosis-prone diabetes, 26
kidney disease, *see* nephropathy
kidney transplantation, types, *202*

L

lactic acidosis, 156, 234
laser treatment, *101*

latent autoimmune diabetes in adults (LADA), 1, 26, 234
    and calorie intake, 160
LDL, *see* low-density lipoproteins
leptin, 46, 234
lipid-lowering drugs, *82*
    and cardiovascular disease, 71–72
lipid metabolism, abnormalities, 39–40
lipids, and nephropathy, 114–115
lipoatrophy, 124, 234
lipohypertrophy, 123–124, *123*, 234
    at insulin injection sites, *200*
lipolysis, 23, 40, 147–149, 234
lipoprotein, 234
lipotoxicity, 234
    and type 2 diabetes, *45*, 46
living with diabetes, 60–63, **60**
long-acting insulin, 184
    analogs, *183*
low-density lipoproteins (LDL), 40, *82*, 234

M

macroalbuminuria, 103, 234
macrosomia, *218*, 234
macrovascular disease, 64
    treatment and management principles, 66–67
maculopathy, 95, 99, *99*, 234
    treatment and management, 101
major histocompatibility complex (MHC), 29, 234
malignant otitis externa, 137–138
    diagnostic criteria, **138**
management, 49, *59*
    of elderly patients, 56–57, **57**
    of young patients, 53–56
maturity onset diabetes of the young (MODY), 7, 53, 234
    some forms of, **8**
mealtime insulin, 195
metabolic disturbances, 146
metabolic fluxes, alterations, **42**
metabolic instability, on insulin, 195–196
metabolic syndrome, 234
    and type 2 diabetes, 40–42, **41**
metformin, 167, 169, 234
    efficacy, *169*
    vs. lifestyle intervention, *169*
    side effects, 169–170
MHC, *see* major histocompatibility complex

Michaelis constant, 16, 234–235
microalbuminuria, 104–105, **105**, 235
   and irbesartan, *114*
microvascular disease, 73
   causes, **73**
   treatment and management principles, 77–78
MODY, *see* maturity onset diabetes of the young
monitoring
   blood pressure, *159*
   glucose in pregnancy, 211, **212**
   ketoacidosis, **151**
monofilament testing, *87*
mononeuritis multiplex, 89, 235
mononeuropathy, 85, 235; *see also* focal sensory mononeuropathies
mortality
   inpatient, *205*
   and type 1 diabetes, 31–32
motor neuropathy
   in feet, 129; *see also* acute motor neuropathy
mucormycosis, 138, *138*
muscle conditions, associated with diabetes, 127–128
musculoskeletal disorders
   associated with diabetes, 124; *see also* Charcot's arthropathy; diabetic foot; hand conditions; joint conditions; muscle conditions; skeletal conditions
mycotic genital infections, 143–144

N

nateglinide, chemical structure, *171*
necrobiosis lipoidica, 120, *120*
necrotizing fasciitis, 141–142, *142*
necrotizing otitis externa, *see* malignant otitis externa
NEFA, *see* nonesterified fatty acids
neonatal diabetes, 8
neonatal problems, 217–219
nephropathy, 103, 235
   diagnosis, 106
   early changes, *104*
   event rates, *108*
   and GLP-IRAs, **113**
   management in primary practice, *107*
   natural history, 103–106
   overt, 105
   screening, 51, **51**
   treatment and management, 107–108
neuroendocrine disturbances, and autonomic neuropathy, 92
neuroglycopenia, 13–14, 235
neuropathic foot, *see* ulcers
neuropathy, 235
   classification, **85**
   clinical patterns, *88*
   diagnosis, 86–87
   in feet, 129
   impact of pancreas transplant, 202
   prevalence, 85
   treatment and management, 92–94; *see also* acute motor neuropathy; acute sensory neuropathy; autonomic neuropathy; chronic sensory polyneuropathy; mononeuropathy; sensorimotor neuropathy; vagal neuropathy
nonesterified fatty acids (NEFA), *13*, 40, 46; *see also* free fatty acids
non-insulin therapies, 166
   injectables, **168**
   injections, 178–180
   oral agents, 167–178, **168**
nonproliferative diabetic retinopathy (NPDR), 235; *see also* retinopathy, nonproliferative
number of people with diabetes worldwide, *3*

O

obesity, 159–160
   and cardiovascular disease, 79
   childhood, *53*
   in developed countries, *34*
   and type 2 diabetes, 40–42, *42*
ocular nerve palsies, 95, 100
onychomycosis, 141, *141*
oral glucagon-like peptide 1 (GLP-1), 177
osmolal gap, 150, 235
osmolality, 154–155, 235
osteomyelitis, *133*, 235
osteoporosis, 128
oxidative stress, 235
   pathways, *75*

P

PAD, *see* peripheral arterial disease
pancreas transplantation, 117, 201
   criteria for, 201
   outcomes, 201–202
   types, 201, *202*
pancreatic β cell deficiency, and type 2 diabetes, 42–43
pancreatic β cell dysfunction, 27, 31
patient care, *see* management
patient education, 59–60
PDR, *see* retinopathy, proliferative
perinatal outcomes, and type 1 diabetes, *210*
perinephric abscess, 143
peripheral arterial disease (PAD), 129, 235
   treatment and management, 133
peritoneal dialysis, 115–116
peroxisome proliferator-activated receptors (PPARs), **172**, 235
Phalen's test, *125*
physical activity, and cardiovascular disease, *163*
PKC-β, *see* protein kinase C-beta
pneumonia, 138–139
polydipsia, 235
polyneuropathy, *see* chronic sensory polyneuropathy
polyphagia, 235
postprandial metabolic responses, *13*
potassium channel, 8, 171, 235
PPARs, *see* peroxisome proliferator-activated receptors
pramlintide, 180
pre-eclampsia, 214, 217, 236
pregnancy
   and diabetes, 208–210, **209**
   glucose monitoring, 211, **212**
   glucose monitoring targets, **212**
   glycemic goals, 211
   and oral glucose-lowering agents, **214**
   outcomes, *215*
   risks, **215**
   and type 1 diabetes patients, 211–213
   and type 2 diabetes patients, 213–214
premixed insulin, 195
pressure, in feet, 130, 133–134
prevention, of type 2 diabetes, 47–48, **48**
proinsulin, 24, 236
   structure of, *19*

proliferative diabetic retinopathy (PDR), 236; *see also* retinopathy, proliferative
protein, 161–162
    restriction, and nephropathy, 115
protein kinase C-beta (PKC-β), 236
    activation, 77
proteinuria, 103, 105, *106*, 108, 114–115, 215, 236
psoriasis, 122, *123*
pupillary effects, and autonomic neuropathy, 92
pyelonephritis, 142–143, 236

R

Ramadan and dietary preferences, 58–59
rapid-acting insulin, 182–183
    analogs, *182*
reactive oxygen species (ROS), 76, 236
referral criteria, for diabetic foot disorders, **131**
regular insulin, 182
regular U500 insulin, 184
renal abscess, 143
renal dysfunction, progression, *115*
renal outcome studies, with SGLT-2i, **109–111**
renal replacement therapy, 115–117
repaglinide, chemical structure, *171*
retinopathy, 95
    grading, **97**
    impact of pancreas transplant, 202
    laser treatment, *101*
    natural history, 95–96
    nonproliferative, 96–98, *98*
    prevalence in type 1 diabetes, 95
    proliferative, 98–99
    treatment and management, 100–101
revascularization procedures, 72–73
risk factors, 49–50
    for diabetic foot disorders, 129, **132**
    environmental, 35–36
    type 2 diabetes, **35**
    in vascular disease, 78
risk reduction, of vascular disease, 78–84, *79*
risks
    cardiovascular, *64*, 78

of diabetic pregnancy, 214–215, *215*
of malformation, *218*
ROS, *see* reactive oxygen species

S

scleroderma diabeticorum, 122, *122*
screening
    for complications, 50–52
    for diabetes in hepatitis C, *140*
    for diabetic foot disorders, **86**, 130
    eye examinations, **96**
    for loss of protective sensation, *52*
    for neuropathy, *87*
    for proteinuria, *106*
    retinal, *51*
    for type 1 diabetes, 32–33
    for type 2 diabetes, 46–47
    urine albumin values, **51**
secondary diabetes, 8, 236
second messenger systems, 24, 44, 236
sedentary lifestyle, and cardiovascular disease, 79
self-management, in young people, 54
self-monitored blood glucose, **159**
sensorimotor neuropathy, 85, 236
sensory neuropathy
    in feet, 129; *see also* acute sensory neuropathy
SGLT2 inhibitors, 177–178
    and genitourinary infections, 144
SGLT-2I, in cardiovascular and renal outcome studies, **109–111**
skeletal conditions, associated with diabetes, 128
skin disorders, 118
    associated with diabetes, 121–122
    associated with diabetes medications, 122–124
    associated with insulin resistance, 118–120
    associated with type 1 diabetes, 120–121
    in type 1 and type 2 diabetes, **118**
smoking
    and cardiovascular disease, 82
    and nephropathy, 115
sodium-glucose linked transporter 2 inhibitors, 236; *see also* SGLT2 inhibitors

sorbitol, 236
    accumulation, 76–77
    conversion, 77
sport, 61
statins
    effect of, *81*; *see also* antithrombotic agents
sudomotor dysfunction, 236–237
    and autonomic neuropathy, 92
sulfonylureas (SUs), 170–171, 237
    action, *170*
    drug interactions and side effects, 171
surgery
    and blood pressure, 208
    and diabetes management, 206–208, **208**
    foot, 134; *see also* bariatric surgery
symptoms, 9

T

TB, *see* tuberculosis
T cell dysfunction, 137
thiazolidinediones (TZDs), 172–174, 237
    and blood glucose, *173*
    and cardiovascular disease, 174
    chemical structure, *173*
    side effects, 174
Tinel's test, *125*
transplantation, 116–117
    failure rates, *117*
    survival, *116*; *see also* kidney transplantation; pancreas transplantation
travel, 61
trigger finger, *see* flexor tenosynovitis
triglyceride, 40, 237
TRIPOD study, *174*
tuberculosis (TB), 139, *139*
type 1 diabetes, 1–2, 7, 237
    causes, 26–31
    development, 31
    disease progression, *31*
    epidemiology, 25–26
    etiological events, *26*
    genes associated with, *30*
    genetic factors, 28–31, *29*
    insulin regimen, 186–190
    mortality, 31–32
    nongenetic factors, *31*
    perinatal outcomes, *210*
    prediction of, 28

and prevalence of retinopathy, 95
screening, 32–33
subtypes seen in adulthood, 25
type 1B diabetes, 25, 237
type 2 diabetes, 1–2, 7, 237
    ADA/EASD management guidelines, *71*, *158*, *167*
    associated conditions, 37–40
    bariatric surgery, 164–165
    cardiovascular outcomes trials with antidiabetes medications, **68–70**
    causes, 35–37
    development, 42–45
    dietary intervention, 164
    epidemiology, 34–35
    etiology, *38*
    genetic *vs.* environmental factors, *37*
    genetic factors, 36–37
    lifestyle interventions, *48*
    metabolic syndrome and obesity, 40–42
    natural history, *38*
    prevention studies, 48, **48**
    remission, 164–165
    risk factors, **35**
    screening and prevention, 46–48
TZDs, *see* thiazolidinediones

U

ulcers, 237
    classification, **130**
    in diabetic foot, **130**, *131*
ultralong-acting insulin, 184
ultrarapid-acting insulin, 183
urinary tract infections (UTIs), 106, 142–143
    diagnosis, *143*

V

vagal neuropathy, 91, 237
vascular disease, screening, 52
vascular endothelial growth factor (VEGF), 76, 101, 237
very-low-density lipoproteins (VLDL), 40, *82*, 237
vitiligo, 120–121, *121*
vitreous hemorrhage, *99*, 237

W

WHO criteria for diagnosis, 2–4, **3**